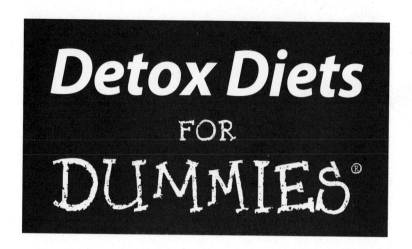

Detox Diets
FOR
DUMMIES®

by Dr. Gerald Don Wootan, DO, M.Ed.,
and M. Brittain Phillips

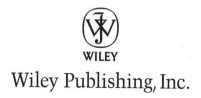

WILEY

Wiley Publishing, Inc.

Detox Diets For Dummies®

Published by
Wiley Publishing, Inc.
111 River St.
Hoboken, NJ 07030-5774
www.wiley.com

WILEY

Detox Diets

FOR

DUMMIES®

About the Authors

Gerald Don Wootan, DO, M.Ed.: Dr. Wootan is an osteopathic physician board certified in family practice and geriatrics. He holds bachelors' degrees in biology, psychology, and medicine, a master's degree in counseling psychology, and a doctorate in osteopathic medicine with board certification in family practice and geriatrics. He is the medical director of Jenks Health Team in Jenks, Oklahoma, a medical practice that specializes in integrative medicine with a strong emphasis on natural detoxification and nutritional supplementation. He is also the Medical Director of Narconon Arrowhead, an inpatient drug treatment facility that utilizes natural therapies. Dr. Wootan is trained in and utilizes the Defeat Autism Now! protocol for treating children on the autism spectrum and is an active member of the American College for the Advancement of Medicine.

M. Brittain Phillips: Brittain didn't used to think much about toxins, but after working with Dr. Wootan on this project he's not putting anything in his shopping cart without checking the label for high fructose corn syrup. (It's everywhere!) He studied biology and English at DePauw University, and he's happy to report that with this project he finally found a way to combine the disciplines. He works and writes in Charleston, South Carolina.

Dedication

Jerry: This book is dedicated to my mother and father, Corrine and Ralph Wootan, and my uncle, Howard Mauldin, MD. My mother showed me true unconditional love and instilled in me a feeling of introspective self-worth that has lasted me my entire life. My father showed me that dreams can be attained and that discipline is the way to get there. From my earliest memories, my Uncle Howard was my inspiration and role model as a physician and as a person.

Brittain: For Mimi. Moderation in all things, indeed.

Authors' Acknowledgments

Jerry thanks his office staff, and specifically Nancy Smith, who did so much to support him and allow him the time to do this work. He also thanks Mike Mahoney, Vice President of Xymogen Exclusive Professional Formulas; his daughter Heather Walters, ND; and his brother, George Wootan, MD, for their support and input on technical aspects of detoxing; and his sister Darla Nesom for being there. He gives a special note of thanks for the staff at Wiley for their assistance during their entire writing process. This book would not have been possible without the guidance and assistance of Brittain Phillips.

Brittain thanks Dr. Wootan for his professionalism and patience throughout this project. He thanks Cindy, who was right about this stuff all along; mom and dad, who set the perfect example; and Sarah, who never ceases to amaze.

Publisher's Acknowledgments

We're proud of this book; please send us your comments at http://dummies.custhelp.com. For other comments, please contact our Customer Care Department within the U.S. at 877-762-2974, outside the U.S. at 317-572-3993, or fax 317-572-4002.

Some of the people who helped bring this book to market include the following:

Acquisitions, Editorial, and Media Development

Project Editor: Joan Friedman

Acquisitions Editor: Lindsay Lefevere

Assistant Editor: Erin Calligan Mooney

Editorial Program Coordinator: Joe Niesen

Technical Editor: Ted H. Spence, DDS, ND

Senior Editorial Manager: Jennifer Ehrlich

Editorial Supervisor: Carmen Krikorian

Senior Editorial Assistant: David Lutton

Editorial Assistant: Jennette ElNaggar

Cover Photos: © Dana Hoff

Cartoons: Rich Tennant www.the5thwave.com

Composition Services

Project Coordinator: Sheree Montgomery

Layout and Graphics: Ashley Chamberlain, Joyce Haughey, Melissa Jester

Proofreaders: Melissa Cossell, Susan Hobbs

Indexer: Potomac Indexing, LLC

Publishing and Editorial for Consumer Dummies

> **Diane Graves Steele,** Vice President and Publisher, Consumer Dummies

> **Kristin Ferguson-Wagstaffe,** Product Development Director, Consumer Dummies

> **Ensley Eikenburg,** Associate Publisher, Travel

> **Kelly Regan,** Editorial Director, Travel

Publishing for Technology Dummies

> **Andy Cummings,** Vice President and Publisher, Dummies Technology/General User

Composition Services

> **Debbie Stailey,** Director of Composition Services

Contents at a Glance

Table of Contents

Chapter 6: Recognizing Toxin-filled and Otherwise Unhealthy Foods 97

Chapter 7: Deciding on the Best Foods for a Toxin-free Dinner Table 105

Introduction

*F*ew things in the world are as pristine as a newborn baby, right? For thousands of years, a brand new bundle of joy represented all that was pure. But just in the last century or so, the world has changed quite a lot, and so have our babies. A recent study showed that an average newborn has detectable levels of more than 200 toxic or cancer-causing chemicals on the day of birth. That's a shocking but very real indication that you are constantly exposed to an enormous amount of chemicals that are toxic to humans. (Is it any wonder that 1 in every 6 children has a neuropsychological disorder? Or that autism, which is associated with exposure to toxins, now affects 1 in every 91 children?)

Quite a lot of damage is done to the environment in the name of progress, and at the top of the list is the spread of toxins into the air, water, and soil. Many people have long had faith that the commercial interests driving the progress would be strict with their pollution policies and work to ensure that toxic substances aren't released into the environment. Beyond that, government entities at all levels have assured us that they are monitoring these developments and keeping us safe from toxic influences. Unfortunately, the facts prove otherwise.

The development of industry has expanded much more rapidly than the resources available to monitor it. As a result, today more than 80,000 man-made chemicals are released into the environment each year, and fewer than 3,000 of them have been tested to determine their toxic effects on humans. Some of the most toxic materials have been banned, but often those bans don't cross borders. That means, for example, that a pesticide may be banned in the United States but used extensively in a neighboring country that ships crops directly to U.S. food providers. Air pollutants travel even easier, and they end up settling on water sources and open land if they don't invade our lungs.

The fact is that the world is more toxic now than it has been since the dawn of mankind, and it's not likely to get considerably less toxic anytime soon. That's the bad news. The good news is that your body is a marvelous machine that does a really good job of taking care of itself. It's able to flush out quite a bit of the toxic material that ends up inside you.

But even the strongest body can't win the fight alone. You have to work hard to limit the amount of toxins entering your system, and you have to take a proactive approach to detoxifying the harmful substances already in your body. If you suffer from chronic illness or autoimmune disease, you simply *must* look at toxic triggers for these illnesses. The process starts with your diet, but several other useful options for detoxification exist. In this book, I include plenty of information on a range of these considerations — from diet to saunas to supplements and more.

About This Book

My goal in this book is to show you how you can cut down on your intake of toxins and detoxify your life so that you can enjoy the best possible health for as long as you're on the top side of the grass.

Your diet is the most important factor when it comes to determining how toxic you are. (You are what you eat, after all.) I spend quite a bit of time providing you with details on how you can shape your diet and eating habits so that you're getting the maximum detox effect. But I don't stop with diet, and you shouldn't either. Given the toxic threats all around us, you'll be wise to consider any and all options for flushing toxins out of your body and out of your life. The truth is that everyone is exposed to toxins on a daily basis, and you need to do everything you can to reduce the damage those toxins are doing on your body and mind.

Embracing the ideas and practices behind detoxification isn't always easy because traditional medicine doesn't usually focus on the presence and influence of toxins. Many doctors and most pharmaceutical companies are lukewarm at best to the idea that toxins are causing a lot of the ailments that are becoming more and more prevalent every year.

That means you need to be your own advocate and take the time to familiarize yourself with all the various threats and how they can affect you. You need to invest time, but by doing so you're investing in your future health — your most important asset. You have to take charge of your own health and assume responsibility for the outcome. Doctors can offer some good information, but in the end the decisions are yours. I challenge you to look at the facts about toxicity and use common sense to determine what remedies you need to incorporate into your life and the lives of your loved ones.

Conventions Used in This Book

Following are a few conventions I use to help guide you through the book:

- ✔ I use a number of medical and health-related terms in this book that you may not be familiar with. In those cases I *italicize* the jargony term and follow it up immediately with a definition.

✔ I also present a lot of acronyms throughout the book. To prevent you from drowning in alphabet soup, I spell out the full words the first time an acronym is used in a chapter.

✔ In Part III, I include several recipes in each chapter. If you're a vegetarian, look for the tomato next to the recipe name that indicates the recipe does not contain meat or fish. (Be aware that the recipe may contain eggs or cheese, however.)

✔ All Web addresses appear in `monofont` so they're easy to pick out.

Keep in mind that when this book was printed, some Web addresses may have needed to break across two lines of text. Wherever that's the case, rest assured that we haven't put in any extra characters (such as hyphens) to indicate the break. So, when using one of these Web addresses, just type in exactly what you see in this book. Pretend as if the line break doesn't exist.

What You're Not to Read

In the interest of full disclosure, I want to let you know that you have to read every word in this book. As soon as you're done I'll give you a call, and you'll have to take an essay test on the topics I cover. Hope you have a flexible phone plan.

Seriously: Each part and chapter in the book contain their own information, and where you may want to jump around from chapter to chapter I've inserted cross references to facilitate your page flipping. Feel free to skip around.

If you have absolutely no regard for my feelings and you're not interested in reading every single word in the book, you may consider skipping the sidebars, which contain interesting but not essential information. Sidebars are contained in the gray shaded boxes.

Foolish Assumptions

I've written this book with a few assumptions about you in mind. Here are those assumptions, in no particular order:

✔ I assume you're on board with the fact that our planet is currently chock-full of toxins and that those toxins can affect your well-being.

✔ I assume you know diet is important to your health.

✔ I assume you're at least willing to consider that traditional medicine doesn't currently have all the answers for the various diseases and conditions plaguing people in increasing numbers, and that medical professionals could very well be underestimating the influence that toxins have on our bodies and our collective health.

How This Book Is Organized

I've divided this book into five parts. Each part covers a different aspect of detoxification, and the information I offer on the impact that diet has on your detoxification is pretty strong throughout. The great news is that you can jump around all you want; you don't have to read Part I in order to understand Part III, for example.

Part I: Getting to the Bottom of Natural Detoxification

If you're new to detoxification, it won't hurt to check out Chapter 1. That chapter is an overview of toxicity and detoxification ideas. Read it if you want to find out what detoxification means and what it can do for you.

The rest of the chapters in Part I clue you in on the many different kinds of toxins that surround you, how they end up in your body, and (perhaps most importantly) how your body manages to flush quite a lot of them out. You'll be surprised at some of the places where toxins are hiding and what they can do to your health. This information is a little scary, but it's also necessary because you have to know where the toxins are coming from if you're going to try to avoid them.

Part II: Working toward a Detoxified Life: Getting Started

Part II gives you the details on how you can get started on a detoxification regimen. It opens with Chapter 5, which fills you in on a few basics (most of them diet-related) for detoxing. The part then proceeds with a couple chapters that tell you how to dodge toxin-filled foods and — even better — what you should be buying at the grocery store to fill up your pantry and fridge with nontoxic options. You may be amazed at the range and amount of toxins that you can find in very common food items.

I wrap up Part II with a quiz that you can take to figure out just how toxic you are. The quiz takes up all of Chapter 8.

Part III: Enhancing Wellness through Detoxification

Part III really gets down to the nitty gritty of how toxins affect various aspects of your health and how you can detoxify — especially with your diet — to keep those areas of your health in top-notch shape. I tell you how to maintain a healthy weight, boost your immune system, increase your energy level, quit smoking, and much more!

Throughout this part you find an excellent feature of this book: wholesome, healthy, detox recipes that you can make yourself to help ensure your diet is contributing to your health in a toxin-free way.

Part IV: Maintaining Healthy Detoxification Habits

Part IV may be small, but it's mighty. In Chapter 17, I explain many of the important aspects of your diet that you need to keep on the front burner if you're going to be successful with any detox effort. From vitamins to essential fatty acids and everything in between, Chapter 17 hammers home the importance of nutrients and how they fit into an effective detox diet (not to mention a generally healthy lifestyle).

Chapter 18 is another one of my favorites. In it you can read all about the various options for detoxification that await you outside the grocery store and kitchen. Check out this chapter to find out how you can really stretch your detox efforts.

Part V: The Part of Tens

If you're familiar with books *For Dummies,* you may flip straight to this part, which is full of interesting (and fun) lists. If you're new to the *For Dummies* series, check out "The Part of Tens" for quick-hitting information that can pique your interest and help you determine where you may want to go next as you dig into the book.

Icons Used in This Book

Throughout the book, you'll notice three icons in the margins that help you navigate the text:

When you see this icon, you can be sure that you're getting an important piece of how-to advice about detox dieting or general detoxification.

This icon lets you know that you should slow down for a moment and really let the information soak in. It's important stuff!

I use this icon to fill you in on potentially toxic pitfalls.

Where to Go from Here

There's no wrong way to use this book. If you're just getting started on your quest to understand how toxins affect your health, you may want to get cracking with Part I (even Chapter 1, if you're interested in covering all your bases). But maybe you already have a good feel for the toxins that are out there, and you really just want to know how you can use detoxification and detox dieting to improve a specific part of your health. If that's the case, I recommend jumping into Part III.

If you want to begin embracing the practices and techniques of detoxification right away, Part II is where you want to be.

Or maybe you want to start with some light fare and ease your way into the subject. If so, check out "The Part of Tens" (Part V).

No matter how you want to start or continue your path toward leading a healthy, detoxified life, you're bound to end up with better health as a result. And that's a destination we should all add to our itineraries.

Part I
Getting to the Bottom of Natural Detoxification

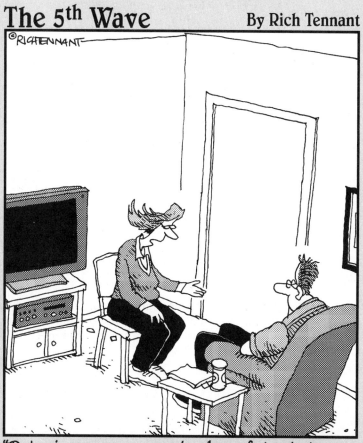

The 5th Wave   By Rich Tennant

"Detoxing means removing harmful substances from the body, so let's start with the remote and the BlackBerry."

In this part . . .

1 kick things off with a good hard look at the toxins that have become a very real (and very harmful) part of our world. There are tens of thousands of toxins in dozens of categories, and they exist in the air, in water, and on land. You really can't escape them, but it's important that you understand where they're lurking so you can at least do your best to avoid them whenever possible.

In this part, you can also read about the efforts that your magnificent body makes to cleanse itself of toxic substances. If you're not already convinced of the wonders of the human body, prepare to be amazed!

Chapter 1

Understanding Detoxification and Detox Dieting

*Y*our amazing body is the most complicated machine on earth. But keeping that complex machine operating at an extremely high level can be surprisingly simple. You can enjoy maximum health for decades if you follow just a few rules, the most important of which are:

✔ Keep your body fueled with the right kinds of food.

✔ Avoid anything that can cause your body harm.

These rules may be simple, but I didn't say they were easy.

The world around us is filled with toxins. In fact, our planet is more toxic now than it has ever been in human history. To be honest, it can be a real challenge to get healthful, toxin-free food and to dodge all the toxins that exist in our environment, just waiting to creep and seep into your body to do you harm. That's the bad news: So many toxins exist at such high levels that you simply cannot escape their reach.

The good news is that you can fight back against the situation. You can make adjustments to your lifestyle — starting with your diet but reaching far beyond — to limit the amount of toxins you're exposed to. And you can make a concerted effort to detoxify the harmful substances that already exist in your body.

Throughout this book I discuss ways that you can give your body the healthful, wholesome fuel it needs, while at the same time avoiding toxic materials and working to remove the toxins that have already built up in your body's systems. If you can stick to the plans that I lay out for you in the pages that follow, you'll enjoy a level of health that many people may hardly believe is possible.

Figuring Out Why Everyone Should Detox

Anyone living in the developed world, and particularly in the United States, is exposed to chemicals and other toxic substances on a daily basis. These toxins are more varied and exist in much higher quantities than ever before. It's scary to think about, but we really don't know what the long-term health effects of all these toxins could be for the human race as a whole. What we *can* see are the health effects of the toxicity that people suffer from now, and the picture certainly isn't pretty. Small doses of toxins usually don't have an immediate effect, but the long-term accumulation can eventually cause entire organ systems to fail with no obvious cause. Thousands of people currently face chronic diseases that weren't even on the books a century ago, and the average child born today comes into the world with more than 200 different toxins already present in her body.

I'd like to believe that people across the globe will stop adding more and more toxins into our surroundings, but we all know that's wishful thinking. Things are likely going to get quite a bit more toxic before they start getting cleaned up, so it's best to start planning now for a toxin-filled future.

I don't want you to panic about the toxins that surround you, but you should at least realize what you're up against. You must also realize that you can take steps to avoid toxins and detoxify your body to counter the toxic trend. And always remember that you're not alone — we're all fighting against the health threats posed by toxins, and the important work of detoxification should be embraced by everyone (or at least everyone interested in living a long, healthy, enjoyable life!).

Defining detoxification

So what is detoxification, anyway? It's any process that removes a substance that is injurious to your body or that changes a toxic substance so it's no longer injurious. Dozens of different detoxification methods exist, and I cover the most useful and important ones — including diet, which is the most critical of all — throughout this book. Broadly speaking, though, you can split detoxification up into two categories: internal and external.

Internal

Our bodies have an extraordinarily complex array of systems that change, break down, attack and destroy, or eliminate threats to our internal environment and health. For thousands of years these systems have helped humans to enjoy relatively good basic health, but for most of those years the exposure to toxins was very low and rarely caused a problem. That's not so today.

The primary internal systems for detoxification are the stomach, intestines, liver, immune system, kidneys, and lungs. Each one works in a different way to keep us as clean as possible, and you can enhance the detox power of each system by taking the steps I describe in this book's chapters.

External

When it comes to external detoxification, your skin is second to none. Your skin serves as an important barrier that keeps many toxins from entering your body. Your sweat glands, which are extremely important sites for detoxification, are also housed in your skin.

Seeing what detoxification can do for you

When you think about toxins, you can consider them poisons. You don't want poisons floating around in your body, do you? Toxins can affect virtually every system and part of your body, causing a massive decrease in efficiency and function. Toxins also cause disease. Removing toxins — and avoiding them in the first place — can have some truly startling positive effects on your health, which I detail throughout Part III of this book. Here are just a few examples:

- ✔ **Increasing energy:** Many toxins directly affect the production of energy in your body, and when your toxic levels are high you have far less energy than you would enjoy if your systems were toxin free (or close to it). The more toxins you can remove and keep out, the more energy you'll have.

- ✔ **Boosting immune function:** Your immune system plays a major part in detoxification. The more it has to work toward getting rid of toxins, the less work it can do on its normal tasks (such as preventing infections and killing cancer cells). Getting rid of toxins makes life easier for your immune system, which allows it to do its job effectively.

- ✔ **Managing stress:** We usually think of stress as an emotional response to an unwanted situation. That's definitely one cause of stress, but toxins can put even more stress on your body, which reacts the same to emotional stress and toxic stress. Stress harms your body in many different ways, including (but not limited to) organ damage and brain problems. Managing toxic and emotional stress can be a major contributor to good health.

✔ **Decreasing fat:** Everyone needs a little stored energy, and fat is one of the ways you fulfill that need. Unfortunately, many of us are storing enough energy (in the form of fat) for several people. That's a medical problem — a very serious one. In addition to the strain obesity puts on your cardio-vascular system, there's a toxic element of obesity that many people don't understand. Fat-soluble toxins are stored in your fat cells, and these cells release toxins into your bloodstream on a regular basis. You have to get the toxins out of the fat cells before you can reduce the fat. Then, with less fat, the toxins have fewer places to hide.

Taking a Look at Toxins

If you start looking around for toxins, you don't have to go very far. Start by looking under your kitchen sink. See those disinfectants and cleaners? They're almost certainly loaded with chemical toxins. Open your pantry. Do you have any processed foods in there? Be honest. If so, check the ingredients lists. If you see any words that you can't pronounce, those are probably toxins. Head into the bathroom next. Chances are your hair spray, deodorant, and other personal hygiene products contain toxic substances. Don't even go into your garage — you could spend all day in there discovering toxins.

If you don't feel like walking around the house, just take a deep breath. The fumes from your carpet or from a freshly painted wall in the next room will add to the toxic list. And toxic influences from outside your house, down the street, or across town — influences generated by places like factories and power plants — are contained in the air you're breathing, too.

To be fair, in many of these cases the amount of toxins you're exposed to at one time is usually small. But toxins are very stubborn; they accumulate in your body and can add up pretty fast. It's kind of like putting a bucket under a slow leak in a faucet. Even though the leak is very slow, before long the bucket is running over.

Knowing what qualifies as a toxin

A *toxin* is any substance that your body can't use in a purposeful way or that requires energy to be removed. Even substances that your body has to have to survive can be toxic if you get too much of them. It's truly a miracle that we can expose our bodies to the vast numbers of toxins in our environment and we don't just drop over and die. But even though your body is resilient, if you push it too hard, something is bound to break. If you have a good grasp of what's out there in terms of toxins, you can more easily identify and avoid them.

Natural chemicals

People often think of toxins as manmade chemicals, but Mother Nature provides plenty of toxins, too. If you've ever brushed up against some poison ivy or been bitten by a spider, you know what I mean. The key to limiting the amount of damage that natural toxins do to your body is avoidance.

Living toxins

In addition to the natural chemicals that act as toxins, plenty of living things can have toxic effects on your health. Bacteria, for example, are all around us. Some types of bacteria are helpful, like the kinds that live in your intestines and help to digest your food, but many other types are extremely toxic and harmful. Yeasts, parasites, and viruses are other common living toxins.

Manmade chemicals

In the past 100 years, man has been really busy creating new things that are supposed to make our lives easier and better. Unfortunately, many of these things contain toxic chemicals and/or are made using some sort of toxic process. The chemical creations include pesticides, petrochemicals, and food additives, to name just a few.

In the United States today, more than 80,000 chemicals are being released into our environment, and less than 3,000 have been tested for toxic effects on humans. The U.S. Environmental Protection Agency (EPA) allows any chemical to be released unless scientific proof exists that it causes cancer or is toxic in some other way. We have the cart ahead of the horse when it comes to manmade chemical toxins.

Finding toxins everywhere

By now you're probably getting the picture that we're really surrounded by toxins and things that can make us toxic. But how do these toxins end up in our bodies, where they can do us harm? Here are the common routes:

✔ **Ingesting toxins orally:** It may seem crazy to stick toxins into your mouth, but we do so every day. Food is the biggest source of toxins for most people.

Processed foods today contain more than 3,000 chemicals that aren't natural. These chemicals enhance flavor and can preserve food for months, if not years. Many food preservatives can have really harmful effects on the body. Some ding up your immune system, and others cause dangerous (even deadly) allergic reactions. Throughout this book I tell you about the toxins that can lurk in your food if you're not making smart, detox diet decisions about what goes in your pantry and on your plate.

And even if toxins aren't *in* your food and water, you may have toxins *on* your food. At the top of this list are pesticides and chemical fertilizers that are meant to help grow food but end up in our bodies, assaulting our organs and tissues.

✔ **Inhaling toxins:** When it comes to airborne toxins, remember this: Anything you smell is getting into your body. If something has a nasty chemical smell, parts of that chemical are entering your body through your mucous membranes and lungs. Even scarier is the fact that many chemicals have no smell, so you don't know that you're breathing them in.

As I note in the previous section, about 80,000 chemicals are released into your environment, many of them in gaseous form. Obviously, the potential for inhaling toxic substances is extremely high. That gentle summer breeze may contain heavy metals, bacteria, mold, viruses, and countless chemicals.

✔ **Taking toxins in through your skin:** Your skin does a very good job at keeping out toxins, but it isn't perfect. Your skin is capable of absorbing chemicals that come in contact with it, and toxins are no exception.

Getting Rid of Toxins

What's the best way to get rid of toxins? Avoid them in the first place. An ounce of toxin prevention is worth far more than a pound of detoxification cure. But you can do only so much when it comes to dodging toxins. You could live in a bubble in the most pristine part of the world, and you'd still end up toxic. Lucky for you, you have a whole host of systems and natural mechanisms that will help you eliminate the toxic substances that course through your veins (and your arteries, and your tissues, and your organs . . .).

Watching your body fight toxins

Your body gets rid of toxins in a couple of key ways that I introduce in this section. The first is the elimination of toxins; you have systems in place that simply flush the bad stuff out. The second is chemical detoxification, which occurs when various parts of your body — the liver is a top example — break down toxins into simpler, less harmful materials that are usually shuttled out of the body in your waste products.

Toxin elimination

When you talk about the natural elimination of toxins from your body, your kidneys deserve center stage. Sure, some organs have a higher profile — your brain and heart come to mind — but when it comes to sorting out toxins and putting them on the first fast train out (usually into the toilet), nothing beats the kidneys. They're especially adept at clearing out water-soluble toxins.

Many fat-soluble toxins that can't be whisked away by your kidneys or broken down by your liver (more on that organ in a moment) get sequestered in your fat cells, where they become a constant source of toxicity. How do you get rid of those toxins? You sweat the small stuff. And the big stuff. And everything in between. Sweating is a remarkable detoxification technique; several different kinds of toxins can be removed from your body only through sweating. (I come back to that topic later in the chapter.)

Chemical detoxification

Chemical detoxification takes place when one of your body's parts breaks down the chemical structure of a toxin so it's no longer harmful. The process starts in your nose and mouth, where immune cells begin busting up toxic substances. The tonsils do a lot of work on toxins before they continue toward your stomach, where some of the most potent acid in the natural world goes to work on a breadth of toxins.

That brings me to the liver. Your liver is a fantastic chemical processing plant, and it can break down toxins that range from ammonia to alcohol. You don't have to read very many pages in this book before coming to a spot where I sing the praises of the liver.

Taking an active role in detoxification

Your body can take care of quite a bit of detoxification on its own, but today's elevated toxin levels demand that you give your body a hand. If you want to enjoy long-term good health, you must work hard to enhance and augment your body's detox efforts by taking these steps:

- ✔ **Choose your food wisely:** You can drastically cut down on your toxicity by making good food choices. If you can eliminate processed foods from your diet, dodge most genetically modified foods, and embrace all things organic, you'll be doing your health an enormous favor. This is important stuff, and I devote many pages of this book (including all of Chapters 6 and 7) to food and detox dieting topics.

✔ **Fill in the gaps with supplements:** The quality of our food has dropped dramatically in the last few decades. As if that weren't enough, your body needs even more essential nutrients than ever before if you expect it to fight off the ever-increasing amount of toxic threats that surround us all. Because of these factors, the vast majority of people — particularly people living in the United States — need to take supplements to ensure the best possible intake of vitamins, minerals, essential fatty acids, and other key nutrients. I discuss supplements throughout this book, particularly in Chapter 17.

✔ **Cleanse through chelation:** Heavy metals are some of the most common toxins, and they're everywhere. Lead may have been banned from paint and gasoline several years ago, but the lead that used to be added to those products is still around. Mercury is extremely prevalent as well and can be found in everything from dental fillings to fish to fluorescent light bulbs.

If you think you may be suffering from dangerously high levels of heavy metals, chelation could be a good choice for you. *Chelation* is a medical treatment that uses a medication to trap and remove heavy metals from your body's tissues. Several variations on chelation exist, which I describe in Chapter 18.

✔ **Use a sauna:** Sweating is an outstanding way to use your body's natural systems to flush out toxins, particularly the fat-soluble ones that contribute to obesity and continually poison us. You should be sweating every chance you get! Exercise is a great way to work up a sweat, but if you really want to sweat it out, nothing beats a sauna. I explain your sauna options and how to use them in Chapter 18.

Dieting the Detoxification Way

If you're not enjoying optimal health, or if you're struggling with obesity, you need to take a good, hard look at the many benefits of a detox diet. Changing what you eat (and how you eat it) so that you're focusing on wholesome, healthy foods and cutting out toxic ingredients is the first and most important step toward ensuring good health and maintaining a healthy weight. The principles for detox dieting are relatively simple, but the changes they require can be pretty tough. (They're not as tough, however, as living an unhealthy and obese life.)

Losing those extra, harmful pounds

Not many people make the connection between toxins and obesity, but clear, proven relationships exist that you need to understand if you want to stay at a healthy weight. Getting on (and sticking with) a detox diet will go a long way toward minimizing your toxicity. And if you can make detox dieting a part of your life *for life,* you'll lose the extra, harmful pounds that weigh you down and damage your health.

Body fat is toxic!

You don't run into many people who are fond of fat, and for good reason. In addition to being unattractive in the eyes of many people, fat is also a storehouse for toxins in your body. Fat-soluble toxins are tucked away in fat cells to prevent them from harming your organs and other vital tissues, and when the toxins are more concentrated, the fat cells get bigger in an effort to keep them diluted. If you can avoid toxins and detoxify the toxins you're already carrying around with you, shedding fat becomes much easier.

Body fat stresses your body's systems

For every pound of fat your body makes, it has to make about 4 miles of blood vessels. Carrying 25 extra pounds of fat means your heart has to pump blood through another 100 miles of vessels. As you can imagine, that's not good news for the most important muscle in your body, and it's just the beginning. Fat wreaks havoc on your joints, contributes to diabetes, and causes too many other conditions to list here. Lose the toxins, lose the unhealthy foods from your diet, and you'll lose the fat. And then your health will flourish. See Chapter 9 for all the details on making detox dieting part of your daily life.

Tackling unhealthy habits

Choosing the right toxin-free foods and ensuring that your eating habits are as healthy as possible will do more than just help you to eliminate excess fat. Giving your body the healthy fuel that it needs can also be a critical factor in helping to kick unhealthy habits like drinking and smoking. What's more, if you really embrace detox dieting, you can greatly enhance the recovery and healing process that takes place after you've put down the bottle and snuffed out your last cigarette. Pair those dietary choices with some more detoxification efforts — saunas, for instance — and you can go from an unhealthy smoker or drinker to a healthy, detoxified person in a fraction of the time.

If you're a smoker (or former smoker), be sure the check out Chapter 14. For information about using detox methods to fight alcohol abuse, see Chapter 15.

Chapter 2

Tackling the Different Types of Toxins and Their Effects on You

*W*hat's the first step for waging a war against toxins and their harmful effects on your body? Know thy enemy. You can't make a concerted effort to cleanse your body of toxins or avoid contact with them in the first place if you don't understand what they are, where they come from, and what they can do to your body. That's what this chapter is all about.

The current presence of toxins is overwhelming. Toxic sources are ubiquitous in our everyday lives, and the effects on your body's complex systems can be devastating. Some of the sources will surprise you; I bet you're familiar with the dangers of lead paint, but how about the presence of arsenic in the treated lumber you used to build your deck, or the antimony in your baby's bedding? I devote a good portion of this chapter to identifying common toxins that we're exposed to every day, so you can understand what's out there and how it could be entering your body.

Humans have some built-in mechanisms that help to rid our bodies of foreign materials that occur commonly in nature. But because dangerous manmade chemicals have become more abundant only in the last 100 years or so, we're not equipped to deal with their threats to our health. These toxins put a serious strain on our natural detoxification mechanisms and can eventually exhaust and overwhelm them. Toxins can damage many of our other systems, as well.

Exploring the Various Types of Toxins

The range of toxic materials that surrounds you every day of your life is dizzying. For the purposes of this book, a *toxin* is any substance that has harmful effects on human biochemistry or tissue. Keep in mind that some chemicals that are usually helpful to us actually become toxic if we get too much of them; vitamin D is an example.

Because the term *toxin* can be used to describe so many different substances, it can sometimes be difficult to focus on the specific toxins that you should be aware of while working toward detoxifying your body. In this section, I fill you in on many of the most dangerous toxic materials that you're likely to face on a regular basis — toxins that are very common and also very harmful.

When most people start thinking about toxins, their minds jump immediately to nasty chemicals. They think about smokestacks spewing poisonous gases into the atmosphere and rusty pipes pouring sludge into a nearby stream. But that isn't the whole picture. Don't get me wrong: Plenty of industrial byproducts and other manmade toxins pose a threat to the wellbeing of millions. But when you're considering the range of toxins, you should also keep in mind things like bacteria and viruses, or even medical materials like chemotherapy drugs.

I cover most of the major types of toxins in this section, so read on to discover the toxins that can creep in silently around you and jeopardize your good health. I also offer some brief insight on what each of these toxins can do to your body, and if you find yourself wanting to know more about toxic effects you can skip ahead to the next section of this chapter.

As you read, you'll probably want to know what you can do to limit your exposure to toxins. Feel free to flip ahead to Chapter 3, which features information on how to dodge toxins. And if you're eager to know whether or not you have dangerously high levels of these toxins in your body, check out the details on getting tested for toxins (by a doctor) in Chapter 5.

Feeling the weight of heavy metals

Heavy metal doesn't just refer to music with blaring electric guitars and thunderous drum solos. The heavy metals I describe over the course of the next few pages can be found virtually anywhere, and they have an extremely toxic effect on the human body.

Heavy metals feature a chemical structure that causes them to harm the human body's normal (and complex) chemical processes. These metals occur naturally in the earth, but they're usually present in very low levels and rarely cause problems for people in those forms. The real trouble begins when heavy metals are used commercially and end up in concentrated amounts in the goods that we purchase, bring into our homes, and incorporate in our everyday lives.

Read on to get a feel for the most widespread and dangerous heavy metals.

Mercury

With the exception of plutonium (which is radioactive), mercury is the most toxic substance on earth for humans. Just one one-thousandth of a gram is toxic, and hundreds of tons of mercury are released into our environment every year in the United States alone. Mercury is a known toxin for nerves and contributes to a wide range of ailments from autism to Alzheimer's to decreased fertility. Estimates from clinical evaluations show that one in eight women have dangerously high mercury levels. Mercury is transferred from mother to fetus during pregnancy, which may help explain why one in six children today has neuropsychological problems. Not only is mercury highly toxic, but it's also very tough to eliminate from the body. Natural removal is so slow that after one exposure it takes 15 to 30 years for half the mercury to be eliminated.

You can be exposed to mercury through several different sources, and the following are among the most common:

✔ **Dental fillings:** The "silver" or amalgam fillings that dentists use to fill cavities are 50 percent mercury. That mercury gradually seeps out of the fillings and into your body. The American Dental Association insists that the mercury is bound to other metals and doesn't typically enter the body, but multiple studies have shown otherwise. In fact, many European countries have banned the use of amalgam fillings in children and women of childbearing age. If that doesn't turn you off to the use of these types of fillings, consider that when dentists receive the material used to make the fillings it comes in packaging made for hazardous materials, and when the fillings are removed dentists must dispose of the remnants using toxic waste procedures! In my opinion, you should completely avoid amalgam fillings, and if you already have them you should consider having them removed. If that's the case, be sure to find a biomedical dentist who knows how to take out the fillings safely, using a rubber dam and a high speed vacuum.

✔ **Coal:** The coal that's mined and burned to generate electricity contains mercury. Coal-burning power plants release thousands of pounds of mercury into the atmosphere each year. Many of the world's quickly developing countries, including China, are building coal-burning plants at an incredible rate, so the amount of mercury released into our air is getting higher all the time. The technology to remove the mercury from power plant byproducts exists, but it's an added expense that would cut into power company profits.

✔ **High fructose corn syrup (HFCS):** High fructose corn syrup is one of the most common sugar substitutes used today, and one of the first steps in making HFCS involves soaking corn in a solution that contains mercury. That mercury can end up in the foods you eat that contain HFCS. A recent study by the Institute for Agriculture and Trade Policy showed that when HFCS was the first or second ingredient listed, half the processed food samples they tested contained mercury.

✔ **Fish:** Mercury from a huge range of sources eventually ends up in bodies of water across the globe, and as a result it also ends up in fish. The problem has swelled dramatically in the past decade, leading the U.S. Food and Drug Administration (FDA) and Environmental Protection Agency (EPA) to release multiple warnings about the dangers of eating fish and shellfish, especially for children and pregnant women. The FDA issued a public warning in 2001 with an update in 2004 that stated that if a pregnant woman eats a single 3-ounce portion of swordfish, shark, tile fish, king mackerel, or tuna, she will ingest enough mercury to damage the brain of her fetus.

Educate yourself about the mercury-related risks associated with eating fish and shellfish by visiting www.epa.gov/waterscience/fish/publicinfo.html.

✔ **Fluorescent lightbulbs:** Many homes and businesses have been switching to fluorescent lightbulbs to help cut down on energy use, but that news isn't all good. Fluorescent bulbs contain mercury, and if a bulb breaks you should treat the situation with extreme caution.

You can and should read the EPA's suggestions for cleaning up a broken fluorescent lightbulb at this Web site: www.epa.gov/hg/spills/.

Mercury can also be found in flu vaccines; flip ahead a few pages in this chapter to read all about those potential threats.

Lead

The toxicity of lead has been recognized for many years, but the widespread use of the metal throughout history means that we'll be forced to deal with lead and its health consequences for the foreseeable future. Federal legislation was enacted in the 1970s to remove lead from paint and fuel, and many people assume that lead levels have dwindled as a result. That's simply not the case because lead doesn't go away — it's a very persistent material.

Lead poisoning causes many health problems, including damage to neurological systems. The developing brains and nervous systems of children can be severely harmed if their lead levels are too high.

Most children today are tested for lead poisoning, but the vast majority of those tests are based on blood samples. Blood tests reveal elevated lead levels in the blood. Here's the problem: Lead is absorbed by brain and other tissues, and blood tests aren't as good at registering high lead levels in the brain. Plus, blood tests reveal only very recent exposure. Luckily, other tests can more accurately detect overall lead levels; to read all about them, flip ahead to Chapter 5.

What are the major sources of lead toxicity today? Lead can be found in all sorts of places, including the following:

✔ **Lead paint:** Most of the paint used on homes prior to 1960 contained dangerously high levels of lead, and lead was still present in paints used on homes up to the late 1970s. Some estimates indicate that 10 million pounds of lead are still on painted surfaces in the United States. As many as 6 million homes, which house about 2 million children, have surfaces covered in paint that includes lead.

When you think of lead paint, you may think only about painted interior and exterior walls of old houses. Unfortunately, that's just the tip of the iceberg. Lead paint can be used on all kinds of surfaces, and believe it or not lead is still used in some paints today. Although it seems unthinkable, some toy manufacturers still use lead paint on toys, even though it's illegal. To get a feel for the scope of this problem, run a search for "toy hazard recalls" on the U.S. Consumer Product Safety Commission's Web site (www.cpsc.gov).

✔ **Water supplies:** Some older homes have plumbing that includes lead or lead soldering. That lead can leach into your drinking water, and the problem is more common than you may think. Some researchers indicate that as many as 16 percent of household water supplies have dangerous concentrations of lead.

✔ **Other sources:** Millions of tons of lead are produced every year for industrial and commercial uses, and the toxin ends up in many items. For example, the glazing used on some types of pottery contains lead, and the supplies used in creating stained glass can be lead-rich, as well. And you know that antique lead crystal decanter that your grandmother passed down to you? It's called *lead crystal* for a reason. Many candles also have lead core wicks.

For more information on lead and lead poisoning, visit the EPA's lead information page at www.epa.gov/lead.

Aluminum

Aluminum is a toxic metal that serves absolutely no useful purpose in the human body. It's also the most abundant metal in the earth's crust. We all have some aluminum in our systems, but because it's a toxin and can have some nasty effects on the body, you need to know where aluminum is commonly found. The following is a list of a few everyday items that are made of or can contain aluminum:

- Aluminum foil
- Antacids
- Antiperspirants
- Baking powder
- Bleached flour
- Cookware
- Municipal water supplies
- Toothpaste

The toxic effects of aluminum are well understood and are being studied more all the time. Aluminum has toxic effects on the brain. It would be next to impossible for you to completely curtail your intake of aluminum, but it certainly wouldn't hurt you to limit your use of products that contain high amounts of the metal.

Some of the ailments that have been linked to higher-than-usual levels of aluminum include neurologic conditions similar to Alzheimer's, colic, rickets, intestinal problems, extreme nervousness, anemia, headaches, memory loss, speech problems, and aching muscles.

Arsenic

Arsenic is an element that occurs naturally in soil, and the concentrations of arsenic existing in the environment vary from location to location. As with some of the other toxins described in this section, small amounts of naturally occurring arsenic are somewhat normal and don't represent a serious health risk.

However, increased exposure to arsenic can have devastating effects on your body. Arsenic can cause intestinal problems, anemia, skin lesions, liver or kidney damage, and even death. The EPA has stated that arsenic can cause several types of cancer in humans. And a study published in the *Journal of the American Medical Association* (a prestigious, widely respected medical journal) found an association between increased arsenic levels and type 2 diabetes in adults.

Arsenic and poultry farming

In recent years, the use of arsenic in poultry farming has become an increasing concern. The debate centers on an arsenic-based substance called *roxarsone,* which is added to chicken feed to help cut down on parasites that live in chicken intestines. Several potential health issues can arise from that practice, the first of which being (of course) the presence of arsenic in chicken meat. A few years ago, the Institute for Agriculture and Trade Policy (IATP) tested 155 samples from uncooked supermarket chicken products and found detectable arsenic in more than half of the samples. The IATP also tested 90 fast food chicken products and found that all 90 contained detectable arsenic. The IATP cautions that its testing is by no means definitive, but the findings are troubling at best.

As a result of some of the public outcry over the use of roxarsone, several poultry producers have stopped using it. If you're concerned about the issue, do some online research to find out which producers no longer use roxarsone. And you can always buy USDA certified 100 percent organic chicken; organic standards prohibit the use of arsenic-based substances.

Even more troubling could be what happens when the arsenic from roxarsone *doesn't* get absorbed by chickens. In that case the arsenic passes out of the chicken in its feces, which is often used as an agricultural fertilizer. When the fertilizer is applied to fields, the arsenic can be washed away and find its way into groundwater, which is a common source of drinking water for many communities.

Clearly it's in your best interest to limit your exposure to arsenic whenever you can, but how can you do that? The first step is to be mindful of where arsenic is present in your surroundings.

Arsenic compounds are used as wood preservatives, so many "pressure-treated" varieties of wood contain arsenic. These types of wood aren't used for residential purposes as much now as they were in the past, but you can still easily find lumber that has been treated with arsenic compounds. Decks and outdoor children's play sets are a couple of prime sources.

Arsenic is also used in paints, dyes, metals, drugs, soaps, and semiconductors. It's added to some fertilizers and animal feeding operations, which can increase the amount of arsenic in food.

Antimony

Antimony is a heavy metal that is used as a fire retardant in many fabrics. It's also a potent toxin that can get into your bloodstream and then into your body's tissues within two hours of exposure. Antimony accumulates in organs and even bone, and it can disrupt the way that your organs function, causing anorexia, fatigue, muscle pain, low blood pressure, fragile red blood cells, mental changes, and heart pain.

Where can antimony be found? You can find it in a variety of fire-retardant textiles: clothes, bedding, and carpet to name a few. It's also present in solders, small arms ammunition, lead batteries, paints, enamels, glass, and pottery glazes.

The EPA doesn't closely monitor environmental levels of antimony, so data on its prevalence is tough to come by.

Tin

Tin is another common heavy metal, and it often combines with other materials to form compounds. Some of these compounds are easily absorbed into the human body when tin is ingested (in food or water), and — fortunately — some of the other tin compounds are less likely to enter your system.

People inadvertently ingest tin in a number of different ways. You can take in tin if you eat or drink something that comes in a tin can that has a damaged liner, for example. Tin is also present in solder, in toothpastes that contain stannous fluoride (check for it in the ingredients list on your toothpaste package), and in other health and beauty products like soap and perfume.

You can also find tin compounds in things like rodent poison, fungicides, wood preservatives, herbicides, and sprays used to control mites and ticks.

Tin toxicity is very hard on the body, causing symptoms like brain swelling, headaches, visual defects, low blood sugar, and decreased immune function.

In addition to the metals I describe in this section, several others are less commonly encountered but can still cause serious problems. These metals include barium, bismuth, cadmium, platinum, thallium, tungsten, and uranium. If you're getting tested for toxicity — read more about that in Chapter 5 — you may want to include tests for these metals just in case.

Living toxins: Getting toxic from the inside

As I mention at the start of this section, a toxin is any substance that has a harmful effect on human biochemistry or tissue. A common misconception is that only chemicals are toxins. There's much more to the story than that.

Toxins can be living things, and it's important that you consider — and act to prevent — the toxic effects of bacteria, viruses, yeast, and parasites.

Certain types of these four categories of living things can be a constant challenge to your body and can negatively affect your health just as much as some of the dangerous heavy metals.

Most of these living toxins enter your body through your mouth, nose, lungs, and stomach. Your immune system puts up a good fight, but it can be overwhelmed — especially if it has been weakened by other toxins along the way — and may not be able to tackle the challenges that some bacteria, viruses, yeast, and parasites present.

Bacteria

Bacteria are microscopic, single-celled organisms that live on our skin and inside our intestines. If they're located anywhere else it's called an *infection*, and the results are toxic. We're covered inside and out with good bacteria that live with us, cleaning up our skin and intestinal tract. But if you get the wrong kind of bacteria in your intestines, the toxic effects can include the following:

- Abdominal cramping
- Body infection
- Constipation
- Diarrhea
- Foul-smelling stools
- Spastic colon

You can also experience neurological symptoms like fatigue, changes in mood, agitation, and decreased attention.

Viruses

Viruses are very basic living things that can reproduce and interact with your body's cells. The types of viruses range from the virus that causes the common cold to the human immunodeficiency virus (HIV). Viruses usually reproduce very rapidly, but your immune system (if it's healthy) can kill most of them off.

The best way to defend your body against viruses and the toxic problems they cause is to maintain a robust immune system. Check out Chapter 10 for lots of useful information on how you can detoxify your body to help your immune system flourish.

Yeast

Yeasts are single-celled fungi, and they're ever-present in our environment. There are plenty of good yeasts (as anyone enjoying a cold beer or a slice of bread can tell you), but some yeasts can act as toxins when present in your body in unusually high numbers. The yeast cells themselves aren't necessarily toxic, but some of the substances produced by yeasts can cause a range of ailments. The more yeast cells living in your body, the more toxic substances are generated. Those toxins can cause the following ailments, among others:

- ✔ **Gastrointestinal problems:** Constipation, diarrhea, indigestion, cramping, excessive gas, heartburn, spastic colon, irritable bowel syndrome, colitis, and chronic gum inflammation

- ✔ **Neurological problems:** Fatigue, depression, psychosis, mood swings, insomnia, drunken feeling, hyperactivity, agitation, and decreased attention span

- ✔ **Respiratory problems:** Asthma, allergies, recurrent infections (sinusitis, tonsillitis, bronchitis), colds, and sore throat

If your diet includes a lot of sugar, you're probably nourishing the yeast cells you're hosting and making it easier for them to live and reproduce. That's not a good thing, and it's one of many reasons to rein in the amount of sugar you eat on a daily basis.

Yeast-related problems commonly crop up after people take antibiotics. The powerful antibiotics used now are great at wiping out the bacteria that cause sickness, but there's a downside: The harmless and good types of bacteria (the types that live in your intestines and aid digestion) get wiped out, too, and in their absence yeasts can grow and reproduce at rapid rates. That's a big part of the reason that women often suffer vaginal yeast infections after taking rounds of antibiotics.

Parasites

Parasites are tiny creatures that live on or inside our bodies — freeloaders that feast on the nutrients we bring in and contribute absolutely nothing to our health or well-being. They range from worms (tapeworms and hookworms, not the worms that you used as fishing bait when you were little) to the critters that cause malaria. Many parasites set up shop in the intestines because that's one of the best places to find a wide variety of available nutrients.

For centuries it was common for people to get a bowel cleanse or some other form of parasite removal once a year. (Perhaps you remember hearing your grandparents or great-grandparents talk about getting "wormed" — that's the same thing.) *Parasite cleanses,* or techniques that help to rid the body of parasite invaders, are far less common now than they used to be, and in most cases that's not necessarily a good thing. For details on how you can use some of these methods to keep parasites out of your system, flip to Chapter 10.

Swallowing the bitter pill: Toxins in medicines

Many of the toxins I explain in this chapter come from sources that aren't surprising. It's not really hard to believe that a massive coal-burning power plant, for instance, may be spewing some toxic materials out into the environment. But some toxins come from sources that most people think of as benign or even beneficial. One of the most surprising areas where toxins are becoming increasingly common is traditional medicine. Some of the treatments and drugs used to cure illnesses can actually cause quite a few others. The culprits range from vaccines to radiation, and I discuss several of them over the course of the next few pages.

Vaccines

Vaccines have been in the news a lot lately, and they likely will continue to be for quite some time. I want to start this explanation by stating that I don't tell my patients to refrain from getting vaccines. Vaccinations can be a good thing, and it would be hard to refute the fact that some vaccines have helped to save many lives in the last 60 years. When my patients ask me about vaccines, I tell them that the best thing they can do is to get informed about the vaccinations they're considering and make a decision that takes into consideration all the related risks and benefits.

That said, here are a few of the vaccines that have been under fire recently:

✔ **Influenza vaccines:** Commonly called *flu shots,* a number of vaccinations for the influenza virus are on the market today. Some of these vaccines include a chemical called *thimerosal,* which contains mercury. (Flip back a few pages in this chapter to read all about mercury.) Thimerosal is used as a preservative in these influenza vaccines, and it's about half mercury, by weight.

The toxicity of the mercury in thimerisol is currently being debated, but no matter which side of the debate you fall on, here's some good news: Some influenza vaccines do *not* contain thimerisol, so you have options if you want to get a flu shot but don't want to also get a dose of mercury. The bad news is that mercury-free shots can be difficult to locate, and some doctors don't know which type they have. In some states, the mercury-free versions are reserved for Medicaid patients.

The FDA has a lot of thimerosal information on its Web site, including a list that shows you some of the vaccines that do not contain the substance. Check out `www.fda.gov/cber/vaccine/thimerosal.htm`.

✔ **Diphtheria, tetanus, and pertussis (DTP) vaccines**: Many forms of the DTP vaccine, which is commonly given to infants, contain both aluminum and formaldehyde. Some people argue that the amounts of these toxins in the vaccine are minimal and don't cause any problems; others contend that the substances are dangerous no matter how small the amount.

✔ **Polio vaccines:** Many of the polio vaccines made today are processed through the cells of Green Monkey kidneys. In previous decades, monkey viruses have contaminated polio vaccine doses, and those doses were given to the general public before the virus was discovered. Many researchers claim that the problem is behind us, but some scientists believe we still need to be concerned.

✔ **Hepatitis B vaccines:** Most of the controversy surrounding vaccines for hepatitis B centers on the use of the vaccine in children. U.S. government data has shown that children under the age of 14 are as much as three times more likely to suffer adverse effects from the hepatitis B vaccine as they are to catch the disease in the absence of a vaccination.

Some of the questions that have been raised about the safety of vaccines can make some people roll their eyes, but the fact is that many of the questions are justified and require quite a bit more research. To get a feel for how serious some of these questions may be, consider the following quote, which is taken from a statement that Dr. Jane Orient, the executive director of the Association of American Physicians and Surgeons at the time, presented to a Congressional subcommittee in 1999:

> *Public policy regarding vaccines is fundamentally flawed. It is permeated by conflicts of interest. It is based on poor scientific methodology (including studies that are too small, too short, and too limited in populations represented), which is, moreover, insulated from independent criticism. The evidence is far too poor to warrant overriding the independent judgments of patients, parents, and attending physicians, even if this were ethically or legally acceptable.*

If you're thinking about getting vaccines for you or your family, make sure you have a candid conversation with a doctor who will listen to your concerns about the risks associated with the vaccinations you're considering.

Chemotherapy

Chemotherapy (also called *chemo*) is a treatment for cancer that uses a combination of drugs to kill or slow the growth of cancerous cells. It can be a very useful way to fight some cancers, but the drugs used are effectively toxins. The side effects of chemo can be extremely uncomfortable or painful and can include hair loss, abdominal pain, weakening of the bones, and even cancer.

Even at its best, chemo is very hard on the body, but it can be made less of a burden if a patient's diet and nutrition are healthy before and during the treatment. Patients who have taken care to eat a healthy diet — the kind of diet I trumpet throughout this book, particularly in Chapter 7 — generally experience less severe chemotherapy side effects than those who have poor eating habits.

If you're facing a fight against cancer and you have to decide whether or not to proceed with chemotherapy, make sure you have an extensive conversation with your doctor about the effectiveness of chemo treatment on the specific type of cancer in question. Some types of cancer can be treated extremely effectively with chemo, but other types don't respond nearly as well. For example, if a certain kind of cancer has a five-year survival rate with chemo treatment and a four-year survival rate without chemo, you may want to consider other ways to treat the cancer. On the other hand, chemotherapy can provide a 90 percent cure rate for some types of cancer.

Radiation

Like chemotherapy, the use of radiation in modern medicine is focused on treating cancer patients. And as with chemo, radiation can be a very necessary evil if you have a cancer fight on your hands.

Radiation treatment involves pointing an ionizing radiation beam at a mass of cancer cells in order to kill the targeted tissue (usually a cancerous tumor). The beam is moved around a focal point in the tumor so that the surrounding tissue receives only a small amount of radiation while the target area is hit hard with the radiation.

Radiation therapy has made terrific strides in recent years, but the process still has a toxic effect on the healthy tissues that surround the cancerous cells. As you'd guess, the healthier the tissue, the less likely it will be damaged by the radiation. And what's the best way to build healthy tissues in your body? That's right — stay away from toxins and eat a healthy diet that focuses on the right (toxin-free) foods.

If you're going to have radiation therapy, do some research on hyperbaric oxygen therapy, which can reduce the damage to your body from radiation.

Exploring the Effects of Toxins

In the previous sections of this chapter, I offer some basic information on how various toxins can harm your body and its many complex systems. It's always good to be familiar with the havoc that a particular toxin can wreak on you, but I think it's also very useful for you to understand some of the more general problems that toxins can cause. The toxic problem in our world is a big one, and you can get a feel for the scope of the issue if you take a step back and view it through a wide-angle lens. That's the point of this section: to clue you in on the broad range of awful effects that toxins can have.

Some toxins affect the body by modifying its natural chemical balance, causing certain systems to break down. Others are less sneaky and can flat-out kill some body tissues. Still other toxins actually alter our genetic material, causing devastating problems like birth defects. I explore all these possible effects in this section.

Cellular damage

The most basic type of harm that toxins can cause you is cellular damage. (No, I'm not talking about what happens when you accidentally drop your cell phone on the sidewalk. This is much more serious stuff.) We are all made of cells, and toxins have a very nasty habit of changing the proteins and other materials in our cells, to the point where a cell's basic functions can be altered or stopped completely.

Some people hear about the basics of cellular damage and think, *What's the big deal? Cells are so small, and I've got trillions of 'em! If a little bit of mercury kills off a few cells, I'll be fine.*

The problem is that when toxins have a negative effect at the cellular level, the scope of the harm done can snowball very quickly. If many cells are damaged, it doesn't take long for an entire section of tissue to fail. If that failure is bad enough, it can jeopardize the health of one of your organs. And when an organ is in trouble, it won't be long until your whole body is in serious danger.

Nerve damage

Nerve tissue — the stuff that makes up your brain, spinal cord, and all your nerves — is very delicate, and it's subject to damage from incredibly small amounts of toxins. The toxins in some insecticides, for example, can cause brain damage in a matter of hours from just a single exposure. Or take some of the heavy metal toxins I describe earlier in this chapter. If you have an acute exposure to one of those substances, or even many small exposures over a long period of time, you can easily end up with damage to your nervous system that extends from your brain to your spinal cord to the nerves that spread out throughout the rest of your body.

Some research even argues that conditions affecting the nervous system — Alzheimer's, Parkinson's, and multiple sclerosis are just three examples — can be partially caused or accelerated by heavy metals and other chemicals that cause toxic nerve damage. As with many medical debates, there are supporters with considerable evidence on both sides of that conversation, and additional studies that will help to shed light on the issue are being published all the time. But there is no question that heavy metals cause nerve damage.

Intestinal complications

You may not think very highly of your intestinal tract, especially if you've had any encounters with a spicy habanero enchilada lately, but your intestines really are marvelous, complicated things. The processes that take place in your intestines are absolutely vital to your health, and keeping that part of your body in tip-top shape can go a long way toward boosting your overall health. Unfortunately, many of the toxins to which we're exposed every day can have an incredibly negative effect on your intestines.

Any unhealthy, unnatural thing (read: toxin) that you eat or drink that isn't broken down in your mouth or stomach can cause irritation or inflammation of the intestines. When your intestines get inflamed, the result may be diarrhea, which is one way that your body tries to rid itself of toxic materials. If the inflammation persists, the intestines will slow down their function, and constipation is the result.

Many people try to override the diarrhea part of the process by taking medicines, but that's not always the best route. After all, your body could simply be trying to clear out a substance that doesn't belong. Before you reach for the antidiarrheal medicine to help solve a minor case of diarrhea, consider the option of drinking plenty of water and enduring the problem to give your body the chance to rid itself of a potentially harmful substance.

Chronic inflammation of the intestines due to toxins can also cause a condition called *leaky gut syndrome*. Leaky gut syndrome isn't often recognized by doctors of traditional medicine, but a growing amount of evidence supports the theory behind the condition. With leaky gut syndrome, your intestines aren't able to maintain a proper barrier between the contents of your intestine and your bloodstream. Materials that should remain in your intestines pass through into your bloodstream, and food allergies and other ailments may result.

Fat cell accumulation

One of the body's mechanisms for dealing with toxins (read all about those mechanisms in Chapter 4) is to store the toxins in fat cells. That works out only if the toxin in question is *fat-soluble*, meaning that its chemical makeup allows it to be stored in fat. When your body sticks a toxin in a fat cell, the fat cell tries to get bigger in order to decrease the concentration of the newly introduced toxic substance. And what happens when your fat cells increase in size? Fat is accumulated, and you gain weight. This process is part of the reason that people suffer from obesity, which of course is a problem of epidemic proportions in the United States, costing us billions of dollars every year.

Chapter 3

Discovering Where Toxins Come From (And How to Avoid Them!)

*T*he toxins that surround us today are many and varied, but the ways in which those toxins enter our bodies are limited to three main routes: our food, our drinking water, and the air we breathe. If you want to live a truly detoxified life, all you have to do is make certain that every morsel of food you eat, every drop of water you drink, and every breath of air you take are toxin free! As you may imagine, that's very difficult to achieve, but if you do you'll be rewarded with a healthier life.

In this chapter, I offer insight on how toxins assault you through food, water, and air. I let you know how toxins end up in these three places, explain a little about what they can do to your body in certain situations, and provide useful tips on how you can avoid eating, drinking, and breathing toxins.

Hungering to Understand Toxins in Food

The food you choose to eat is one of the most important factors — some people would argue *the* most important — in determining your overall health. It's such an old cliché, but you really are what you eat. If you want to be toxin free, you have to eat toxin free (or at least as toxin free as possible).

In this section, I tackle a couple key questions:

✔ How does food end up loaded with toxins?

✔ What basic steps can you take to avoid toxins in food?

You may be shocked by the many toxic hurdles that your food has to clear before it ends up on your dinner table, but after reading about all the potentially toxic influences you probably won't be surprised to find out that quite a lot of your food contains some sort of dangerous material. And you're sure to wonder — if you don't already — how you can begin to take steps to limit the amount of toxin-filled food that ends up on your plate. That's why I finish this section with some very basic recommendations for how you can start that process. (I dive into much more detail on that topic in several of the chapters you can find in Part II.)

Digging up details about toxins in soil

Soil is the starting point for a huge number of food products that we eat today. The plants that make up a substantial part of our diets — from basic grains to exotic fruits — get their start in the soil. And plenty of the other materials we consume, such as meats, either eat plants that were grown in soil, are in constant contact with soil, or both. Good ol' dirt really is the starting point for a lot of the calories we take in every day.

The troubling part about the importance of soil in helping to grow and support the things we eat is the fact that soil can be extremely toxic. Many thousands of tons of toxic materials are released directly onto the earth each year, and many thousands more make their way to the soil after first being pumped into the air or into bodies of water.

When it comes to toxins in the soil, one of the top offenders is a group of substances that are supposedly added to the soil to improve the food we eat: fertilizers. Fertilizers can contain all sorts of toxic materials, and the ways in which these materials end up in common fertilizers may cause you to cringe.

One example is the practice of mixing industrial wastes into fertilizers. Yes, you read that right: Industrial waste is sometimes "recycled" and used as a component in fertilizer. The general idea behind this process is that some industrial byproducts, including zinc and nitrogen, are key ingredients in certain types of fertilizer. So instead of trying to dispose of the byproducts, why not just use them to create the fertilizers that make our soil more productive? Well, for starters, the byproducts don't contain only zinc and nitrogen. They can also contain toxins like the heavy metals that I explain in Chapter 2.

You may wonder how this practice is allowed to continue. Put simply, some people argue that the amounts of toxins in the industrial waste that eventually ends up in the soil aren't necessarily any higher than the levels that are normally found in the soil. (Remember that many toxins, particularly heavy metals, do exist in nature in small amounts.) But the truth is that we don't fully understand what this practice is doing to our soil and to our food, and there's no question that the fertilizers are much more toxic than what naturally occurs in soil.

You may also be wondering why farmers would knowingly add toxins to the soil through the use of fertilizers. The truth is that many fertilizers don't list the toxic materials they contain because fertilizer producers aren't required to list all the ingredients used to make their products — only the active ingredients that make plants grow faster or bigger.

Another fertilizer-related source of toxins in our soil are *biosolids*: the waste materials removed from our water at water treatment plants. Biosolids are commonly sold or given away for use as fertilizer. The idea is that the biosolids are a somewhat more natural alternative to chemical fertilizers, which is all well and good. The problem is that biosolids have their own toxic components, like hormones, detergents, pesticides, carcinogens, antibiotics, and other pharmaceuticals. Basically, anything that ends up in our water supply can end up in biosolids, and that includes plenty of toxins. When you get right down to it, biosolids aren't really a more natural alternative to chemical fertilizers.

Investigating insecticides and pesticides

The use of pesticides on fruit and vegetable crops can often result in increased amounts of dangerous toxins in your food. (*Pesticides* are chemicals used to kill insects, fungi, and even rodents.) The goal of most pesticides is to wipe out pests but not harm other living things. Unfortunately, the majority of pesticides contain toxins that endanger the health or even the lives of many animals — humans included.

Children are especially vulnerable to the toxins in pesticides, even when amounts are extremely small. If you're buying or serving food for kids, try to cut down on the amount of pesticides that end up on their fruits and vegetables. Check out Chapter 7 for details.

Pesticides contain so many different toxic ingredients that poisoning can affect any body system. The most common effects are on the nerves: Acute poisoning can cause tremors, shakes, and severe psychiatric and behavioral changes, not to mention brain tumors. And you don't have to be exposed to a large amount of these types of toxins to get sick from them. Very small doses over a long period of time can result in severe damage to your health. The National Academy of Sciences estimates that in the next 70 years, pesticide residue on food will cause 1 million additional cases of cancer in the United States.

More than 3,000 active toxic ingredients are used in pesticides, and U.S. Environmental Protection Agency (EPA) records show more than 100,000 registered pesticide products in the United States. That massive number includes pesticides that are used on the largest farms down to the pesticides you buy for your lawn or garden.

If you want to buy pesticides to use on your garden at home, make sure you know which pesticides are the most dangerous. How? Pay close attention to pesticide labels. Pesticide products each have one of three labels, as follows:

- ✔ **Caution:** Mildly toxic. Anything more than an ounce is a lethal dose for a human. (Even smaller amounts will kill a child.)

- ✔ **Warning:** Medium toxicity for a pesticide. A teaspoon to a tablespoon is enough to kill an adult.

- ✔ **Danger:** Highly toxic. A very small amount is enough to kill an adult. (Look for the skull and crossbones symbol to identify a pesticide in the "Danger" category.)

I strongly suggest cutting out the use of pesticides at home. You can find natural, nontoxic products that will rid your house and yard of pests; a quick online search will yield several options. But if you choose to use chemical pesticides, please try to stick to products in the "Caution" category.

Of course, most of the food you eat doesn't come from your garden, so what can you do to ensure that you're limiting the amount of pesticide toxins that ends up on your food? You can take several steps, from washing fruits and vegetables thoroughly to making wise decisions when you're buying your food. I include suggestions at the end of this chapter, and you can find more detail in Chapter 7.

Picking out problems with processed food

When I talk about *processed* food, I mean food products created using practices that range from genetic modification to food additives. To me, processing includes anything that's done to food outside of natural conditions. And at this point, all kinds of strange and dangerous things are done to our food long before we take a bite.

Genetic modification

The processing of food starts very early, even before the food is grown or raised. *Genetic modification,* which involves tinkering with a plant or animal's genes to make it easier to grow as a food source, is done on about 70 percent of the food in the average grocery store. Genetically modified foods aren't usually created to provide better nutrition but rather to increase production (so we can grow more tomatoes or raise more beef, for example).

I know it doesn't sound like such a bad thing to grow more food, but we don't fully understand the long-term effects that genetically modified foods can have on our bodies. For example, some vegetables are genetically modified to cause them to produce a toxin that acts as a pesticide so insects and other critters aren't as likely to feast on the crops. There's currently a debate on what effect that toxin can have on humans when the vegetables eventually end up on our plates. At the very least, I think we can all agree that what's going on is not a natural process, and there's real potential for negative effects on our health that we don't yet fully understand. For a much more detailed discussion of this subject, see Chapter 6.

Food additives

In total, food companies add 2,800 substances to their products in an effort to save a buck, boost sales, and ensure that their food will last on the store shelves for a very long time. If I covered all 2,800 of these substances here, *your* shelf life probably wouldn't be enough to get through them all. So instead I provide a snapshot of some of the toxins that are intentionally added to processed foods:

- ✔ **Aspartame:** One of the most toxic substances we are exposed to nearly every day, *aspartame* is a blend of toxic chemicals that's used as a sugar substitute in processed foods. You can find it in everything from diet soft drinks to chewing gum. It took the U.S Food and Drug Administration (FDA) 16 years to approve aspartame, and now millions of pounds of it are added to our food each year.

    Aspartame can act as an *excitotoxin* — a chemical that causes nerve cells to fire rapidly. Some studies have shown that excitotoxins cause nerve cells to fire so unusually fast that they do themselves irreparable harm.

    This substance can cause dizziness, visual impairment, disorientation, muscle aches, numbness, and more. At 86 degrees Fahrenheit, aspartame breaks down into wood alcohol, formaldehyde, and then formic acid — all toxic. Some women also report that aspartame worsens the symptoms of premenstrual syndrome (PMS).

    Aspartame is often used as a sugar substitute in so-called "diet foods," even though no conclusive evidence links aspartame (or any other sugar substitute, for that matter) to weight loss.

- ✔ **BHT:** You don't need to know the long chemical name that is abbreviated as *BHT,* but you do need to know that it's a common additive in many processed foods. In many ways the jury is still out on BHT, but the International Agency for Research on Cancer (IARC), which is an arm of the World Health Organization, considers BHT to be a possible carcinogen. To me, even a possible carcinogen is worth avoiding.

✓ **High fructose corn syrup:** This is a big one. High fructose corn syrup has become the primary sweetener in all kinds of foods, from soft drinks to cereals. You'd have a hard time walking more than a foot down any grocery store aisle before running into a food that includes it. Unfortunately, high fructose corn syrup contains mercury, which is one of the worst toxins for humans and one that I write about quite a bit in this book. This chemical form of fructose has also been linked to tooth decay, migraines, diabetes, obesity, and cancer. My advice is to start cutting down on the amount of high fructose corn syrup you're eating and drinking now, and keep cutting down until you're consuming very little or none of it.

✓ **Monosodium glutamate (MSG):** A huge range of processed foods include MSG — an additive that enhances food taste. MSG is an excitotoxin that can cause symptoms like nausea, cramps, dizziness, rash, heart palpitations, numbness, and even mood swings and confusion.

✓ **Olestra:** Olestra is essentially a fake fat. It's used in place of fat in processed foods to make the nutritional information look a little better for people who are trying to lose a few pounds (although no evidence proves it can help with dieting). How does it work? Simple: Olestra molecules are too big for our digestive systems to absorb, so this substance just moves on down the line instead of ending up in our bodies like normal fats. But here's the problem: You must have some real fats in your diet for you to absorb key vitamins like A, D, E, and K, not to mention *carotenoids* (nutrients that protect us from cancer).

✓ **Sodium benzoate:** This substance is a food preservative and a common additive in soft drinks. Also known as *benzoic acid,* it is thought to form benzene in soft drinks, especially when it can combine with vitamin C. Benzene is a very nasty toxin and a known carcinogen.

✓ **Splenda:** Splenda is another artificial sweetener that can cause toxic effects. It's made by adding chlorine to a natural sugar. The result is a material in the same chemical family as DDT and chlordane — two extremely toxic substances. Studies conducted on animals have shown Splenda to cause swelling and damage to the liver in moderate doses, as well as tumors in some animals.

When food additives are evaluated to figure out how toxic they can be for the human body, they're tested one at a time. This is a real problem because just like most other toxic situations, the combination of two or more food additives can multiply the toxic effects of all the additives. In other words, the food additive combo can be more toxic than the sum of its parts! For example, if certain blue food colorings (which you can read about next) are added to MSG, the toxic effect is seven times as potent as it would be if the additives were kept separate. And remember than many processed foods contain several additives, so it's not uncommon to find a toxic mix in a single product.

Food coloring

Artificial food coloring may make processed foods look bright and (for some strange reason) appetizing, but the toxins that make up these additives don't belong in your body. Most artificial food colors are derived from coal tar and petroleum. It doesn't take a nutritionist to tell you that coal tar doesn't belong in the human diet. You'd expect to see food coloring as an ingredient in things like junk food and soft drinks, but it also pops up in some less obvious places, like salmon and fresh cherries. Here's a quick rundown of a few common food colors:

- **Blue 1&2:** Used in baked goods, candy, and beverages. Both dyes have been linked to cancer in tests using mice.

- **Green 3:** Used in sauces, jellies, and more. This one has been linked to bladder cancer.

- **Orange B:** Approved for use in only hot dog and sausage casings. This dye has been associated with urinary obstruction.

- **Red 3:** Sprayed on fresh cherries and used in fruit cocktails, baked goods, and candy. Studies have shown it causes thyroid tumors in rats.

- **Red 40:** Used in snack foods. This dye has been linked to hyperactivity disorders.

- **Yellow 5:** Used in soft drinks, potato chips, jams, jellies, and more. This dye is strongly associated with hyperactivity and tantrums in children.

- **Yellow 6:** One of the most commonly used dyes in sausage, gelatin, baked goods, candy, and beverages. It has been linked to tumors of the adrenal glands and kidney.

Many of these color chemicals also contain heavy metals. (Flip back a chapter to read all about heavy metals and their effects on your body.)

Paying attention to packaging

If you read any of the last few pages, you can plainly see that our food is exposed to many different kinds of toxins through soil contamination, pesticide use, and food processing. As if that weren't enough, the packaging that surrounds our food can introduce toxic chemicals as well.

Hundreds of harmful chemicals are either included in or used to make food packaging materials, and I don't have the space here to discuss them all. But it's important that you consider packaging as a source of toxins, so in the next couple of pages I provide a quick look at a few of the most common toxins found in food packaging.

BPA

Some common varieties of plastic — including several that are used to make food containers — contain a chemical called *Bisphenol-A* (BPA). BPA is a synthetic sex hormone that has been linked to cancer, miscarriage, obesity, reproductive problems, heart disease, early puberty, and hyperactivity.

BPA is very harmful and particularly troublesome because it's found in so many different types of containers, from the linings of food and drink cans to baby bottles. You can find BPA in plastic food containers, sippy cups (specialized drinking cups for infants and toddlers), and even the IV tubes used in hospitals. (Okay, that last one is not technically food related, but it's still a pretty scary place to find a dangerous toxin.)

How widespread is BPA? The EPA states that 20 percent of the U.S. diet comes from foods that are packaged in plastics that contain BPA. And the BPA present in all that packaging material is clearly finding its way into our bodies: The Centers for Disease Control and Prevention (CDC) recently reported that 93 percent of Americans it tested have BPA in their systems.

To help cut down on your exposure to BPA, do the following:

- Use glass containers for food storage whenever possible.
- Limit your use of plastics stamped with a #7 on the bottom for any food-related purposes. (Not all #7 plastics contain BPA, but this is still a good general rule.)
- Don't microwave or heat your food in any plastic containers; heating plastics that contain BPA makes the chemical leach out into food at a much faster rate.

As with many toxic chemicals, the debate about the harm that BPA can do to us continues to rage on. My advice? Stay away from BPA whenever you can.

Phthalates

Phthalates are another dangerous class of chemicals found in food packaging. You rarely see the word "phthalate" listed anywhere, but the individual chemicals included in the group are easier to spot: DINP, DEHP, BBP, DBP, DUNP, DIDP, DNOP, and DIBP are some common examples. You can find these chemicals in many kinds of plastic materials, including plastic food containers and plastic food wrap.

What do phthalates do to the human body? The chemicals are suspected of causing cancer, reproductive problems, liver disease, and kidney disease, among other problems. To get an idea of how nasty phthalates are, take a look at the following wording, which appears on the label for pure DINP (the kind you'd use in a lab if you were a chemist):

May cause cancer; harmful by inhalation, in contact with skin, and if swallowed; possible risk of irreversible effects; avoid exposure; and wear suitable protective clothing, gloves and eye/face protection.

All the effects of phthalates like DINP aren't fully understood yet, but do you really want a substance that requires such a scary warning label coming in contact with the food you eat and the food you feed your family? I doubt it. To limit your exposure, avoid products that include one or several of the phthalate acronyms in their ingredients. Also, avoid the use of plastics stamped with a #7, and heat up your food in glass or porcelain containers instead of plastics.

PFOA and PFCs

Perfluorooctanoic acid (PFOA) and *perfluorochemicals* (PFCs) are in a class of chemicals used to make nonstick cookware and utensils, and they're also found in grease-resistant coatings for food packaging. If you don't limit the discussion to food-related materials, you can also throw in stain-resistant carpeting and fabrics and waterproof clothes as sources for the chemicals. Both PFOA and PFCs are toxic. It looks like the EPA will eventually classify PFOA as a carcinogen, and 19 EPA studies show PFCs to be a substantial risk for human health.

Dodging toxin-heavy foods

Nothing would make me happier than to tell you that you can completely avoid toxins in your food. Unfortunately, I don't think it's possible to cut out every single toxin from your diet. The best you can do is work hard to limit the amount of toxic exposure you and your family get from the food you eat. If you do that, you'll be light-years ahead of the majority of people. Understanding the problem and working to correct it are both enormous steps in the right direction.

In this section, I don't cover every detail of how you can fill up your grocery cart (and your dinner plate) with toxin-free foods, but I do provide basic tips on how to start the process. You can find some useful information on how to avoid specific types of food-related toxins in the first several pages of this chapter, and you can read much more on the topic in Chapters 6 and 7.

Reading food labels

It's easy to jot down a list of food items you need at the grocery store and then just cruise up and down the aisles until your cart is full and the foods on your list are all crossed off. The way that foods are produced, marketed, and put in front of you on the shelves has been streamlined to the point that you can fill your pantry quickly, easily, and cheaply without giving much thought to the process. The downside is that the path that toxins take to your food — and your body — has been streamlined too, and if you want to work toward limiting your exposure to toxins you have to insert some thought back into the process. One key way to do so is to read food labels carefully and completely when you're making choices about what foods to buy and eat.

Here are three steps for reading food labels to help you spot and avoid toxins:

1. **Don't buy a food if it contains ingredients that you don't know or can't pronounce.** I know that sounds incredibly simplistic, but it's a good general rule. For example, if you see a label that features ingredients like "100 percent organic pepper," "100 percent organic carrots," or "salt," you can feel pretty good about the lack of toxic materials that are added to the food as ingredients. However, if you see things like acesulfame-K — one of hundreds of common toxic ingredients — you want to pass on buying or eating that food product. (I discuss this rule in more detail in Chapter 5.)

2. **Pay attention to the order in which ingredients are listed.** Ingredients are listed according to the amount of each ingredient in the food. The ingredients that make up most of the food are listed first, and the ingredients that are present in smaller amounts are listed last. If you really believe that you have to buy a food product that contains a potentially harmful ingredient, try to buy a variety or brand that lists that ingredient at or near the bottom of the ingredients list.

3. **Watch out for different variations of the same toxin.** Food companies commonly list questionable ingredients under different (yet suitable, according to regulations) names or words. For example, forms of MSG can be listed as "calcium caseinate," "textured protein," or "glutamic acid," to name a few variations. You can't be expected to memorize every variation of every toxin, so use this rule in combination with rule #1 in this list. If you think an ingredient may be a different name or variation of a toxin and you can't pronounce it, don't buy it.

Some similar (and potentially harmful) ingredients can be listed with very different names and in multiple places within an ingredients list. Take sucrose, dextrose, and maltose, for example. They're common substitutes for sugar, and some processed foods contain two or even all three of them. A food label may list the three near the bottom of the ingredients list because technically they're different substances, but if you add up all the amounts of each contained in the food, it would be more like the first or second ingredient on the list. This technique is called *stacking,* and it's a common method for making an ingredients list look a little better than it really is.

Knowing the most common toxins in food

If you wanted to remember all the toxins that can be found in or on food products today, you'd probably have to quit your job and work on memorizing toxins full time. Realistically, you can't know everything about toxins in food, but you can do yourself (and your family) quite a bit of good if you just avoid the most common food toxins. Keep your eye out for these top toxin-containing ingredients:

- Artificial colors
- Aspartame
- High fructose corn syrup

Thirsting for Toxin-free Water

What's more important to life than water? Every living thing that we've ever discovered has required liquid water to survive, and humans are certainly no exception. The human body can go a few days without water, but if you're like me, you'd rather not go more than a few hours without a tall glass of it.

Our need for fresh water and the fact that most materials will dissolve in water make it particularly troublesome as a vehicle for spreading toxins. You need to be aware of the many toxic threats that your drinking water can pose, and you also need to consider the steps you can take to ensure that your water is as toxin-free as possible. I provide information on both fronts here.

Figuring out how toxins end up in drinking water

Many of the toxins pumped into our air and onto our soil end up in our water supply. Rain and the movement of water on and in the ground have a way of picking up substances — toxins included — and moving them all together toward a nearby body of water. These bodies of water include the various reservoirs that make up our drinking water supplies. So it shouldn't shock you to find out that the water that comes out of the tap in your kitchen sink isn't sparkling clean and toxin free.

Drinking water can contain all kinds of toxins. Read on to find out about a few of the most common.

Pharmaceuticals

The prescription and over-the-counter drugs we take don't all get absorbed into our systems when we pop a pill or drink a spoonful of syrupy medicine. A good portion of those pharmaceuticals passes virtually unchanged through our bodies and gets flushed (quite literally) down the toilet. More than 100 different kinds of drugs have been detected in water supplies all over the world, so we're not talking about an isolated problem here.

You may assume that the water treatment processes used to clean up our water take care of these wandering pharmaceuticals, but that isn't the case. The most common water treatment techniques don't remove or change pharmaceutical compounds. So if you think about your municipal water supply, the antibiotics your postal worker has been taking for his sinus infection, the painkillers your coworker took after her recent surgery, and the antidepressants your neighbor has been taking could be ending up (in small quantities) in your water supply. And then there are the veterinary medicines used on pets and farm animals. (The hormones used in raising beef cattle have been found in many water supplies and have been causing quite a stir in the media lately.)

The amounts of pharmaceuticals present in our water are small, but the whole idea behind most of these medicines is for a relatively small dose to have an effect on your entire body, so even tiny amounts can cause changes to your body's systems. Even more troubling is the threat of drug allergies: If a person has an extremely strong drug allergy, he could potentially suffer an allergic reaction just by drinking water from his community's water supply.

Commercial waste

Trillions of tons of toxic waste are released into our environment every year through commercial and industrial processes, and toxic materials have a tendency to collect in water.

Chemicals are usually assumed to be harmless unless proven otherwise, so most of the 80,000 chemicals used in or in the making of the products that surround us haven't been through a government-sanctioned safety review. Most of these chemicals aren't even monitored until someone notices patterns of illness, disease, or death resulting from exposure. Unfortunately, sometimes it takes years of exposure to a toxin before the effects show up and cause a real health problem, and by then it can be too late.

The watershed effect

A *watershed* is an area of land where all the water under it or on it goes to the same place. There are 2,110 watersheds in the United States, some of which cover thousands of square miles. Toxins can have a devastating effect on a watershed because small amounts of a toxin spread over a large area can be carried by moving water within a watershed and concentrated where the water eventually collects. You may not live close to a manufacturing plant that releases toxic chemicals, but if that plant is within your watershed there's a good chance that it — and any other toxic source in your watershed — is contributing to the contamination of your area's water supply. (Many areas use reservoirs or lakes as their primary water supply.) The same is true of the toxic fertilizers and pesticides used on farmlands. You may not live right next door to a field that is sprayed with these materials, but if that field is located in your watershed, your water supply could be at risk.

The millions of Americans who depend on private wells for their water aren't immune to the problem. Toxins can be transported by groundwater, and as a result toxic chemicals can be dumped on the ground and turn up in well water many miles away.

Processing

The processing of wastewater is designed to turn water that has been used into water that can be used again — to purify and clean it so it's safe for drinking, bathing, and so on. However, many water processing operations don't do a great job of removing chemical toxins, and known toxins are often added to the water supply.

The focus of most water processing efforts is to remove large solids from and disinfect the bacteria in the wastewater. Steps are also taken to remove a number of dangerous chemical toxins, but thousands of other toxins aren't taken into account.

What's even more disconcerting is the common practice of treating water supplies with toxic chemicals like chlorine for the purpose of killing bacteria. Chlorine has an unquestionably toxic effect on the human body, causing irritation and damage to the respiratory system among other things. The EPA contends that the levels of chlorine in drinking water that result from the chemical's use as a bacteria killer aren't high enough to harm the people who drink and bathe in it, but many people disagree. If you're not crazy about having a sip of chlorine with your drinking water, read on to find out how you can seek out a solution.

Avoiding toxin-tainted water

Water, water everywhere — but what is safe to drink? The barrage of toxic threats to our water supplies makes that a tough question to answer.

Local and municipal water supplies are regulated by the EPA, but the overall quality of water from place to place within the United States can vary greatly. Bottled water is regulated by the FDA, but the quality of bottled water can vary as well. In the next few pages, I clue you in on how you can flatten out some of that variation and help to ensure the quality of the water you're drinking by figuring out your local water report, getting your water tested, filtering your tap water, and buying bottled water that meets your standards.

Analyzing your local water report

Municipal water departments are required to make a public notice of water quality on an annual basis but don't have to test it every year. Your local water department can provide you with that information upon request, and the folks managing the water supplies in many areas send out the reports each year as a matter of course. In larger communities the information is also available online, so do a little online research to find out if the details of your water quality may already be at your fingertips.

It's great that water departments are required to make public the analysis of the water supply, but reading one of those documents can be quite a task. You usually find a lot of information on just a few pages, and the details can be both technical and confusing. Taking a good look at the report is certainly worth your time, though, and you can make the process easier by keeping a couple things in mind:

✔ Take note of all the toxins I talk about in this book that are *not* included in the report. That means your water department is not testing for them.

✔ Pay special attention to footnotes or asterisks. As in reports from any other government or industry group, these notes can allow important information to be stashed away in the fine print.

I once received a report from our local water department that had a footnote symbol in the section on the arsenic levels in our water. The footnote said that the arsenic data was based on a water sample from three years ago. It didn't explain why the arsenic data was from testing that took place three years earlier. (You would think that the water department could secure a sample of its own water for a new test.) I tried to get an answer that would clear up the situation, but the water department never provided any solid reasoning for the footnote. I can only conclude that the arsenic data was from the last year the water actually passed the EPA guidelines, which didn't give me a whole lot of confidence in the quality of the water coming out of my tap.

Getting your water tested

Everyone should consider getting their water tested for these six different categories of dangerous materials: microorganisms, disinfectants, disinfection byproducts, inorganic chemicals, organic chemicals, and radionuclides. (It's not critical that you understand all the details about these categories. Just know that any comprehensive water test should include all six.) A water test is particularly important for families that rely on well water, but even if you're connected to a municipal or local water supply, don't rule out the idea of getting some tests run on the water that comes out of your taps.

The National Institutes of Health (NIH) recommend that well water be tested at least once each year for dangerous chemicals and bacteria. It also recommends that testing be done even more frequently if an infant is drinking the water or if there's a chance that the well's structure was recently damaged in any way. If you're on a well, you also want to know if any oil, gas, or mining operations have ever been present in the area; if the land has ever seen heavy pesticide use; and if a junkyard or landfill is (or has been) nearby. If any of these activities have taken place on or near the land, make sure you opt for extremely thorough testing.

If you're on a municipal water supply, you may think it strange to have your water tested. But even if your city water supply is pristine, a lot can happen to the water between the city's pipes and your tap. Your house's plumbing, or even some of the city's pipes, could contain lead or other metals that can leach into your water, and water tests can detect those toxins.

In addition to these general testing recommendations, specific conditions merit water tests, including the following:

- If anyone in your home has recurrent gastrointestinal problems, have your water tested for toxic bacteria.

- If you notice strange stains in sinks, toilets, or clothing that you've washed at home, test for copper, manganese, and iron.

- If your water has a foul smell or taste, test for hydrogen sulfide, acidity, copper, lead, iron, zinc, and sodium.

- If you're getting an usually large amount of soap scum residue in your tubs, sinks, and toilets, have your water checked for hardness (heavy salt content).

- If you're thinking about moving into a new house, have the water tested before you make the commitment to move in.

- If you live in a rural area, you may want to get your tap water tested. Some rural areas don't have the funding to carry out the more expensive types of water treatment. Also, there's a greater likelihood that the water has been contaminated by runoff from agricultural fertilizers and pesticides.

- If you are planning to get pregnant, make sure your water is pure.

When you make the choice to have your water tested, the first step is to contact your local and state health departments. Some departments will test your water free of charge, although in most cases those tests are pretty limited. After you've exhausted those possibilities, you can turn to private water testing companies. You can find a listing in your phone book or online.

When selecting a private water testing company, make sure you use only those companies that are licensed in your state to conduct water testing. Also, make sure that the company you choose is willing to speak with you in depth about the results of the water tests. Much of the information that comes out of the testing process is technical, so you'll need someone to talk you through it.

For more information on water purity and testing, check out the EPA's Web page for ground water and drinking water: www.epa.gov/ogwdw.

Removing toxins from your tap water

If you're concerned about toxins in your tap water, look into setting up a system for filtering or purifying your water. Dozens of options for water filtering and purification are available, and you can find many of them online or at your local hardware or home improvement store. A perfect system doesn't exist, but with a little research you can select one that fills your specific needs. Most of the units fit under your sink or on your countertop, although some are meant to be installed where the incoming water pipe enters your house. Here's a rundown of the most common options:

- **Carbon water filters** are easy to install and inexpensive. They absorb many toxins and microorganisms while letting most minerals pass through. Carbon filters don't change the acidity of the water (a good thing), but they're subject to developing mold if left unused for long periods of time (a bad thing). I think carbon filters are a good, basic option for water filtration.

- **Water distillers** definitely produce water that is free of impurities, but the distillation process also removes minerals from water. Your body needs many of the minerals found in tap water, so if you go the water distiller route you need to make sure you're getting plenty of minerals elsewhere in your diet. Water distillers also tend to produce more acidic water, which isn't the healthiest.

- **Ceramic filters** are adept at filtering out microscopic particles and microorganisms. The filters can be renewed by brushing them under running water. One downside: Ceramic filters tend to noticeably decrease the flow of water.

- **Reverse osmosis (RO) filters** are readily available in a variety of sizes and are relatively inexpensive. Your local home improvement store probably has several options. A system with a 1-gallon reserve costs about $150. Most RO filters are easy to install. (I speak from experience —

I recently installed one.) They remove almost all toxins, but you must remember that the good minerals are also removed.

- ✔ **Ultraviolet (UV) radiation systems** use a special lamp to kill all living organisms and leave the minerals untouched, but the lamp loses its effectiveness over time and you can't tell whether it's still working without testing the water. Another big downside: UV systems don't remove heavy metals and other chemical toxins from your water.

Buying clean water

If you want to skip tap water altogether for drinking purposes, you can turn to bottled water as your primary source. If that's your choice, you're certainly not alone: Americans drink more than 7.5 million gallons of bottled water each year.

Bottled water can seem pristine and pure, but don't let those pictures of peaceful springs and snow-capped peaks on the labels fool you. In many cases, bottled water is just as likely to contain toxins as tap water, so you need to do your research to make sure the bottled water you're buying is as toxin-free as possible. Forty percent of bottled water is straight tap water with no additional treatment. Do your research to guarantee that the water company does proper treatment.

The bottled water industry is regulated by the FDA under its food safety program, but the FDA doesn't do any active testing. You can find bottled water quality reports on the Web sites of many of the largest bottled water companies, and most of the other companies will provide you with information on their water's quality if you request it.

In addition to water that comes in bottles that you simply buy off the shelf, many grocery stores now have in-house reverse osmosis (RO) water systems that you can use to fill large (usually 5-gallon) reusable containers. RO water is probably the most consistently clean water you can buy, but it contains few if any natural minerals. It's worth noting that the large containers used in this process are almost always made of the type of plastic that doesn't leach toxins into your water.

A Breath of Not-So-Fresh Air: Inhalable Toxins (And How to Avoid Them)

Thus far in human history, we've had a tough time figuring out a good way to live without breathing. Good, clean air is critical for people to live healthy, happy lives. If you're hoping for a way around that fact, all I can tell you is don't hold your breath.

The good news is that we're not in any danger of running out of air. There's plenty of it to go around, so we're definitely in good shape on the quantity front. The problem with our air is the quality. In our centuries-long quest to make human civilization bigger and badder all across the globe, we've done quite a lot of damage to the quality of our air. Despite the efforts of many people to cut down on air pollution, we're still spewing untold amounts of toxins into the atmosphere every year.

Toxins in our air can cause just as many health issues as toxins in our water and in our food. If you're committed to detoxifying your body, you need to figure out what's floating in the air around you and what you can do to keep airborne toxins out of your system.

Understanding airborne commercial and industrial toxins

You can't blame commercial and industrial processes for all the rampant air pollution that has taken place in the last couple centuries, but our plants and factories are responsible for more than their fair share. Many of the toxins I describe in Chapter 2 are released into the air (usually as byproducts) in some form by industrial operations just as often as they're dumped into our water and on our soil. Several other toxins seem to be particularly problematic when it comes to air quality.

In the next couple pages, I describe in some detail the most common and dangerous toxins that are released into our air every single day. I hope that through reading this section, you can better understand what we're up against as we work toward cleaner air for ourselves, our families, and everyone else sharing this planet.

If you want to see specific information about the air quality in your area, visit the EPA's air quality information page at www.epa.gov/air/data/geosel.html. You can plug in your zip code or select your state from a map of the United States to see a report on the quality of the air you're breathing right now.

Carbon monoxide

We release huge amounts of carbon monoxide into the atmosphere every year, and most of it can be traced back to automobile engines. When you inhale carbon monoxide, it attaches to your red blood cells where oxygen is supposed to attach — a huge problem. It can cause brain damage and death, among other horrible things. To help protect yourself and your family from this common toxin, make sure your home's heating system is running properly and avoid situations in which you're inhaling large amounts of automobile exhaust.

Ozone

When you hear the word *ozone,* you may think of the ozone layer and the hole that we put in it over the course of a few decades in the twentieth century. Ozone is a gas composed of three oxygen atoms stuck together. Yes, this gas makes up the ozone layer, which blocks many of the harmful effects of the sun. But when ozone is present lower in the atmosphere — at or near ground level, for example — it's a potent toxin that contributes heavily to the formation of smog. Ozone has a very harmful effect on the lungs and lung tissue. It causes coughing, shortness of breath, and chest pain, and it's particularly rough on people who suffer from asthma. Like carbon monoxide, ozone is released in automobile exhaust, and when it gets together with other airborne pollutants to form smog, your best bet is to steer clear.

Many large cities now make ozone alert announcements when levels of ozone in the area's air become dangerously high. If you live in a metropolitan area, look for ozone alerts in your local news sources. When an alert is announced, do your best to stay in a controlled-air environment. You don't have to hole up in your house until the alert is lifted. But if you have an outdoor activity planned and you see an ozone alert, consider switching your outdoor plans to a different day. Chances are your picnic or bike ride will be a lot more enjoyable if you're not breathing in elevated toxin levels all day.

Lead

I cover lead in detail in Chapter 2, but I include it here also because it's a common airborne toxin. I know it may seem odd to think of lead (which is a very heavy material) floating around in the air, but lead dust is released into the atmosphere all the time by waste incinerators, smelters, and makers of batteries that contain lead. If you live near any of those types of operations, be sure to get tested for lead. And if you have children, make doubly sure they are tested regularly as well. (Check out Chapter 5 for more information on seeing a doctor about your toxicity levels.)

Nitrogen dioxide

Nitrogen dioxide is another airborne toxin present in automobile exhaust. It has toxic effects on the lungs and can be especially harmful for people who have asthma or lung disease. If you spend time near major roadways, your exposure is likely 30 to 100 percent higher than if you live and work away from heavily trafficked roads. Unfortunately, about 16 percent of homes in the

United States are located within 300 feet of a major roadway, so millions of Americans are exposed to high amounts of nitrogen dioxide. If possible, keep that in mind when it comes time to move to a new area or into a new home.

Sulfur dioxide

Sulfur dioxide is one of many sulfur chemicals that easily dissolves in water and forms acid. These chemicals are released by all sorts of industrial processes, and they can have extremely detrimental effects on your lungs and other organs. They also help to create acid rain, which is damaging to many different aspects of our environment and health.

Acrolein

Acrolein is a prevalent but not very well-known toxin that has many uses in industry; it may be most commonly used as a multipurpose pesticide. (You can read all about the dangers of pesticides a little earlier in this chapter.) The harmful effects of this toxin include serious complications for your mucus membranes and respiratory tract.

Manganese

Manganese is an essential element for good health — you'll likely find it listed in the ingredients for your multivitamin — but excess levels can be very toxic. Manganese poisoning can cause symptoms similar to those of Parkinson's disease, including tremors, difficulty walking, and facial muscle spasms. The most common source of toxic problems with manganese is welding. If you're involved in welding or have a welder in your family, be sure to include manganese when you get tested for toxicity.

Mercury

I write about the horrible toxic effects of mercury throughout this book. (Flip back one chapter for lots of basic information.) When it comes to airborne toxins, mercury comes into the picture in what can seem like a very peculiar setting: the dentist's office. Airborne mercury is created every time a dentist makes, applies, drills, or removes an *amalgam* (often called *silver*) filling. These fillings are half mercury, which means dentists and their staff are usually exposed to quite a bit more mercury than the rest of the population. In all my years of practicing medicine, I have never tested a dentist for mercury who didn't have toxic levels in his or her body.

If you think you may have been exposed to airborne mercury because of amalgam fillings, you should get tested for mercury toxicity. This is especially true if you work in a dentist's office where amalgam fillings are created, handled, and removed on a regular basis.

Having dental fillings removed

If you need or want to have amalgam fillings removed, you and your dentist should follow these protocols to limit your exposure to the mercury they contain.

The patient's protocol

As the patient, you should take the following supplements starting before your fillings are removed:

- Cilantro: Helps with mercury removal
- Vitamin C: Improves immunity and detoxification
- Alpha-lipoic acid: Aids liver health
- Garlic: Boosts immunity and has sulfur
- Kidney formula (with juniper and uva ursi): Strengthens kidney health
- Liver formula (with milk thistle and olive leaf): Boosts liver health
- Vitamin D: Aids kidney function and bones
- Turmeric: Helps immunity
- Vitamin B complex: Aids liver function

You should also take detox baths once a week while the fillings are being removed. This aids the removal of mercury and other heavy metals from the skin. In the bath water, add

- 2 cups Epsom Salt (which contains magnesium sulfate)
- 1 cup baking soda
- 2 to 3 teaspoons of powdered vitamin C
- 2 to 3 teaspoons of yellow mustard powder

These substances will help pull heavy metals from the skin. Yellow mustard contains sulfur, for example, which bonds to mercury and pulls it out of the skin.

Soak in the tub for 15 to 20 minutes, and then scrub your skin with soap. The bath water will begin to turn dark gray and cloudy. The discoloration will leave a ring around the tub, which lab tests have found to contain aluminum, lead, and mercury.

For additional assurance, you can have an IV with vitamin C before the filling removal and a chelation treatment with DMPS after removal (see Chapter 18 for details).

The dentist's protocol

The dentist should use a certified mercury removal protocol, which includes these measures:

- Clean air filtration in the room where fillings are being removed
- A rubber dam to prevent mercury pieces from being swallowed or inhaled
- Water coolant to keep the filling from heating up (because heat releases toxic mercury vapors)
- High-speed suction or vacuum for removing toxic vapors and debris
- Filtration masks for all employees in the room while the procedure is performed

If your dentist won't follow this protocol, search for a dentist who will. Online, look for *biological* or *holistic dentists* at these Web sites:

- The **International Academy of Oral Medicine & Toxicology:** www.iaomt.org
- The **International Academy of Biological Dentistry and Medicine:** www.iabdm.org
- The **Holistic Dental Association:** www.holisticdental.org

Formaldehyde

Many people think of formaldehyde as embalming fluid, and they're sometimes shocked to find out that the toxic chemical is used widely in the production of things like leather goods, plywood, particle board, paper, foam insulation, and even pharmaceuticals and vaccines. It's a gas at room temperature, and exposure can cause eye and throat irritation, nausea, headache, and fatigue. High levels of exposure can cause swelling of the lungs, which can result in death. Formaldehyde has a distinctive odor that you may remember from the frog dissection portion of your high school biology class. If you work in a setting where formaldehyde is used, insist on being given a respirator — it can save your life.

Benzene

Like formaldehyde, benzene is used across a wide range of industries and applications. It is generated by burning coal, gasoline, and oil, and it's used in the making of products like inks, rubber, plastics, and pharmaceuticals, to name just a few. Benzene causes eye, skin, and respiratory irritation, along with headache and dizziness. Short-term elevated levels can cause unconsciousness and death, and if you're exposed to benzene over a long period of time it'll wreak havoc on your body. It has reproductive effects, damages your blood, and is (according to the EPA) a likely carcinogen. If your job puts you in contact with benzene, make sure you have a good respirator and use it whenever exposure is probable. If you're worried about benzene levels in your body, check out Chapter 18 for information on how you can utilize saunas to help rid your body of benzene (and other toxins, as well).

Getting a feel for the inhalable toxins in your home

If you think that most airborne toxins come from factory smokestacks and hang in the air only in the smog that envelops some cities and industrial areas, think again. Your home could be a hotbed of airborne toxins.

Many household products, particularly cleaning products, are loaded with toxic chemicals. Take a quick look at the ingredients of some of the products you have in your home, and compare that list with the toxins described in Chapter 2 and elsewhere in this book. Not only are these products toxic if you have skin contact or (heaven forbid) accidentally ingest them, but the fumes they put off are also toxic.

A recent study looked at the toxins present in 120 homes on Cape Cod, which probably isn't an area that springs to mind when you think about toxic environments. The study focused on the air and dust present in those homes, and the findings were hair-raising. Every single house had more than 20 toxic compounds known to cause cancer, neurological problems, and birth defects. There were even traces of some substances that had been widely banned years before (like DDT), and plentiful amounts of toxins like phthalates (which I describe in detail earlier in this chapter).

What are the sources of the inhalable toxins that are present in the homes of many Americans? Following are a few examples:

- ✔ Paint fumes
- ✔ Dry cleaning
- ✔ Air/carpet fresheners
- ✔ Detergents and fabric softeners
- ✔ Household insecticides
- ✔ Lawn and garden chemicals

Do yourself (and your family) a favor and work toward limiting your exposure to these toxic materials.

Chlorine is a very common inhalable toxin in many homes. Use bleach cleaners and detergents containing chlorine sparingly (if at all), and remember that if you can smell chlorine, that means you're being exposed to more than you really should be.

Cleaning the air around you

The threats presented by inhalable toxins are serious and tough to avoid. So how can you clean up your air and limit the amount of toxic materials that you're breathing every day? The following are a few excellent first steps:

- ✔ **When you're outside, be mindful of the quality of the air around you.** Pay attention to air quality measurements on your local weather report, and spend your time outdoors on days when the air is relatively clean. Avoid being outdoors near manufacturing plants, refineries, and major roadways.

- ✔ **When you're moving to a new home, keep air quality in mind.** You probably won't end up buying or renting a new home based on the air quality in the area — there are usually many other pressing matters to consider. But if you can factor in the home's proximity to sources of airborne toxins, your lungs (and the rest of your body) will thank you.

> ✔ **Cut down on the inhalable toxins you keep in your home in the form of household products.** The first things to go should be insecticides, pesticides, and anything that says "danger," "poison," or even "caution." This includes cleaning supplies, so please don't insist on trying to hang on to toxic cleaners.

There are many excellent alternatives to toxin-filled household cleaning supplies. A knowledgeable staff member at your local health food store can probably suggest all sorts of choices or even tell you about ways that you can make your own safe cleaning supplies. If you can't find suitable replacements for your old products, use them sparingly and always in well-ventilated areas.

Here are some tips to get your household moving in the right direction:

> ✔ **Use natural cleaning products.** For example, vodka or other grain alcohol makes a great cleaning spray.

> ✔ **Pay special attention to your carpet.** Carpet accumulates and holds dust and toxins. If you must have carpeting, clean it often and use a vacuum with a filter that does not spray the dust back into the air.

> ✔ **Change your filters frequently.** Air conditioning filters and ducts can be a source of toxic accumulation and exposure. Change your filters according to the recommendations set out by the manufacturer, and use quality filters. You can also have your ducts inspected and cleaned professionally, especially if you live in an older house.

> ✔ **Use a quality HEPA air filter.** HEPA stands for *high efficiency particulate air,* and HEPA filters do a great job of removing airborne toxins from indoor environments. Hundreds of HEPA filters are on the market, so do some online research and even consult with your doctor before choosing the one that is right for you and your family.

Chapter 4

Understanding How Your Body Detoxifies Itself

*T*he wonders of the human body never cease to amaze me. When you really think about what your body is capable of doing, I bet you're amazed too. One of the most impressive things your body does is deal with the influx of toxins.

From your mouth to your skin to your kidneys — and many places and parts in between — your body is set up to help you avoid and cleanse yourself of toxins. I think it's critical to grasp all the ways in which your body deals with toxins so that you can play an active role in helping it out and augmenting its detoxification processes. That's what I focus on throughout this chapter. Take a spin through the next several pages to find out what's going on inside your body to help maintain your health against an environment that continues to get more toxic with each passing year.

Your Mouth: Chewin' It Up

All digestion starts in the mouth. Food and liquids enter your body through your mouth, and some extremely important things occur there. Successful and healthy digestion requires that the mouth is doing its job, and your body's ability to detoxify itself can be greatly aided if you make an effort to allow your mouth to do its important work.

Remember when your mom told you to slow down and chew your food? That was excellent advice. When your teeth tear and grind your food into smaller bits, your food is better prepared to go through the various steps in digestion. Chewing your food well allows your stomach and intestines to break down the food and extract its nutrients with a higher degree of effectiveness. The result is a healthier you all across the board, and it's a heck of a lot easier for your body to fight off toxic threats if it's healthy. But that's not the only detoxification value that chewing your food offers.

When you chew thoroughly instead of swallowing larger bits of food, you make it easier for the acid in your stomach to break down the food. Stomach acid is a terrific toxin fighter, and you want to see that your body is taking full advantage of its powers, so be sure to chew your food thoroughly before swallowing it.

In addition to chewing, the mouth adds an ingredient that's critical for digestion: saliva. This super fluid does all sorts of great things:

- **Binds and lubricates:** The mucus in saliva makes the food you eat very slippery, and it binds the food together in a soupy mixture that slides down your esophagus without damaging the lining of that important tube, which runs from your mouth to your stomach.

- **Allows you to taste dry food:** Without saliva, it would be virtually impossible to taste dry food. If you were eating something with toxins that can be tasted — food spoiled by harmful, toxic bacteria, for example — you probably wouldn't even know it.

- **Decreases acidity:** When you eat highly acidic food, there's always a chance that the acid could damage your mouth (including your teeth) and esophagus. Saliva contains *sodium bicarbonate,* which is a chemical that reduces acidity. Sure, your stomach is highly acidic, and after your food gets there it gets fully soaked in acid. But your stomach lining is equipped to handle acids in a way that your mouth and esophagus just can't.

- **Starts the digestion of starches:** Saliva releases a chemical that begins to break down starches into basic sugars. That's a good thing because your body can't do much at all with starches, while it absolutely has to have sugars (for energy) to survive.

- **Kills bacteria:** This is a big one. Saliva contains a substance called *lysozyme* that can kill off bacteria in your food and even the bacteria that try to grow in your mouth and on your teeth. If you read Chapter 2, you know that some types of bacteria can be just as toxic as the worst chemical toxins, so it's of the utmost importance that you're not bringing high levels of bacteria into your body when you put food in your mouth. (A side note: Bacteria cause bad breath. Healthy amounts of saliva kill more bacteria, thereby helping you to avoid bad breath.)

- **Improves oral hygiene:** Saliva constantly flushes away food debris, which is a major cause of poor oral hygiene.

This advice really surprises some people, but you shouldn't drink fluids with your meals. Doing so simply isn't good for digestion. If you need to wash down your food with liquids, you're not chewing your food enough, and you're not allowing the food to be penetrated by and covered in saliva. You're also diluting the acid in your stomach, which is an important component in the process of killing toxic bacteria before it enters your intestines. Many pharmaceutical drugs reduce saliva and can cause a really dry mouth; if you have this problem, talk to your doctor. My advice is to wait a couple hours after a meal before drinking fluids. After that, you can drink all the water you want.

Your Stomach: Breakin' It Down

If your body had a trash can, it would be your stomach. When your sinuses use mucus to trap particles of dust, viruses, mold, and bacteria, where does that mucus end up? In your stomach. When your mouth takes in food and liquids that could contain dangerous, toxic bacteria, where does that material end up? In your stomach. When the tubes leading down to your lungs trap foreign materials in the air you breathe before they get down to your sensitive lung tissue, where do they send those materials? That's right — up your windpipe, into your esophagus, and then down into your stomach.

Your stomach is rough, tough, and ready to take on just about anything you put into it. Can you blame it for growling every once in a while?

Death to the microbes!

The key to the stomach's wonderful ability to handle almost everything your body throws at it is stomach acid. This isn't some weak acid like the kind in your orange juice. If your stomach acid were sitting on your kitchen table instead of in your stomach, you'd soon be in the market for a new kitchen table. It's even strong enough to eat away metal, so you can imagine the number it does on many toxic materials that end up in your stomach when you inadvertently eat, drink, or breathe them in. Your stomach acid breaks down many types of dangerous toxins, and the health of your stomach is an important factor in keeping your body as toxin-free as possible.

Stomach acid can kill almost anything that's living when it reaches the stomach. As you can imagine, this ability has major benefits for your immune system. It's a whole lot easier for your body to simply kill off things like harmful bacteria, mold, and parasites in your stomach than to deal with the effects of those critters compromising your immune system.

Interfering with your stomach's work

When stomach acid is potent and present in healthy amounts, it can be very difficult for potentially harmful living things to pass through the stomach and enter your intestines. However, many people today take medication — both prescription and over the counter — for stomach pain or indigestion, thereby lowering the amount and strength of acid in the stomach. These medicines can help to relieve stomach pain, but they also make it a lot easier for living threats to survive in your body and eventually give your immune system fits.

If you're experiencing frequent stomach pain or indigestion, make sure you and your doctor consider several possible causes before you start taking medication that weakens the acid in your stomach. The pain can be caused by a number of different things, and you don't want to compromise the important acid in your stomach if you don't need to.

When one of my patients experiences a burning feeling in her stomach or symptoms of acid reflux, I always test the levels of acid in her stomach. I don't expect to find extremely high levels of acid; in fact, in most cases (and especially with older patients) the problem is a *lack* of stomach acid. Hard to believe? Here's how it works.

When it's working correctly, your stomach won't let food enter your intestines until the food is at least partially digested. If you don't have enough acid in your stomach, the food isn't digested well enough and your stomach hangs onto it instead of sending it on down the line. Soon your stomach begins to contract on the stalled food in an effort to try to mix it with the small amounts of acid present. If it's five hours after you've eaten a meal and you're lying down with a stomach full of food, and your stomach begins contracting, you're bound to have pain or acid reflux.

This sequence of events is most common in older patients. A higher percentage of older people are taking potent acid-reducing medication than ever before. If that were the right solution, the cause would have to be that older people are producing higher amounts of more powerful stomach acid as they age. That would mean that the cells in the stomach are working better in their effort to produce more acid. But let's be honest: Hardly anything works better as we get older — stomach cells included. In these situations it could very well be that acid-reducing medicines are a counterproductive treatment. If you think you may be making your stomach problems worse by taking medicines that cut down on your stomach acid, be sure to bring up the question with your doctor before taking any action. The bottom line is that most acid reflux is cause by low acid — not high acid.

The good news if you're acid deficient is that the problem is relatively easy to correct. You can take an old medicine called *sucralfate* that doesn't lower acid levels but does help to cover any raw spots in your stomach lining that could be causing you pain. (The most common brand name for sucralfate is Carafate.) You can use this drug in combination with *betaine HCL,* which helps acidify your stomach to the right levels when you're eating a meal. That combination will correct stomach pain problems in many people. But again, please don't take these steps until consulting your doctor.

Breaking down good and bad proteins

In addition to killing off harmful organisms, the acid in your stomach works to break proteins down into amino acids, which your body has to have in order to survive and thrive. (You can read a bit about amino acids and their important nutritional value in Chapter 5.)

Without the stomach's processing of protein into amino acids, you wouldn't be able to digest and absorb those materials into your bloodstream, and you'd have a hard time staying healthy for very long. Keeping up healthy levels of acid in your stomach is key here. If you use acid-reducing medications unnecessarily, you could be putting your nutrition at risk.

Your Intestines: Thirty Feet of Detox Action

It's hard for some people to believe, but your large and small intestines are a combined 30 feet in length. That's the length of a football field's end zone! And the sheer size of your intestines pales in comparison to what they do when it comes to sorting out toxins and absorbing the right nutrients into your body. They really are fantastic body parts, and much of the detoxification effort put forth by your body takes places all along that 30-foot length.

Your intestines have thousands of little folds called *villi.* They add a huge amount of surface area to the intestines — so much, in fact, that they make the total area of your intestines that's available for absorption roughly the same size as a tennis court! Villi are responsible for absorbing different materials out of the partially digested food that passes by them. Whatever they absorb is passed into your bloodstream and therefore made available for your body to use. They're not supposed to absorb toxins, of course — anything your body doesn't need should pass by and out with your stool — but some toxins have a chemical structure that allows them to get past the villi and into your bloodstream.

As a rule, your intestines do a masterful job of absorbing the nutrients you need and shunning the toxins that can harm you. But if you don't get enough of the former and you're bringing in far too much of the latter, you can cause some major problems for your intestines. I shouldn't have to tell you how important it is to maintain the health of a 30-foot organ that is responsible for the absorption of almost all your body's nutrients.

Bringing up the barrier

When you think about it, the wall of your intestines is really the only thing between your body's tissues and your stool. It's an amazing and very protective barrier, and it's almost magical in its ability to let the good stuff pass into your body while keeping the bad stuff moving through with your waste.

In addition to providing a wonderfully dynamic physical barrier, the intestines also include a lot of important elements of your body's biological barrier against disease: your immune system. It's a little-known fact that about 80 percent of your body's immune system is located in your intestines. The *GALT* (gut-associated lymphoid tissue), located mostly toward the end of your small intestine, is the final barrier that separates the inside of your body from your stool, which at that point usually contains harmful things like toxins, bacteria, yeast, mold, and parasites.

Taking in too many toxins through your diet can compromise the health of your intestines, including the GALT. That situation makes it difficult to maintain the integrity of both the physical barrier and the immune barrier, and disease is often the result. If you want to keep your intestinal barriers working like they should, do what you can to eliminate toxins from your diet.

Considering normal flora

Your intestines perform some critical functions, but they also act as a boarding house for most of the beneficial bacteria living in your body. The normal, healthy bacterial flora in your intestines play an important role in digestion, breaking down several different kinds of food that your body isn't able to break down on its own.

The normal flora in your intestines also provide you with another service. When present in healthy amounts, the beneficial bacteria take up space and nutrient resources that could otherwise be used by harmful, toxic organisms like bacteria, yeast, and parasites. I provide some details on normal bacterial flora in Chapter 5, so flip ahead if you'd like to read more.

Eliminating the mess

The chemical processes and reactions that take place in your intestines when nutrients are absorbed and toxins are shut out are as complex and elegant as anything you'd find in even the most technologically advanced chemical company. On top of that, your intestines also have a very complicated way of moving your partially digested food and stool through at a proper rate, so that all the processes can take place in the right amount of time. This function helps to keep toxins moving through and eventually out of your body. If your intestines move things too fast, diarrhea (which can have a disastrous effect on your nutrition and hydration levels) is often the result. If your intestines move things too slowly, constipation can occur. When your stool spends more time in your intestines than it should, you're just giving the toxins in your stool more time to hang around and get inadvertently absorbed into your system.

There are many intestinal diseases that conventional physicians typically treat with medication that helps to control the symptoms but doesn't do anything to address the cause of the problem. Many of these ailments, like Crohn's disease, ulcerative colitis, and irritable bowel syndrome, can be greatly exacerbated by the presence of too many toxins in your diet, and detoxification diets often go a long way toward providing relief.

Your Skin: Touchable and Functional

Your skin is the largest organ you have. In terms of avoiding toxins, the role your skin plays is indispensable. Your skin is the first line of defense against any toxins that you don't eat, drink, or breathe.

The skin has three layers:

- ✔ **The *epidermis*:** This is the outer layer that you can see. It gets a lot of wear and tear, and it regenerates very rapidly if you're healthy.
- ✔ **The *dermis*:** Your dermis is the next layer down from your epidermis, and it contains all sorts of useful things like blood vessels, hair follicles, oil glands, and sweat glands. (I clue you in on the importance of sweating a little later in this section.)
- ✔ ***Subcutaneous fat*:** This layer gives you some insulation and padding, but fat cells are often locations for toxin storage.

Now that you have a basic understanding of the structure of your skin, let me explain what it does for your body in terms of aiding in detoxification and helping you to avoid taking in toxins in the first place.

Putting up a barrier

Like the intestines, which I describe in the previous section, the skin creates a barrier between your body's tissues on one side and potentially toxic influences and conditions on the other. But the skin isn't as receptive to allowing some substances to cross the barrier into your body. Skin works to keep most of what's outside on the outside. If you take care of your skin and don't expose it to an overwhelming amount of toxic threats, it does an excellent job.

Some toxic chemicals are very rapidly absorbed, and you should never allow those materials to touch your skin. If you're handling any potentially toxic substances, make sure you wear the proper safety clothing, gloves, and eye protection.

As a mechanical barrier, your skin makes your body waterproof. Because many toxins are water soluble, this means that your skin keeps out some of the toxins that may be dissolved in the water that you bathe in or swim in. One of the other terrific aspects of skin is that it takes care of itself. If you injure your skin and compromise its barrier, making it more likely to allow various toxins to cross over into your body, your skin will heal itself. It has to be tough but flexible, and it includes oil glands that help it to flex and bend as you move. If it needs to get tougher, then over time calluses develop to keep the barrier intact in places where you really put it to the test.

Skin is a versatile barrier that keeps many toxins from gaining access to the inside of your body. But like many other body parts, it can only do so much. If you don't make an effort to keep your skin healthy and free from excessive toxic threats, it can be compromised, and increased toxicity is the result. Making an effort can be as simple as avoiding swimming in water that could have elevated toxin levels or wearing gloves when handling potentially toxic materials. It's also important to give your skin all the nutrients that it needs, especially vitamin C, sulfur, and omega-3 fatty acids (fish oil).

Giving a nod to natural bacteria

If you read about your intestines earlier in this chapter, you know how useful it can be to have natural, beneficial bacteria around. The same holds true for your skin. Having enough good bacteria present can prevent bad bacteria from growing and building up.

Hundreds of types of bacteria are present on your skin, and several of them are considered good bacteria. One of the most prominent is *Staphylococcus epidermatis,* which plays a key role in keeping toxic, harmful bacteria in check on your skin.

You can help the good bacteria on your skin to keep its upper hand on the bad bacteria simply by washing your body. Don't go overboard, though, because excessive washing with harsh soaps can wipe out the good bacteria and also break down the skin's natural oils, which can serve as an additional layer of protection against bad bacteria.

Sweating (out) the small stuff

I can't say enough about the importance of sweating in detoxification. It truly is one of the most effective ways our body can get rid of toxins.

As a natural detoxification process, sweating is one of the best ways to rid your body of toxins that can be present for many years. Under normal conditions, we sweat about a quart of liquid a day, and it's estimated that sweating can remove about a third of the toxins that your kidneys can. Not bad!

I know it's a little creepy to think that some toxins can hang around your body for several years, but that is indeed the case. When toxins end up in your bloodstream or in your tissues, your body tries to protect your organs by stuffing fat-soluble toxins into fat cells to isolate them. If your body doesn't know how to process or get rid of a toxin, it just stores it away in a place where it's not as likely to damage your organs as it would be if the toxin were floating around in your bloodstream. After a toxin is stashed away in a fat cell, it can remain there for many years. This process can result in the buildup of fat and weight gain, because fat cells have a natural mechanism that makes them grow in an effort to try to dilute the toxins within them. Bigger fat cells mean more fat and an increased likelihood that you'll gain weight. You can read much more about this topic in Chapter 9.

Sweating aggressively — that is, more than what you typically sweat on an average day — mobilizes the toxins from your subcutaneous fat cells to your sweat glands, where they can be moved outside your body as you sweat. When that happens, the concentration of toxins in your fat cells is much lower. The cells aren't as likely to try to grow to dilute the toxins, so you may be able to lose weight and clear out excess fat.

Less than a hundred years ago, most people were sweating aggressively every day, and in the summer they were in somewhat of a sauna for a good part of the day. The advent of air conditioning changed all that (at least in many parts of the developed world), and we sweat quite a bit less as a result. That's nice for keeping shirts clean, but it undercuts your body's efforts to detoxify itself through sweating. To make sure that you're getting the full detoxification benefit of sweating, exercise regularly and consider using a sauna to enhance the frequency and intensity of your sweating. (You can read more about saunas in Chapter 18.)

Your Liver: A Detoxification Powerhouse

Your liver is a very complicated organ, and it performs many essential functions. (Some researchers estimate that the liver performs as many as 500 different functions for your body!) Much of what the liver does is complicated, and you don't really need to understand all the ins and outs to grasp its importance and its role in detoxification. Here, I'd like to give you a basic understanding of some of its crucial processes:

- **Toxin processing:** All the materials absorbed by or inadvertently leaked into the intestines go into a special vein that leads directly to your liver. The liver processes the blood by removing and breaking down many of the toxins. I dive a little deeper into the details of this process later in this section. Your liver processes about two quarts of blood per minute.

- **Bacteria destruction:** Your liver is loaded with immune cells, which kill many of the bacteria that manage to work their way through the intestinal wall.

- **Cholesterol creation:** Cholesterol is made in the liver. You may not think of cholesterol as a good thing, but cholesterol is very important for your body; cholesterol is the basic molecule used to generate several of your most critical hormones.

- **Blood protein production:** Ninety percent of your blood proteins are made in the liver. That's extremely important for you, and also for all those vampires out there.

- **Blood clotting:** The clotting of blood doesn't actually take place in the liver if everything is working as it should, but several of the materials your body uses for blood clotting are made in the liver.

- **Antioxidant production:** An antioxidant called *glutathione* is one of the most important for your body's healthy function, and it's made and stored in your liver.

- **Blood sugar control:** Your liver helps control your blood sugar by converting glucose to *glycogen* (a form of glucose that your body can store) and vice versa.

- **Vitamin storage:** Vitamins A, D, and B12 are stored in the liver. So is iron.

- **Bile production:** *Bile* breaks down fats in your intestines, and it removes toxic waste from your liver. Your liver makes bile (as if it weren't doing enough already!).

So the liver really is a jack of all trades. You can thank your liver for breaking down many, many toxins in your body (although you might avoid doing that in public — people tend to think it's strange when you talk to your liver outside of the privacy of your own home). There are two main ways that your liver breaks down toxins, and I present the broad strokes of both next.

Phase 1 detoxification

Two major types of detoxification occur in the liver: *Phase I detoxification* and *Phase II detoxification.* Phase I either breaks down a toxin (rendering it pretty much harmless) or changes it somehow to prepare it for Phase II. (More on Phase II in a moment.)

During Phase I detoxification, your liver first tries to use enzymes to break off pieces of a toxic chemical's structure. This process often works and results in a substance that is far less toxic and more water soluble, so it's less dangerous to your health and easier to move out of the body with one of your waste products. If that doesn't do the trick, the next step is the addition of antioxidants. Sometimes that process works where the first step failed. If step two doesn't work, it's time for Phase II detoxification.

Before moving on to Phase II, I want to take a moment to tell you about several substances that can help to enhance Phase I detoxification:

- ✔ **Nutrients:** These include niacin, vitamin B1, vitamin C, and glutathione.
- ✔ **Herbs:** Caraway and dill seeds are two of the best.
- ✔ **Foods:** Cabbage, broccoli, oranges, grapefruit, tangerines, and Brussels sprouts are especially helpful.

For the sake of full disclosure, I'll also admit that some drugs — narcotics, alcohol, nicotine, steroids, and phenobarbital — also increase the activity of Phase I detoxification. But as you can imagine, that's only because the liver has to step up its game to deal with the influx of toxic materials that correspond with drug use.

A number of things also slow down Phase I detoxification:

- ✔ **Some herbs:** Curcumin and capsaicin are examples.
- ✔ **Certain foods:** Clove oil, hot peppers, and grapefruit juice are among the top offenders.
- ✔ **Drugs:** Antihistamines, medicines that block acid secretion in the stomach, and certain antianxiety medications are culprits.

✔ **Aging:** Getting up in years slows down your liver's Phase I detoxification. This is another good reason to try to limit your use of prescription drugs: They often have to be broken down by your liver, which puts a strain on it as you get older.

✔ **Diet:** As you'd expect, your diet can have a major impact on your liver's health and ability to detox your body. Eating too many processed foods chock full of additives (and coated in pesticides) puts stress on your liver.

Studies have shown that the Phase I detoxification your liver is able to carry out is based heavily on genetic factors. Because of their genes, some people are fortunate to have livers that can process many more toxins than others. In some cases a person can conduct Phase I detoxification at more than five times the capacity of a similar person (in terms of age, sex, and so on) with different genetic makeup. This difference is one of the main reasons that certain people's bodies are able to detoxify themselves in a much more efficient way than others.

Phase II detoxification

Phase II detoxification is often a continuation of Phase I, but it can happen on its own as well. Phase II detoxification works when the liver attaches toxins together or attaches other substances to toxins to make the harmful materials less harmful and more water soluble (easier to flush out with urine and bile).

Phase II detoxification is a very nutrient-intensive process, so consider including the following foods and supplements in your diet if you want to bolster your liver's efforts:

✔ **Food:** Spinach, black beans, animal protein, legumes, pumpkin seeds, lentils, asparagus, broccoli, cabbage, and other leafy greens.

✔ **Supplements:** Fish oils, milk thistle, and alpha-lipoic acid. (Ask for details at your health food or supplement store.)

If you work on including these types of foods and supplements in your diet, you'll make it a lot easier for your liver to carry out effective Phase II detoxification, and your health will get a nice boost. It's more important now than ever because the amount of toxins you're faced with on a daily basis continues to go up, so your liver's ability to cope is extremely important.

Make sure you're getting plenty of fiber in your diet. In addition to all the other useful things fiber can do for you, it helps your intestines clear out the toxins that your liver has processed. Without ample amounts of fiber, some of those toxins can be reabsorbed, and your liver's hard work will have been for naught.

The liver cleanse

No section on the liver would be complete without mentioning the liver cleanse. It's a process that involves taking a mixture of food ingredients that are purported to help clear out excess toxins from your liver. The mixture usually includes olive oil, Epsom salt, and grapefruit, among other ingredients. Some people report very dramatic results like passing multiple gallstones, and others claim to see a marked improvement in general health after the liver cleanse is complete. Many proponents recommend doing a liver cleanse twice a year to combat the elevated levels of toxins that we're faced with today. I think liver cleanses are a good idea for most people, although you need to be aware of a couple potential side effects:

- Doing a liver cleanse will activate your colon, so if you choose to do one be ready to make multiple trips to the toilet.

- If you're like many people and you pass a gallstone during a cleanse, there's an outside chance that it could get stuck on its way out. (However, I can report that hundreds of my patients have done liver cleanses, and this problem has never occurred.)

If you begin to feel abdominal pain while doing a cleanse, make sure you stop the cleanse immediately and get in touch with your doctor.

Your Kidneys: Major Detox Players

Most people give their kidneys a whole lot of abuse and not much credit. All of the water-soluble materials that end up in your blood eventually find their way to the kidneys, where they're removed and sent out with your urine. The truth is your kidneys are very sophisticated organs that never stop filtering your blood to remove toxins, keep salts and protein levels in check, and adjust your blood pressure. When it comes to detoxification, your kidneys are a major player.

If you want to keep your kidneys running at tip-top shape, try to limit your exposure to toxins (a no-brainer, I know) and make sure you drink lots of clean water without chlorine or fluoride in it. Your kidneys don't stand a chance if you're not drinking plenty of water, because in this case the solution to pollution is dilution!

To keep your kidneys — and the rest of your body, for that matter — healthy, try to drink enough water to keep your urine clear. Clear urine is a sign of a hydrated body. The only times your urine should have a darker yellow color is first thing in the morning and after you've taken vitamins, which can alter your urine's tint.

Part II
Working toward a Detoxified Life: Getting Started

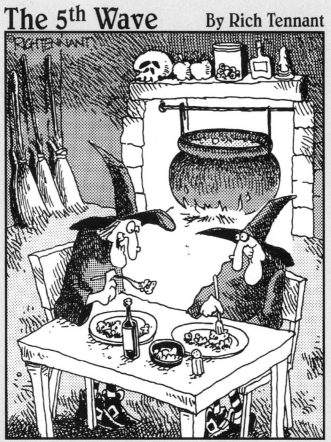

The 5th Wave   By Rich Tennant

"I substitute tofu for eye of newt in all my recipes now. It has twice the protein and doesn't wriggle around the cauldron."

In this part . . .

Chances are good that you're reading this book at least partly due to the fact that you want to improve your diet. (Most people do, right?) If that's the case, you've come to the right place. Two of the most important features of this part are the breakdown of the various types of foods that contain toxins (so you can cut them out of your life) and my explanation of what you need to eat in order to make yourself as toxin-free as possible. Your food choices and eating habits will do as much to influence your overall health as anything else, so you need to make sure you're doing the right (toxin-free) things.

I also use this part to clue you in on a few other detoxification basics so you can begin to employ a rounded approach toward ridding your body of toxins. Finally, I include a quiz at the end of this part to help you figure out the toxicity of your body's systems. Don't worry — I won't be grading it!

Chapter 5

Taking the Detoxification Initiative: The Basics of Detoxing Your Body

In This Chapter

▶ Recognizing how crucial your diet is

▶ Using exercise to help reach your detox goals

▶ Exploring your options for supplements

▶ Making sure your intestinal flora has the right balance

▶ Picking a good, open-minded doctor

*y*our body is well equipped to maintain health and to detoxify an enormous number of chemicals and toxins. It really is a marvelous natural machine. But your body does have its limits, and the world around you now is pushing those limits and in many cases exceeding them.

If you want to keep your health moving in the right direction despite the ever-present threat of toxins, you have to make an effort to augment your body's natural detoxification mechanisms. That's what this chapter is all about. I take you through the basics of several types of active detoxification methods, from diet (which is perhaps the most important battle in your war against toxins) to exercise, supplements, and maintenance of your bowel flora. I even offer some advice on how you can find the right kind of doctor to support and enhance your detoxification.

You won't find lots of specifics in this chapter — the details are in other chapters of this book. But if you're looking for an overview of what you should do if you're serious about detoxification, you've come to the right place.

Detoxing through Diet

Imagine a toolbox that contains all the detoxification techniques and methods you have at your disposal. The toolbox has a place for saunas, one for *chelation* (the process of using a chemical that can attach to and then remove a toxic substance), and on down the list. (I cover these and other detox options in Chapter 18 and in other spots throughout the book.) In this toolbox, you'd need a whole separate compartment for diet. Maybe even a whole drawer. You know what? You may even need another toolbox just to fit all the important dietary components of a healthy, detoxified lifestyle. The right kind of diet is critical for effective detoxification.

Because diet is so critical, I certainly don't skimp on the detox diet details in this book. But before you can grasp the finer points of adjusting your diet to accomplish detox goals, you need to feel comfortable with the basics, and that's what this section is about. (If you'd rather dive right into the nitty gritty details about detox dieting, I recommend Chapters 6, 7, and 9.)

In order for your body to function and maintain health over the course of your life, you must ensure that you continually provide it with a number of nutrients. You don't need these nutrients in any spectacular amounts, and you can even go without some of them for a period of time. I see this all the time in my practice. To be honest, after hearing about the diets of some people I'm surprised they're still alive. (Nowhere is this more evident than in children with autism. I've treated some children who have eaten only chicken nuggets, cheese pizza, and sugary cereal for years.)

Denying your body the essential nutrients it must have to operate is a way of inflicting malnutrition on yourself. Think about that: If you're not giving your body the right amounts of the right nutrients, you're basically creating a problem for yourself that we spend billions of dollars to fight in developing countries every year. There's really no excuse for it!

Over the next few pages, I tell you all about the most important nutrients for your body. I let you know a little about the roles these nutrients play in your system, and I provide a good look at some of the food sources you can include in your diet to make sure you're getting what you need in the right amounts. Filling up your diet with key nutrients is just as important as ridding it of toxins. (If you're craving more information on how to keep toxins out of your food, flip back to Chapter 3 or ahead to Chapter 7.)

Eating the essentials

Your body needs certain substances that it can't make on its own. You have to get these substances in the food you eat (or sometimes in the water you drink) if you want to enjoy long-term health. Here's a basic look at these substances:

- ✔ **Essential amino acids:** *Amino acids* are the building blocks that make protein. There are ten amino acids that we must have, and we can't make them on our own. You can't store amino acids in your body, so you have to get them in your diet every day.

- ✔ **Essential fatty acids:** These include omega-3 fatty acids and omega-6 fatty acids.

- ✔ **Minerals:** Your body needs 16 minerals to operate at an optimal level. You can get all the minerals you need from vegetables and water, but only if you eat 100 percent organic. (Check out Chapter 7 for my thorough explanation of organic foods.)

- ✔ **Vitamins:** We can't make them, and we can't live without them. There are 14 essential vitamins, and each one is unique. As with minerals, you can't get all the vitamins you need from vegetables unless the vegetables you eat are all 100 percent organic.

To read about all of these substances and find out how you can make sure you're getting them in your diet, flip ahead to Chapter 17.

Eating colors for antioxidants

The next time you're in the produce section of a grocery store, take a second to stand back and look at all the colors. Fruits and vegetables seem to be painted from a lush, comprehensive palette that ranges from deep, rich greens to eye-popping bright yellows.

You can use the colors of fruits and vegetables to help guide your dietary levels of antioxidants, which is another extremely important component for your diet.

Antioxidants are substances that help to cut down on *oxidation* — a process that occurs normally in the body but can run rampant and damage your body's cells (especially in the presence of toxins). Antioxidants help keep oxidation under control, and an overwhelming amount of research shows that including plenty of antioxidants in your diet will make you healthier across the board.

Join me for the following look at the rainbow of fruit and vegetable options and the antioxidants that you can find in each color.

Red

Plenty of red fruits and vegetables are available, and many can provide you with wonderfully healthy antioxidants. Take red kidney beans, for example. They're loaded with antioxidants! Red kidney beans have antioxidant levels that are as high as or higher than many berries that are commonly regarded as antioxidant powerhouses. Of course, that doesn't mean that you should skip red berries and other red fruits; raspberries, cherries, red apples, and strawberries are excellent sources of antioxidants, too.

Red tomatoes have a specific kind of antioxidant that is particularly important for men. You can find abundant amounts of *lycopene* in tomatoes, and lycopene has been shown to contribute to the health of the prostate gland. That doesn't mean that women should discount the health benefits of eating tomatoes, of course — just that men should keep it in mind when deciding whether or not to put a slice of tomato on their sandwiches or add another spoonful of sauce to their pasta.

Here's one other specific antioxidant that you can find in red fruits: *resveratrol.* Resveratrol has been shown to decrease the growth of cancer cells, help nerve cells stay healthy in diabetics, and also decrease heart disease by helping to maintain blood vessels. You can find resveratrol in red grape skins and also in red wine.

Blue and purple

Fresh vegetables and fruits that are blue or purple may not be as common as those in shades of green or red, but a few blue and purple foods can provide you with some terrific antioxidant benefits.

Start with plums and their dried counterparts, prunes. Both make great snacks, and they're packed with antioxidants. You can also go for blackberries; they're a little tough to find out of season, but when they're available try to mix them into your diet for an antioxidant boost.

The king of the antioxidant-rich blue foods is the blueberry. You often hear blueberries referred to as one of the "superfoods," and that's not just clever marketing. Blueberries are chock-full of beneficial antioxidants, and they also contain many of the vitamins you need to stay healthy. Load up on blueberries when you can, and keep in mind that the darker the blueberry, the more healthy materials you can find inside.

On the vegetable side of things, try eggplant for a blue or purple food that can provide you with an antioxidant kick.

Orange

Orange (and yellow) members of the fruit and vegetable groups are famous for containing *beta-carotene,* an antioxidant that is thought to help protect against eye disease and some forms of cancer. If you're looking to give your beta-carotene levels a boost, try orange foods like carrots, pumpkin, and winter squash. Orange and yellow fruits that contain ample antioxidants include nectarines, oranges, lemons, peaches, and grapefruit.

Green

Green vegetables make up a big part of the produce section, and they should also make up a substantial part of your diet. From peas to turnip greens to Brussels sprouts and even sea vegetables like kelp, green vegetables help you give your body all sorts of healthy substances, antioxidants included.

I want to give special treatment to broccoli, which packs an extremely healthy punch. Broccoli contains lots of *sulforaphane,* an antioxidant that has been receiving a lot of attention from researchers lately because it helps the body get rid of toxins, supports the immune system, and can even slow down tumors.

Eating raw

The preparation of your food — from processing to cooking — has an impact on its nutrition. Processing foods with chemicals has the most negative impact because those methods often add toxins and rarely (if ever) conserve important nutrients. Applying heat to food is less damaging, but it can still break down some of the really beneficial substances. For these reasons, it's useful to get plenty of raw foods in your diet, particularly plant foods like vegetables, fruits, and nuts. It's really hard to beat fresh produce for nutritional value; there's no better way to get essential nutrients than to load up on all the tasty things that don't get fooled with much (if at all) on their route from the tree (or bush or vine or root) to your plate.

Some people go so far as to eat only raw foods, but that's a practice that can be difficult for most of us to sustain. Chances are you currently cook your food and plan to continue doing so. With that in mind, I provide some simple analyses of a few cooking methods:

- **Frying:** Nothing good happens when you fry food (except the taste!). As you'd probably guess, pan frying is better than deep frying, which is really one of the worst things you can do to your food. Skip deep frying whenever possible.

- **Pressure cooking:** Antioxidant levels in most foods are reduced more through pressure cooking than through any other cooking method. If you're eating specific foods for antioxidant value, be sure you're not pressure cooking them or you're shooting yourself in the foot.

- **Boiling:** Boiling food can be fine for short amounts of time, but boiling for extended periods can really decrease the nutrient value of many foods.

✔ **Baking:** Generally speaking, baking is a good way to cook food without compromising the nutritional value too much. It's a problem only if you're baking foods to the point where they're mushy; if that happens, you know you've lost at least some of the nutrients.

✔ **Steaming:** I'm a big proponent of steaming, particularly for vegetables. It's easy, quick, delicious, and helps to maintain most of the nutritive value of vegetables.

Some fans of raw food diets insist that all vegetables and fruits are better raw than any other way, but that isn't completely true. The nutrients in some foods are actually enhanced through cooking. One example is the lycopene (an antioxidant) found in tomatoes. A recent study showed that one type of lycopene in tomatoes actually increases 35 percent when the tomatoes are cooked for 30 minutes at 190 degrees Fahrenheit. Another study showed that the antioxidant beta-carotene increases when carrots are cooked. Other examples include spinach, mushrooms, asparagus, cabbage, peppers, and many other vegetables, which also provide more antioxidants when cooked.

There's always a trade-off, of course, and in this case it's vitamin C. Most types of cooking break down vitamin C, so while you're cooking some of these vegetables to increase their antioxidant levels, chances are you're decreasing the amount of vitamin C you'll get from them. However, it's pretty easy to get vitamin C in your diet by eating fresh fruits, so in this case you're probably just fine doing a little cooking to up the antioxidant ante.

Avoiding ingredients you can't pronounce

If you want a nearly foolproof way to make sure you're getting what you need and avoiding what can harm you in food, stick to this simple rule: If you can't pronounce an ingredient in the food, don't eat it. I know that sounds remarkably simplistic, but for the most part it really does work. Foods that contain bizarre ingredients with huge names and pronunciations that only a chemist could love don't have any place on our plates.

This rule is a no-brainer when it comes to fresh foods like fruits and vegetables. Produce doesn't have ingredient lists, but if it did you wouldn't have any problem pronouncing all the words. Lettuce. Carrots. Apples. Spinach. Easy enough, right? But go a few aisles over in your grocery store and take a look at the ingredient lists on the food that comes in boxes, pouches, and cans. You'll see ingredients like butylated hydroxyanisole, potassium metabisulfite, and erythorbic acid. Huh? Can you pronounce those ingredients? Do you have any idea what they are? If you answer no to both questions, it's safe to say that those chemicals don't belong in your body. The fact is that you don't need them to survive. So why would you eat them, when it's just as easy to fill up your shopping cart with foods that contain things like rice, cabbage, broccoli, and cherries? Stick with the basics.

Spicing up your life

One of the biggest knocks on eating a healthy diet is a lack of flavor. Some people think about eating healthy and immediately assume that if they fill their diets with nutrient-rich foods, they'll look down at their dinner plates and see nothing more than a few kale leaves and chunks of celery.

In fact, the opposite is true. Healthy, nourishing diets — including detox diets — can and should include a wide variety of flavorful components, particularly spices and herbs. You can get a world of flavor and an excellent array of nutrients just by adding spices and herbs to your diet.

Spices are made from flowers, berries, bark, seeds, and roots, and herbs are usually plant leaves. Both are readily available, and both can be an integral part of a detoxification-focused diet.

Pound for pound, spices have more antioxidants than fruits or vegetables. The antioxidants you can find in spices are varied, and their contributions to your health can be substantial. To give you an idea of how impactful spices can be, a recent study showed that adding lemon balm and marjoram to a diet could increase antioxidant levels by 150 percent and 200 percent respectively.

You probably include some herbs and spices in your diet, but there's always room for more. There's no better way to improve the quality of your recipes and your health all at the same time! To help encourage you in that direction, I offer the following list of spices and herbs and some of their health benefits:

- **Cayenne pepper:** Contains *capsaicin* (a potent antioxidant), beta-carotene, and vitamins A and C.

- **Cilantro:** Contains potent antioxidants and can be useful in the removal of mercury from the body. Coriander is the seed of cilantro.

- **Cinnamon:** Acts as an *antimicrobial,* decreasing the growth of fungi and yeast. It also helps to prevent blood clots, and a recent study has shown it to help decrease blood sugar in diabetics.

- **Cloves:** Helps to reduce nausea, vomiting, indigestion, and stomach ulcers.

- **Coriander:** Offers strong antioxidant effects and contains vitamins A and C.

- **Garlic:** Includes potent antioxidants, decreases blood pressure and cholesterol, and has historically been used to prevent the common cold.

- **Ginger:** Provides antioxidants and can help decrease nausea, vomiting, and morning sickness. A truly dynamic spice, ginger is twice as effective as many common motion sickness drugs and can lessen the side effects of chemotherapy.

✔ **Oregano:** Provides four times the antioxidant activity of blueberries, which are a powerful source of antioxidants.

✔ **Parsley:** Contains strong antioxidants (including beta-carotene), folic acid, and vitamins A and C.

✔ **Red chili powder:** Includes capsaicin and has been used to help reduce inflammation, clear mucus, boost immunity, and decrease cholesterol.

✔ **Saffron:** Loaded with antioxidants and has been used to treat dysentery and improve eye health.

✔ **Sage:** Contains antioxidants and can generate anti-inflammatory effects.

This list is really just the beginning. Most herbs and spices offer some sort of health benefit, and hundreds of different varieties are available. You can use them to boost your health, detoxify, and spice up your meals all at the same time. Your imagination is your only limitation!

Embracing Exercise

For most of human history, exercise consumed a big part of our daily lives. We were physically active for much of the day just doing the work of staying alive. Only in the last 100 years or so have most people stopped doing daily vigorous exercise. And exercise isn't the only thing we've stopped doing since the advent of twentieth-century technology. Until the 1950s and the development of air conditioning, most of the world's population was used to spending all summer in a natural sauna, day and night.

Our bodies are built for physical activity; we simply can't be healthy without exercise and sweating. Virtually every part of our body is dependent upon exercise to work at maximum efficiency, and any effort you make to detoxify your body is greatly enhanced if you make regular exercise part of your plan.

If you're not exercising regularly, you need to start now. If you can get 30 minutes of exercise each day, you'll do wonders for your body. And don't think that you need to be jogging steep mountain trails or pumping iron in an expensive gym to get a workout. For many people there's no better exercise than walking at a fast pace. Even if you're not currently exercising, you should be able to walk briskly for a half hour, but it's always a good idea to check with your doctor before starting an exercise regimen. Don't be afraid to start out slowly and increase your speed gradually until you're walking about 2 miles in 30 minutes. The important thing is to exercise regularly — daily is by far the best — so that it becomes a ritual instead of a chore.

If you want to sleep better at night, exercise in the early morning. Multiple studies have shown that early morning exercise helps keep our day–night cycle stable. Exercising in the morning gives you far more energy during the day and better sleep at night. Exercising in the evening tends to wake up your body when it's trying to prepare itself for sleep. If you think that your schedule, climate, or some other factor prevents you from exercising in the morning, take another look. You may just have to get up 30 minutes earlier, which is something that most of us can do in the interest of promoting long-term health.

If you dread the idea of getting started on even a simple exercise plan, try getting someone else involved to make things more enjoyable. Why not get your spouse or a good friend to walk with you? It's a great way to spend time together, and you may be surprised what some sidewalk and a pair of comfortable shoes can do for a relationship or friendship.

Maximizing detox with your muscles

An obvious benefit of exercise is strengthening skeletal muscles, and going through a regular workout will inevitably improve your muscle strength and endurance. When you use your muscles regularly, they become more toned and utilize energy more efficiently. This means you can get more work done with less energy expended. Exercise also extends the length of time that a muscle can work without getting tired.

In addition, the following are other, less obvious benefits to working out that can help you use your muscles to maximize your detoxification efforts.

Revving your lymph system

One of the most important functions of exercise relates to stimulating your *lymph system,* which is a key body system for detoxification. You may not have ever heard about the lymph system. I bet you've heard about the circulatory system, right? That one involves your heart, arteries, and veins, and it circulates blood throughout your body in a *closed system* (meaning the blood stays in your blood vessels). The lymph system is another body system for moving around liquid substances. It's twice as large as the circulatory system and consists of tubes called *lymph vessels.* The lymph vessels are connected like limbs on a tree, and the small ends are open.

After your body's tissues use the nutrients that are delivered by the blood in your circulatory system, the waste products — including many toxins that your body has to get rid of — are released and travel into the lymph system. Waste products move through larger and larger lymph vessels until they're eventually dumped back into the circulatory system, which carries them to the liver and kidneys to be processed and later expelled from your body.

Your heart works as the pump for your circulatory system, but what's the pump for the lymph system? There isn't just one. The lymph system depends on contracting muscles and the movement of your lungs to move wastes through your system and eventually out of your body. The stronger and more active your muscles and lungs, the more activity your lymph system will enjoy and the more waste products you'll clear out of your body. Taking time for regular exercise helps keep your lymph system in tip-top shape, and it goes a long way in helping you clear your body of toxins.

Muscling out blood sugar problems

Too much sugar in your body can have a variety of toxic effects. I know it can be a little hard to think of sugar as a toxin, but if you have doubts just ask someone who suffers from diabetes.

The control of blood sugar is another vital benefit of exercise. When you exercise, your muscles have an increased demand for energy, and they're more than happy to take sugar directly out of your bloodstream to get the energy they need to keep moving. That process is a huge help in keeping your blood sugar under control, and it also helps to prevent diabetes. The problems caused by diabetes affect millions of people each year, and the cost to treat all those conditions is in the billions of dollars. Think about all the suffering we could prevent and the resources we could save if we all just made it a point to take a brisk walk for 30 minutes every day!

Working your heart, lungs, and brain

Exercising is an awfully important part of total body health, and some of the most crucial advantages of regular exercise affect your heart, lungs, and brain. (I think we can agree that these are three pretty useful body parts.)

Making your heart happy

The heart is a muscle, but it's one that performs feats of stamina and longevity that put most of your other muscles to shame. Like all muscles, it functions much better if it's exercised regularly — preferably on a daily basis. You can exercise your heart muscle simply by engaging in a physical activity that makes it beat more actively than when you're not doing anything physically active. The amount and intensity of that physical activity depends on your age. You can use your age to figure out your maximum heart rate (MHR), which you can therefore use to figure out how hard you need to work your heart muscle. Subtract your age from 220, and the result is your MHR in number of beats per minute.

You don't want to exercise to the point where you're raising your heart rate to your MHR and leaving it there, because doing so would be dangerous. You really want to shoot for various percentages of your MHR, ranging from 50 to 60 percent (when you're just getting started on an exercise regimen) up to 80 percent of your MHR (when you've been exercising regularly for a few weeks and you're trying to build endurance). If you can't maintain 80 percent, try maintaining 60 percent and adding in a few short bursts that take your heart rate up to 80 percent. (Keep in mind that these are just general figures, and your ideal heart rate may be quite different if you have medical problems.)

Don't wait until you have heart trouble to begin an exercise program. Use exercise as a preventative measure, and you'll keep your heart healthier and happier than you ever could with prescription drugs and surgeries — common treatments for patients with established heart conditions.

Letting your lungs breathe easier

Getting a regular dose of exercise keeps your heart pumping along happily, but it also helps you to build stronger lungs. During a session of physical activity, your lungs have to work harder to keep enough oxygen in your blood to fill the needs of all your moving muscles. That increases your lung capacity and contributes to making your breathing easier and more effective. It also has a positive effect on the muscles that you use to expand and contract your lungs, which in turn increases endurance.

Boosting your brain function

And let's not forget about how exercise can benefit your mind. Here's what working out regularly can do for your brain:

- Grow new nerve cells.

- Improve mood and even help reverse depression.

- Release natural chemicals (called *endorphins*) that create a sense of euphoria and reduce pain.

- Improve cognitive function (especially in older people).

- Possibly prevent and treat Alzheimer's and Parkinson's diseases. (Some studies suggest this benefit, but at this point the evidence is inconclusive.)

Supporting Your Health with Supplements

Most of our diets are downright deplorable. Our food choices are often lousy, and even when people make good choices, the actual food items are of a poor quality. In the days before commercial food processing, a person's usual intake of food was rich in vitamins, minerals, and essential fatty acids. The result was generally good health. But all the various methods for processing — from homogenization to radiation — have reduced a lot of our foods to nutrient-depleted masses of empty calories and harmful fats.

I truly believe that you can't be healthy in the Western world today without using supplements to increase your intake of vitamins, minerals, and essential fatty acids. Even if you eat only organic foods, you're not likely to get the extra amounts of antioxidants that are necessary to fight off all the environmental toxins that assault us on a daily basis.

Not everyone in the medical community shares my love and support of supplements. You'll hear some doctors say that taking supplements just makes expensive urine because your body doesn't absorb enough of the key ingredients to have an effect. I simply don't agree.

The recommended daily allowance (RDA) for most vitamins is established by the U.S. Food and Drug Administration (FDA), and in most cases the recommendations are absurdly low. The FDA tends to set RDAs at a level that helps you avoid certain diseases but doesn't help you to improve your health much beyond that. For example, the FDA says that you need 90 milligrams of vitamin C per day, but that measly amount won't do much for you beyond fighting off scurvy. Vitamin C can have wonderful effects on your health, but not in such paltry amounts. (I list my recommended dosages for all the necessary vitamins in Chapter 17, if you're interested. You can also flip to Chapter 22 to read about ten supplements that I recommend everyone take on a daily basis.)

In this section, I use a two-pronged approach to provide you with basic supplement information: I let you know some general rules for selecting supplements, and I clue you in on the ways in which you can avoid a few common supplement mistakes.

Selecting supplements smartly

If you've decided that you're going to begin taking supplements regularly, it's time to go to the store to pick out a supplement product. That sounds easy enough, but in most stores you find an intimidating wall of choices. It can be difficult to choose the right bottle of supplements among all those options. How can you know which supplements are good quality? What do you need to look for before buying? How can you tell, when you're standing there in a store aisle, how a supplement is going to perform when it's in your system? Let me help you sort through some of those questions.

The most expensive supplement you buy is the one that doesn't contain any active ingredients. If all you're buying is a glorified sugar pill, you can save a lot of money by just buying a bag of sugar! Be prepared to consider and analyze several options before making a supplement purchase.

Many supplement companies will tell you that their supplements are more effective because they're administered as dissolvable tablets that you place under your tongue, as patches that you put on your skin, or even as rectal suppositories. The truth is that a good oral supplement (with some legitimate studies that back its effectiveness) is the best option.

Looking for supplement certification

Vitamins and other supplements aren't required to have any testing done before they're sent out into the marketplace. No government entity sets industry-wide requirements that supplement makers have to meet. If a product does not contain as much of the substance as its label says, nothing prevents the manufacturer from selling it anyway. To be honest, in terms of initial obstacles, not much stops someone from bottling sugar pills and selling them as vitamin C. The whole operation can be backed up with a marketing plan, Web site, and multilevel sales scheme.

That said, some supplement manufacturers *do* conduct their own in-house tests to make sure their products are legit. The extent and frequency of the testing varies from company to company.

Make it a practice to check any potential supplement for confirmation that it was made in a *GMP approved* plant. The Good Manufacturing Practice (GMP) regulations are specified by the FDA, and they cover the quality of the actual manufacturing processes by which supplements are made. To achieve the designation, a supplement maker pays a third-party testing firm to come into the plant where it makes supplements. That firm conducts a series of tests to make sure that the plant is operating in a clean, safe, and accurate way. If the testing firm's results are within the guidelines set by the FDA, the supplement maker's plant becomes GMP approved. A supplement made in a GMP approved plant may not be perfect, but at least you know the product was made in a good environment.

Before I recommend any supplement, I confirm it was made in a GMP-certified facility. But I also go a step further. I make certain that the supplement company sends a portion of every lot of its product to an outside independent lab for *assay* (molecular analysis). The supplement company must allow me to contact the lab directly to confirm the test results on any particular lot of product. This testing will include making sure that the supplement dissolves in the stomach or intestines. Exceedingly few companies do these tests.

At the very least, take the following two steps before buying a supplement:

✔ Look for a seal from USP (United States Pharmacopeia) on the label. This designation indicates that the company has made some effort to be credible, but its testing is only random.

✔ Read the label carefully to make sure that the manufacturer, packer, and distributor have addresses in the United States. Some supplements are made in other countries — where manufacturing processes are even more of a crapshoot than they are in the United States. The supplements are then repackaged in the United States, and those products can be dangerous. Even if the supplement brand is familiar, take the time to confirm the addresses of its operations. Some of the best known and advertised names are the worst in quality.

Checking out supplement ingredient lists

Another key to supplement selection is making sure the ingredients that are combined in one product have a valid reason for being put into the same product. Some companies do their own research to validate the effectiveness of a particular combination of ingredients. An enormous amount of data is available on the effectiveness of vitamins, herbs, supplements, and minerals. If you're going to spend your money on a product, make sure you know the scientific rationale for the combination of ingredients you're getting.

When you find a company that does third-party testing before shipping and allows access to the outside lab directly, you can be assured that its products are well formulated and high quality. This type of quality company will also be more than glad to give you the research material to support its use of product combinations. Keep in mind that some of the best products are sold only through physician's offices.

Avoiding potential supplement snags

Supplements are big business. Annual supplement sales are $23 billion, and about 40,000 supplement products are on the market. In an industry so large, it's tough to avoid the occasional subpar or even harmful product. And, as I mention in the previous section, the supplement industry is loosely regulated at best. So you can imagine how many questionable products are floating around.

The biggest problem with supplements is that many of them don't actually contain what the label claims. Depending on the estimate you choose to believe, as many as 70 percent of the supplements on the market either don't have ingredients that match their labels or contain contaminants of some kind. The results can be disastrous: Recently, more than 200 people were sickened when a selenium supplement had 200 times the amount of selenium indicated on the label, for example.

Cases of spiked supplements have also occurred. Not long ago the FDA had to get involved in a situation in which a questionable supplement manufacturer had been adding a drug similar to the powerful male erectile dysfunction medicine to its supposedly all-natural dietary supplement.

With all the potential pitfalls, how do you separate the wheat from the chaff? You need to do some legwork. Here are some pointers:

✔ **If a product claims to guarantee results and help to alleviate all sorts of ailments from headaches to hemorrhoids, save your money.** Reputable sources that produce high quality supplements know better than to advertise that way.

✔ **Look for supplements that are derived from food sources whenever possible.** Synthetic production often eliminates the natural mix of substances present in the natural food source, making them less beneficial and sometimes of no benefit at all.

✔ **Request analyses from the companies that make the supplements you're considering.** The best manufacturers have a litany of evidence to support their claims and verify the integrity of their products, and some of them will provide that information upon request. Don't hesitate to call or e-mail a supplement maker to ask for detailed information about its products. (You can usually find all the contact information on a company's Web site.) Above all, do not accept lab analyses that companies perform in their own labs.

While these suggestions apply to any supplements, you should also be aware of problems specific to certain types of supplements, which I cover next.

Minerals

The big problem with some mineral supplements is that they're not easily absorbed. To confirm that the minerals you're buying will actually end up in your body and not in your toilet, look for *chelated* minerals. Chelating is a somewhat complicated chemical process, and I won't bog you down with the details. The take-home point is that chelated minerals are much more likely to be absorbed by your body than minerals that haven't been put through the process. The process is patented, and you can spot it easily by looking for the company name *Albion* on the supplement's label.

You should also be aware of one other mineral-specific concern. In addition to the active mineral ingredient, some mineral supplements include other substances, including — believe it or not — toxins. What's even harder to fathom is that mineral products that contain these types of materials often list them as ingredients on their labels. Many mineral products are simply ground-up clay. So keep your eyes out for minerals that list lead, silver, antimony, or tin as ingredients! (Yes, I'm serious.)

Probiotics

Probiotics are supplements containing live bacteria that are taken to boost the amount of beneficial bacteria living in your body (the good bacteria living in your intestines). Here are two common problems with probiotics:

- ✔ **Live bacteria levels:** Some probiotics don't have as much live bacteria in them as the label states. A study of 50 products taken from health food store shelves showed that the *most* any product contained was 5 percent of the live bacteria the label stated.

- ✔ **Stray bacteria:** The same study found that 8 out of 50 probiotic supplements tested contained harmful bacteria in addition to the good bacteria advertised on the label.

To dodge these problems, do what you'd do for any supplement: Request some third-party analysis from the supplement company.

Herbs

Because herb supplements are derived from plants, sometimes they contain nasty things like mold, bacteria, heavy metals, and pesticides. This disturbing trend will probably continue as some herb supplement manufacturers aim to cut costs and look overseas for raw materials. Reliable supplement makers test all incoming herbs and reject contaminated shipments, and the purity that results is obvious in the reports that they will send you upon request.

Vitamins

Vitamins are perhaps the most commonly used supplements, and I wish I could report that their widespread use means you won't find problems with the many different vitamins on the market. But that's simply not the case. Like the other supplements I discuss in this chapter, vitamins can sometimes fail to meet label claims. All too often a vitamin maker cuts the amount of vitamin material that's included in each pill without changing the label; recent independent lab analysis confirms that this has been and is currently a significant problem.

I apologize if I'm starting to sound like a broken record, but if you want to make sure your vitamins contain what their labels swear they contain, be sure to contact the manufacturer for some documentation to support those claims.

Omega-3 fatty acids

Here's one more supplement problem to be aware of before I wrap up this discussion: Supplements that contain omega-3 fatty acids usually come in fish oil products like liquids or softgel capsules, and because these things are fish-based they're prone to mercury contamination. I can't imagine that you would want to take a dose of mercury — a deadly toxin — with your fish oil supplement, so be sure to buy fish oil products that have been distilled. Distillation does an excellent job of removing all the mercury.

If you're considering taking a fish oil supplement to up the amount of omega-3 fatty acids in your system, be sure to contact the supplement company first to ask it for analysis that confirms its fish oil doesn't contain anisidine, DDT, dieldrin, or PCBs. These are all toxins, and all have been found in fish oil supplements in recent years.

Changing Intestinal Flora: Gut Check Time

How often do you think about your bowels? Chances are you really consider what your bowels are doing only when something is wrong with them — when you have constipation, diarrhea, or some kind of pain. That's not enough! You need to put some thought into what's going on in your intestines, because the condition of those parts of your body — and what's living inside them — can have a tremendous impact on your total health, from ensuring good nutrition to avoiding disease.

Less than a century ago, most people in the developed world did a much better job of keeping up with their bowels than we do today. Getting a colon cleanse used to be an annual ritual for much of the population, but the practice fell out of favor by the mid-twentieth century. The timing couldn't have been worse, as the advent of processed food was on the horizon and world travel was starting to become a possibility for more people. (Both trends have caused major problems for millions of intestines.) Colon cleanses went the way of the dodo just when we really needed to keep up with them.

In this section, I first explore what lives inside your gut — both the good and the bad. Then I explain how to get tests done that reveal what's going on inside your intestines. Finally, I walk you through the process of cleaning out the bad elements and boosting the good.

Checking out what's living inside you

The bacteria living in your intestines outnumber the cells in your body. *Billions* of organisms are living in your intestines, many of which play a key role in boosting your health, from nutrition to your immune system. Some of them can also play a role in damaging your health in nasty and painful ways. You should definitely understand the various things that live in your gut, so read on to explore the details. I can't fill you in on all the varieties, so I've lumped them into two very broad groups: the good and the bad.

The good

The good types of organisms that live in your intestines are beneficial bacteria that break down your food so the nutrients are more easily absorbed. Good bacteria also make vitamins for you, including B12 and K. As if that weren't enough, they stimulate your immune system (in a good way) and help protect you from disease. When good bacteria are present in the right amounts in your intestines, it's very difficult for harmful bacteria and yeast (which can damage your body) to survive. The most common types of good bacteria in the human intestine are Bifidobacterium and Lactobacillus.

To help boost the amounts of good bacteria that you have living in your gut, you can eat plain yogurt with active bacterial cultures. You can also take bacteria in supplement form (called *probiotics* — read more earlier in this chapter), but you really have to do your homework on the supplement quality to make sure you're getting good value for your money.

Good bacteria are very sensitive to the antibiotics administered when people get sick. Approximately 80 percent of good bacteria are killed when you take a single round of antibiotics! After the good bacteria are gone, it's easier for harmful bacteria and yeast to multiply. That's why diarrhea and vaginal yeast infections are common after someone takes a round of antibiotics — yet another reason to use antibiotics only when absolutely necessary.

The bad

The organisms that you can regard as bad when they're in your intestines include harmful bacteria, yeast, and parasites. Bad bacteria commonly create byproduct gases, and they can cause inflammation and excessive, foul bowel gas. They also cause stress on your immune system, and they can give you chronic intestinal problems.

Antibiotics kill the good bacteria in your intestines and allow the bad bacteria to multiply rapidly. After the bad bacteria multiply, they can easily cause trouble in your intestines. The symptoms of these ailments can persist for years after just a single round of antibiotics. The effects aren't always localized, either — some types of bad bacteria release toxins that can be absorbed in your bloodstream and damage distant organs, including the brain.

You also usually have a small amount of yeast in your intestines. Just like the harmful bacteria, the yeast is kept in check when the good bacteria are present in the right amounts. Good bacteria also help to thwart parasites, many of which love the intestines and can wreak all sorts of havoc on your body. For more details on the problems that yeast and parasites can cause, flip back to Chapter 2.

With its extremely high acid levels, your stomach also helps to control the amount of harmful bacteria, yeast, and parasites that end up in your bowels. If you overuse acid reducers, the stomach loses its acidity, making it easier for these damaging organisms to pass through to the intestines.

Considering useful tests

You can have two types of tests done to help determine what types of critters are living in your intestines: stool tests and urine tests. Both tests need to be administered by professionals, so if you're interested you need to consult your doctor to get the process started. Both tests can be pretty expensive, so be prepared.

Stool tests involve providing a stool sample, which is sent to a lab that examines parts of the sample under a microscope and also runs some chemical tests to find out what is present in your stool. The test is relatively easy, although you may have to stop taking some medications a couple weeks beforehand. (Your doctor will fill you in on those details.)

The process for urine tests is similar: You simply provide a urine sample, which is sent off to a lab for analysis. It's not possible to actually see what's in your intestines by looking at your urine, of course. But labs can run chemical tests on the sample that reveal the presence of byproducts of certain types of bacteria, yeasts, and parasites that commonly set up shop in your intestines and release chemicals that enter your bloodstream and eventually end up in your urine.

Cleansing your bowels

I'm a big proponent of colon cleanses, and I suggest that doing a cleanse once a year is an excellent practice to help you rid your body of abnormal flora and put you on the path to better health.

If you're starting a detox diet or any other detox program, you need to see to it that your intestines are healthy and have the right amounts of the right bacteria living inside them. Doing so involves removing the bad bacteria, yeast, and parasites; eating food and supplements that help your intestines to heal; and replacing the good bacteria. You usually need to take some prescription medications, but they're very easy on the body. It often takes a month to get the intestines back in optimal condition.

To do your bowel cleanse, first find some good intestinal detox supplements. A supplement maker you rely on for quality products should have some in its product line. (See my discussion on choosing supplements earlier in this chapter.) Look for a product that includes wormwood, black walnut hulls, garlic, and pumpkin seeds. I also recommend adding in some clove supplements and a Vermox prescription because both are good for killing off parasite eggs. You should usually take such a supplement for a month in order to kill off the majority of the organisms that live in your bowels.

At the same time, you need to take a product that kills yeast cells. That supplement usually contains barberry, grapefruit seed extract, lavender, and other herbs. I usually add a prescription drug — either Diflucan or Nystatin — to augment the yeast-killing process. It generally takes about three weeks to rid your intestines of harmful yeast cells.

After you've taken a round of supplements and perhaps prescription medications to kill off the harmful bacteria, yeast, and parasites in your intestines, it's time to start building up your intestinal health and adding back in the good bacteria. Do that by eating a diet that's rich in the foods I describe in Chapter 7, and be sure to include lots of bacteria-containing yogurt and probiotic supplements.

If you and your doctor conclude that you're suffering from irritable bowel syndrome (IBS), you should strongly consider doing a colon cleanse. In my practice, I've found that a significant number of patients with IBS have complete relief of symptoms after doing the complete bowel detoxification that I describe here.

Getting a Professional Check-up

For many of the ailments caused by toxins, you need a doctor or other healthcare professional to help you diagnose and in some cases treat the problem. If you want to make a concerted effort to detoxify your body and treat that effort as a top health priority, you need a doctor who understands and is sensitive to more than just the standard practices and beliefs of traditional medicine.

Deciding on a doctor is an intensely personal and important choice, so if you're looking for a doctor or considering whether to stick with the one you currently use, be sure you're as honest with yourself as possible. If you want to consider solutions that fall outside the range of traditional medicine, you need to feel confident that your doctor will hear you out and be willing to work with you. Few things in life are more important than your health, and it's critical that you find someone who will work toward bettering your health without dismissing your input or forcing an agenda on you.

Finding an open-minded doctor

If you want to pursue natural healing, supplementation, or any other form of integrative or alternative self care, you may very well end up butting heads with your doctor. Many doctors aren't as receptive to these ideas as they should be, but you can rest assured that it's not totally their fault. Physicians today are overwhelmed by the influence of pharmaceutical companies. Every medical journal I receive is paid for by drug companies. Every speaker at every traditional medical seminar at the local, state, and national level is paid for by drug companies. Every representative who comes in my office is paid for by a drug company. It isn't in a drug company's best interest for physicians to recommend solutions for their patients that don't involve prescription drugs, and they bombard doctors with information and propaganda accordingly. That situation can make it extremely hard for you to find a doctor who is open to alternative options.

But there's good news, as well, in the form of an ever-growing group of physicians who consider a wide range of disease treatments and health enhancements that go beyond taking a prescription medication.

Two good resources exist for finding open-minded physicians who are keen on considering nontraditional solutions to medical problems: the American College for Advancement in Medicine (www.acam.org) and the International College of Integrative Medicine (www.icimed.com). I strongly recommend visiting their Web sites for a wide range of information on integrative medicine and for physician lists that will help you find an integrative doctor in your area.

Integrative medicine is a concept of medicine using natural treatments when possible but using medication and traditional therapies when necessary. This approach is also called *complementary medicine.* Alternative practitioners (discussed in the next section) are usually not licensed to use traditional medical therapies and therefore use only alternative therapies.

Seeking out an alternative practitioner

Alternative practitioners are healthcare professionals who specialize in medicine that doesn't necessarily fall within the range of what is currently regarded as "conventional." They can be of great help in detoxing and seeking out good health. These types of professionals include chiropractors, naturopaths, and acupuncturists, and they also include some medical doctors (MDs) and doctors of osteopathic medicine (DOs).

MDs and DOs have the benefit of access to traditional medical treatments and prescriptions, which may be required at times. (Keep in mind that not all traditional medicine is bad!) For the best medical care, find an MD or DO who combines traditional medicine with an integrative approach. A doctor who uses natural therapies when possible but also calls upon traditional medicine when necessary is an excellent option.

MDs and DOs have equal medical privileges and very similar training. DOs receive training in manual medicine that MDs don't receive. *Manual medicine* involves working directly with muscles to improve function or reduce pain.

Another difference is that about 80 percent of DOs are primary care doctors and 20 percent are specialists. MDs typically have the opposite split.

A *naturopath* is a professional who uses natural and physical tools to treat various conditions. Naturopaths are alternative practitioners, and they're a varied group that includes acupuncturists and chiropractors as well as a host of practitioners who don't have standardized training. Some alternative practitioners may have limited formal training but are still very talented in their particular field. Be careful, though, because some of these folks can practice bogus medicine (see the next section for details).

Your selection process for your alternative practitioner should be rigorous. Be sure to check credentials, years of experience, and word of mouth references, and also set up an initial interview to make sure you're comfortable with your choice before beginning any medical evaluation or treatment.

Keeping an eye out for bogus medicine

It's sad but true that a number of people claim to be practitioners of alternative medicine who don't offer much useful treatment or analysis at all. Put simply, there's some bogus medicine out there, and you need to keep that fact in mind to avoid getting burned and putting your health (and your money) at risk.

Here are a few key questions to ask yourself when considering an alternative practitioner:

- ✔ Do any state laws govern this profession?
- ✔ Are standardized training and tests required to gain credentials?
- ✔ Do any local, state, or national organizations exist for this practitioner's type of medicine? If so, is the practitioner in good stead with the organizations?
- ✔ Does the practitioner have reliable word of mouth support?
- ✔ Has the practitioner moved around frequently? If so, does he or she have a good reason for those moves?

Chapter 6

Recognizing Toxin-filled and Otherwise Unhealthy Foods

*T*he foods that are available on most grocery store shelves are often loaded with toxins, or they're made using toxic processes, or both. It's tough to eliminate the toxin-containing food from your pantry and refrigerator, but if you're going to get serious about detoxification and detox dieting, you have to take that step.

To begin cutting out toxin-filled foods, you first need to be able to recognize them. That's the aim of this chapter: to show you how to spot toxic foods. I start with a look at genetically modified foods, give you a few tips for how you can grow some of your own toxin-free foods, and call your attention to several types of processed foods that you may not realize pose a toxic threat.

Being Wary of Genetically Modified (GM) Foods

I touch on the prevalence and potential threat of genetically modified foods in Chapter 3, but there's much more to the story. I provide you with a lot more detail in this section. Foods that have been *genetically modified* — often called *GM foods* — include plants and animals with genes that scientists have played with, usually with the goal of increasing food production.

I want to make it clear that we're not talking about selective breeding here. That process involves identifying positive traits in a couple of plants or animals of the same species and breeding them so that their offspring are likely to have those positive traits. The key phrase there is *of the same species.* In genetic modification, genes from lots of different species — from fish to insects to bacteria — are spliced together using biochemical processes in a lab.

In many cases the results sound appealing at first blush. Who wouldn't want a tomato that stays ripe longer or corn that is less likely to get damaged by pillaging insects? The problem is that most foods created using genetic modification haven't been around for very long, and it's extremely difficult for even the savviest scientists to say what GM plants and animals will do to our environment — and, perhaps more importantly, to our bodies and health — in the long run. We may be creating and consuming foods that could damage ecosystems and harm our bodies in ways that haven't been identified yet. Symptoms of these problems could take quite a while to surface, and when they do they may not initially be attributed to GM foods.

To better understand the impact of GM foods, consider what some people within the scientific community have said about the general process of genetic modification of food:

✔ In a recent public statement, the American Academy of Environmental Medicine (AAEM) called for "a moratorium on GM foods, long term independent studies, and labeling." The AAEM went on to say that "several animal studies indicate serious health risks associated with GM food, including infertility, immune problems, accelerated aging, insulin regulation, and changes in the major organs and the gastrointestinal system." The AAEM's conclusion? That "there is more than a casual association between GM foods and adverse health effects. There is causation."

✔ Pushpa A. Bhargava, a world-renowned biologist and former director of the Centre for Cellular and Molecular Biology (one of the Indian government's top science departments), reviewed 600 scientific studies on GM foods and came to the conclusion that GM organisms are a major contributor to the sharply deteriorating health of Americans.

✔ The British Medical Association, which represents more than 100,000 physicians, has called for an outright banning of all GM foods and a requirement for labeling in countries where GM foods still exist.

Clearly, there's cause for concern when it comes to GM foods. With the rest of this section my aim is to finish bringing you up to speed on GM food basics and to let you know how you can identify (and avoid, if you choose) GM food products.

Understanding GM food basics

I don't want to overload you with too many details on how GM plants and animals are created in a lab. However, to help you figure out exactly what I'm talking about here, an example would be useful.

There's a bacterium that lives in soil called *Bacillus thuringiensis*, and it produces a toxin that kills many of the insects that destroy food crops (corn, for example). You might say that the bacterium contains a kind of natural pesticide. At a certain point, some people familiar with genetic modification realized that they might be able to take the gene from that bacterium that helps to produce the natural pesticide and insert that gene into plants that are grown for food. The result would be a crop that produces the insect toxin on its own and is much more resistant to attacks from hungry insects. That's just what happened; the corn you eat today was modified in this way.

You may wonder, *What's the problem? Corn that doesn't get eaten up by insects in the field sounds like a good thing.*

The problem is this: The toxin that is now being produced by the corn ends up in our bodies, and it's difficult to say what effects that toxin could have on us in the long run. What's even more troubling is that the genes that cause the corn to produce the toxin can be transferred to the good bacteria that live in your intestines, and those bacteria will continue to make the toxin for years.

And the potential problems don't stop there. In many instances, GM foods have been shown to cause health problems, including the following:

- ✔ Genetic material from GM foods has been found in the brains of animals that have been fed those foods.

- ✔ Foreign proteins that end up in some GM foods can cause allergic reactions. For example, the United Kingdom saw a 50 percent jump in soy allergies after it started allowing GM soy products to be sold to consumers.

- ✔ A few years ago, a GM form of a supplement was released for public use without being tested. Before it was taken off the market, the product was linked to 37 deaths and 1,500 other reports of adverse affects.

I hope you'll think hard about the impact that GM foods can have on you and your family, and consider trying to limit the amount of GM foods that end up in your diet.

Trying to identify GM foods

GM foods don't necessarily look different from other foods, so it's not always easy to tell which foods are GM and which aren't when you're shopping for food in the United States. That's the exception, though — not the rule. In many countries (including all countries in the European Union), all GM food must be labeled to let consumers know that the food contains GM organisms.

When you're trying to figure out which foods in your grocery store contain GM ingredients, it's useful to know which plants and animals are most commonly modified. At the top of the list are corn and soybeans — two of the biggest sources of our calories in the United States. Recent estimates indicate that roughly 75 percent of the soybean crops and about one-third of the corn crops in the United States have been genetically modified. That's an enormous amount of food! Both vegetables are used to make many different types of ingredients that show up in processed foods (ingredients like soybean oil and high fructose corn syrup, which you find on a huge variety of labels in the processed food aisles of your grocery store). Some researchers say that when you add up all the genetically modified foods and ingredients that are based on GM foods, about 75 percent of the food for sale in a run-of-the-mill grocery store in the United States is genetically modified.

The GM food blitz doesn't stop at corn and soybeans. Several other crops are often tinkered with at the genetic level, including cotton and cotton seed oil (check your candy bars for that one), papaya, tomatoes, potatoes, canola, sugar cane, sugar beets, rice, alfalfa, squash, cantaloupe, and flax. That's not an all-inclusive list by any means, because it's very difficult to obtain information on which crops are actually genetically modified. The regulations and review processes of genetic modification are sparse and lax at best.

And the problem isn't limited to plants. The big genetic modification companies are now genetically modifying animals, too. To date, pigs, goats, fish, and cows have been genetically modified, and in the short term it doesn't look like that trend is going to slow down. As is the case with GM plants, very few regulations or rules exist to limit the use of GM animals for food in the United States, so it can be extremely tough to tell what has been modified and what hasn't.

So what is a health-conscious consumer to do when he's faced with a grocery store full of foods that very well may have been tinkered with?

At this point in the United States, no requirements exist for labeling GM foods. The only surefire way to make sure you're not buying or eating GM food products is to stick to foods that are labeled "100 percent organic." That's actually a good practice to follow whenever possible, and I cover all the ins and outs of eating organic in Chapter 7.

Many people are very concerned about genetic modification and the impact it will have on this and future generations. Right now, no studies exist to tell us what kinds of changes are likely to happen to us and our environment as a result of the GM revolution. But I encourage you to seek out new information about GM foods so you can find out quickly when certain products are revealed to be dangerous, either for your health or for our environment.

Growing Food in a Toxic World

Even if the seeds used to grow many of our foods aren't genetically modified, it's still tough for them to sprout, grow, produce fruit, get harvested, and end up in our grocery stores without being poisoned with fertilizers and insecticides. These chemicals are very widely used, and it's getting difficult to escape their influence on our food. The days of the small-time farmer and his attention to detail are almost gone. Today, large commercial farms with genetically modified seeds, fertilizers, and insecticides are the norm.

Because of these toxic influences, many Americans are trying to grow their own fruits and vegetables so they can be certain that the foods they're eating don't come with a built-in side of poison. I'm a doctor, not a master gardener, so I won't try to tell you how you can turn your backyard (or even a few pots on your patio) into an organic vegetable or herb garden. But as an expert on toxins, what I can offer is an overview of the ways you can cut out the toxic fertilizers and insecticides that many people turn to when they endeavor to grow some of their own food.

If you'd like to read more about how to grow fruits, vegetables, and herbs in a truly organic way, check out *Organic Gardening For Dummies* by Ann Whitman, Suzanne DeJohn, and the National Gardening Association (Wiley). It contains loads of basic but extremely helpful information on how to set up and succeed with a toxin-free garden.

Focusing on fertilizer

Picking out a safe fertilizer can be a daunting task because much of what's available now contains at least a few toxic ingredients. Making matters much worse are the labeling conventions for fertilizers. For instance, a product marketed and sold as a fertilizer is required to list only the plant nutrient ingredients that are included in the formula. The other ingredients — which can and often do include toxins — don't have to be listed.

Fertilizer is usually sold as a mix, and the bags are prominently labeled with three numbers. A common example is "10-10-10." This means that the fertilizer contains 10 percent nitrogen, 10 percent phosphorus, and 10 percent potassium. Here's the obvious (yet unaddressed) question: What makes up the other 70 percent of the product? The truth is that the 70 percent can be anything from municipal sewage sludge to toxic waste. Some unethical fertilizer manufacturers even go so far as to label their products with the word "organic" when many of the non-nutrient ingredients are based on byproducts from water treatment facilities.

If you want to dodge all the possible toxic fertilizer pitfalls, do the following:

✔ Look for fertilizer that is labeled "100 percent organic." That "100 percent" part is important because sometimes "organic" can be used by itself in inappropriate and misleading ways.

✔ Try fertilizers that come from animals. These can include blood or bone meal and manure.

✔ Look into mineral fertilizer options like Epsom salt and limestone.

Investigating insecticides

Generally speaking, insecticides are as loaded up with harmful toxins as any products on the market. Most of the bottles of insecticides in your hardware or home improvement store have enough toxic material to kill you pretty easily. (If you want to discover more about the threats posed by insecticides and see a breakdown of the three different levels of toxicity that are used to categorize these substances, flip back to Chapter 3.) Why does it make sense to spray these materials onto the plants that will produce food you plan to eat?

The good news is that lots of formulas for safe organic pesticides exist, and many good products are available at health food stores and on the Internet. Here are a few examples.

✔ Concentrated garlic rids plants of a multitude of damaging insects.

✔ Soap mixed with *pyrethrum,* an extract from the pyrethrum flower, thwarts a wide range of aphids, whiteflies, mites, and a number of other pests.

✔ A liquid or wax made from hot peppers wards off quite a few insect species. You can even use hot sauce!

✔ You can make an effective fungicide at home by mixing baking soda with a little vegetable oil.

I strongly advise against using chemical, commercial pesticides. But if you do choose to use them, please do so sparingly. Make sure you're working in well-ventilated areas, and be sure to at least wash your hands (or, better yet, take a shower) when you're finished. Be sure to also keep these materials in a safe place (away from children). And make certain that the containers are extremely well marked and identified as poison.

Working around Processed Foods

In Chapter 3, I provide quite a lot of information about processed food. Just about everything I cover there supports this statement: Don't eat processed foods if you can help it. We were meant to eat fresh, healthful, simple foods — not brightly colored, shrinkwrapped mystery foods that are loaded up with high fructose corn syrup and other toxin-laden ingredients.

It usually isn't too difficult to identify processed foods in your grocery store, and if you're honest with yourself you probably know when you're putting a potentially harmful processed food in your shopping cart. But if you need help, here's a very simple and virtually universal rule for avoiding the processed food aisles at the store:

When you're grocery shopping, select most of what goes in your cart from the store's perimeter aisles. The outer aisles are almost always where you find produce, fresh meat, and a lot of the other foods that haven't been ruined by common food processing techniques.

You should be able to dodge most processed foods with just a little effort. However, some food processing methods can be harder to detect but still surprisingly dangerous to your health. I cover the top two here.

Keeping your hands off homogenized food

Many dairy products, including almost all the milk that you find in the average grocery store, have been homogenized. *Homogenization* is a process that involves forcing a liquid through a very fine filter at really remarkable pressures — sometimes as much as 4,000 pounds per square inch. (That's more than a lot of pressure washers, which are used to clean caked-in and baked-on dirt from sidewalks, among other things.)

Milk is homogenized to keep the cream that it contains from separating when you leave it sitting in your refrigerator. (It's done more for aesthetic reasons than anything else.) The problem is that the homogenization process alters the milk, making it less healthy for humans.

Multiple studies show an increase in cardiovascular disease among people who drink larger amounts of homogenized milk. Further examinations into these connections have been historically poorly funded, so we're not exactly sure why homogenized milk may contribute to cardiovascular ailments. One theory involves a substance called *xanthine oxidase* (XO), which is present in milk. XO in milk that hasn't been homogenized isn't absorbed in our intestines, but XO *is* absorbed when the milk has undergone homogenization. Elevated levels of XO in your blood have been implicated as a cause of damage to the blood vessels that can result in plaque development in the arteries, which can lead to blocked arteries and heart attacks.

If you're wary of homogenized milk — and I think you should be — ask at your local health food store for milk that hasn't been put through the homogenization process. You can also find it through local dairies and farms, and some of them will even allow you to come and tour their facilities. That can be a good way to see what is done to the milk you may be consuming to make sure you're seeing the udder truth when it comes to the safety of your milk.

Passing on pasteurization

The *pasteurization* process has been around for about 150 years, and it involves raising the temperature of a food or liquid to a very high level in the interest of killing off bacteria, parasites, and other dangerous organisms. That's not necessarily a bad thing, of course, but a problem arises because heating food up to such extremely high temperatures can destroy many of the beneficial substances that may be present, like vitamins, nutrients, and enzymes. Pasteurization destroys plenty of dangerous critters, but it also limits the good stuff that your body needs to get out of the foods you eat.

These days, pasteurization is most commonly associated with milk. Almost all milk is pasteurized even though the process isn't nearly as necessary now that milk farms and dairies are much cleaner and more sanitary than they used to be. Pasteurization ruins a lot of the good vitamins that milk can provide.

While milk is the most familiar pasteurized food, many others exist, including almonds, apple cider, beer, canned food, cheese, crabs, cream, eggs, fruit juice, honey, maple syrup, soy sauce, sports drinks, vinegar, water, and wine.

You'll often see "Pasteurized" notes on the labels of food products that have been put through the pasteurization process. If you're concerned that your food may have lower nutritional quality because it has been superheated, keep your eye out for that notation.

Chapter 7

Deciding on the Best Foods for a Toxin-free Dinner Table

*O*ne of the greatest things about detoxifying your body and getting started on a detox diet — beside the fact that it can have a fantastic impact on your overall health — is that you don't need to buy all sorts of expensive equipment, take a class, or read 15 books before getting started. (I do recommend reading this book, of course, but I hope that's not too difficult of a task!)

Detox diets can be simple and relatively easy if you understand the basics, and that's what I give you in this chapter. If you're in the right frame of mind and you're willing to make the best choices about your food — both where you buy it and how you prepare it — you'll soon be on your way to cutting toxins out of your diet and building a stronger, healthier body.

Gathering What You Need for a Detox Diet

Toxin-free, healthy food is the most important part of a detox diet, but it's not the only part. In order to stay on a detoxified path, you need to have some specific equipment and a few cooking staples that are chosen with detoxification in mind. I'm not talking about loads of expensive gear and a pantry full of bizarre ingredients that you have to get flown in from some far-away country. Most of what you need will be available locally, and you may already have several of the necessary items at home.

Make sure you don't skip the critical preparation steps I explain in this section. Neglecting them and moving straight on to focusing on the food you'll incorporate in your detox diet can start you off on the wrong foot.

Buying the correct equipment

You can buy the most organic, toxin-free food in the world, but if you're cooking it with the wrong equipment you're shooting yourself in the foot. You need pots, pans, and other essential cooking gear that don't add toxins to your meals.

To be certain you aren't adding toxins to your food while you're cooking it, invest in some good stainless steel pots, pans, and other cookware. Non-stick cookware, which is coated in a chemical that's supposed to prevent food from sticking to the pot's or pan's surfaces, can leach toxins into your food over time.

You also need to consider the potential toxicity of the materials that you use to store and serve your food. If most of your dishes, plates, cups, and food storage containers are made of plastics, you could be inadvertently adding harmful toxins to your food over time. (My discussion of toxins like BPA and phthalates in food packaging from Chapter 3 is relevant here, so flip back and take a look if you want to know more.)

So what can you use to serve and store food if plastic is potentially harmful? Look for options made of glass, ceramic, or stainless steel. (Keep in mind that if you choose ceramic containers you need to confirm that they're lead-free before buying and using.)

A juicy detoxification option

If you're looking for a practical addition to your kitchen that will give you some flexibility in the way you prepare your detox diet foods, look no further than a juicer. The idea of drinking your fruits and vegetables has become more and more popular in recent years, which is really no surprise. Juice recipes that incorporate fruits from apples to apricots and vegetables from carrots to kale can be quick, easy ways to give your diet a healthy boost, and many of them are downright delicious.

Several effective, affordable juicers on the market are perfect for use at home. They range from under $100 for a basic model to well over $1,000 for a juicer with every last bell and whistle, so do your research and let your budget be your guide.

Keeping the right supplies on hand

Every kitchen needs a few staple ingredients that serve as the basis of a wide range of recipes and meals. If you want to work toward making your kitchen an effective home base for a detoxification diet, you need to sort through the staples you have now, get rid of the potentially toxic ones, and bring in new ingredients that don't pose a toxic threat. Here are a few of the basics:

- ✔ **Flour:** You need an all-purpose whole wheat or white flour. Shoot for 100 percent organic. (Check out my discussion of the various levels of organic food in the next section of this chapter.)

- ✔ **Corn meal:** Make sure you get a 100 percent organic option.

  For dry ingredients like flour and corn meal, be sure to use glass containers for storage. You'll likely have these ingredients on hand for a while, and you don't want them to pick up toxins from plastic containers over time in your pantry.

- ✔ **Butter:** I can't say that I recommend eating lots of butter on a daily basis, but it is better than a lot of the options. I definitely suggest using real butter rather than butter substitutes like margarine. Just make sure the butter is 100 percent organic.

- ✔ **Cooking oil:** I discuss your cooking oil options in detail a little later in this chapter, but generally speaking I recommend using coconut oil or olive oil for cooking whenever possible. Again, buy 100 percent organic if possible.

- ✔ **Spices and herbs:** If you're at all concerned that a detox diet has to be a bland diet, banish that thought immediately. Some of the most flavorful ingredients in the world — spices and herbs — are an integral part of any healthy diet, especially one that shuns toxins and emphasizes good things like antioxidants. Stock up on spices and herbs, and flip back to Chapter 5 for a lengthy discussion about which ones you can choose for specific effects.

Going Organic

Organic foods are plants or animals that are grown or raised without toxins. That means they're not sprayed with toxic pesticides, injected with antibiotics or hormones, processed with toxic additives or processes, or packaged in toxic containers. Organic foods have become increasingly popular in recent years; sales of organic foods have increased by 20 percent in each of the last seven years. Overall, that trend is a very good thing because it means the public has begun to recognize the importance of cutting out toxic materials like pesticides and harsh chemical fertilizers from our food, as well as the need to limit our intake of genetically modified food.

I encourage you to eat organic foods whenever possible, although I need to explain several caveats before you start loading up your shopping cart.

First, several different categories of organic foods are available, so you need to be a real label hawk when examining organic options. Here's the breakdown:

- **Specific Ingredients are Organically Produced:** This designation is nothing special because it can be used on a label for any product that has only one organic ingredient.

- **Made with Organic Ingredients:** Foods in this category have to contain only 70 percent organic ingredients. Needless to say, a lot of nasty stuff can exist in the remaining 30 percent. Don't make the mistake of thinking foods with the Made with Organic Ingredients label are toxin-free.

- **USDA Organic:** This categorization can be confusing. In order to qualify for a USDA Organic label, a food must be made of 95 percent organically produced ingredients. The obvious question: What's up with the other 5 percent? Therein lies the problem. The non-organic 5 percent can contain all sorts of materials that don't fit very well at all in a detox diet, including food colorings and animal intestines. Buying USDA Organic foods is generally a little better than buying foods that aren't organic in any way, but it's nothing to shout about.

- **100% Organic:** This is the best of the best. The 100% Organic label is reserved for products that are wholly and completely organic. This means that you don't have to worry about artificial fertilizers, pesticides, genetic modification, antibiotics, or sewer sludge fertilizer.

If you want to buy truly organic food, make sure you look for "100% Organic" on the label.

Making an effort to buy organic foods also usually means that you'll be spending more money. Growing and raising organic food is typically more expensive than growing and raising mass-produced, conventional food. But if your budget allows you to go organic, rest assured that it's money well spent. Eating 100 percent organic foods will benefit your body in ways that no medication ever could. If you can't afford to eat organic all the time, try to do so when you can.

When it comes to produce, the scale of healthiness goes like this (from healthiest to least healthy): fresh organic (100 percent), fresh, frozen organic, frozen, and at the very bottom processed or canned.

Planning Out Your Protein Source

In order to thrive your body needs *amino acids,* which are the building blocks of protein. Your body can make 12 amino acids on its own, but 8 other amino acids can't be made by humans so you need to get them through the food you eat. These eight are called *essential amino acids,* and to get them you need to be certain that you're including sources of protein in your diet, including your diet that focuses on detoxification. Many forms of protein are available to you, but not all of them are appealing to everyone.

Animal sources of protein such as meat, poultry, eggs, fish, milk, and cheese can provide all the amino acids that you require. If you're vegetarian, you have to try just a little bit harder to make sure you're giving your body what it needs to succeed, but with planning and attention to detail you should be fine. Allow me to tell you about the protein sources that fit in detoxification diets for meat eaters, vegans, and everyone in between.

Fleshing it out

If you eat meat, you should have no problem at all getting the essential amino acids your body needs. A diet that includes meat, poultry, milk, cheese, fish, and eggs is flush with amino acids. The problem is that these protein sources can also contain all kinds of toxins. So if you're a meat eater, be sure to keep in mind the following toxic threats as you decide what meats to include in your meals.

As with produce, try to choose meats and dairy products that are labeled "100% Organic" if you want the highest quality foods with the lowest amount of toxins.

On the hoof

Beef is a powerhouse source for amino acids. You can get all the essential amino acids you need by eating beef. But much of the beef you find at the deli and in the cooler at your local grocery store contains a range of toxins — particularly antibiotics and hormones — and you need to be sure you're shopping smart in order to dodge those threats.

Most of the commercially available beef at the grocery store was raised in a *feed lot environment,* which is basically a mega farm for cows that keeps them cramped in very tight quarters and feeds them endlessly on grains, which aren't part of a cow's natural diet. These harsh conditions can result in larger cows that provide more beef, but because that environment is so unnatural and hard on the cows, they have to be given antibiotics and hormones to keep them alive and growing. The antibiotics and hormones given to cows have a toxic effect on the human body. Two of the most commonly used hormones are estradiol and zeranol. *Estradiol* is also a human female hormone, and it can have feminizing effects on both men and women. *Zeranol* is similar to the female hormone progesterone and can produce similar effects in humans, in addition to being suspected of increasing your risk for cancer. Many other substances are also given to feed lot cattle, and most of them wreak havoc on the human body.

If you eat beef, the best way to avoid these toxins is to eat only grass-fed beef. Cattle raised on grass — their natural diet — don't have to be given hormones and antibiotics because they're naturally healthy, and the conditions in which these cows are raised allows them to grow up healthy and full of nutrients that you can obtain when you eat them. Grass-fed beef contains higher levels of essential fatty acids, vitamins, and minerals, and lower levels of saturated (harmful) fat.

The rules are slightly different for pork. No hormones have been approved for use in pork production, so if you're picking out pork you don't need to worry about the presence of hormones in the meat. You do need to consider the use of antibiotics on your pork, though, so look for labels on pork products that say "no antibiotics added" when you're shopping.

But here are the larger worries about pork: Fried pork puts off toxic chemicals. Bacon, for example, puts off 15 times as much toxin as beef. Also, worm cysts can be found in pork so you must cook the meat thoroughly. Bottom line: It's best to leave pork on the grocery shelf.

Birds of a feather

You can get plenty of the amino acids you need from bird sources of protein like chicken, turkey, and duck. Turkey, for example, is a good source of protein that includes seven of the essential amino acids. One of those amino acids is *tryptophan,* a building block for serotonin, which is important for the onset of sleep. Many researchers indicate that the high levels of tryptophan in turkey are the reason so many people get drowsy after eating Thanksgiving dinner each year!

Chicken and duck are even stronger when it comes to essential amino acids; they have all eight and can be good sources of protein for your body. Other types of fowl like pheasant, quail, and dove are suspected to have similar levels of amino acids, but there's not yet enough data for complete confirmation.

When you're picking out bird sources of protein like chicken or turkey, make sure you select 100 percent organic products and preferably those labeled "free range" or "cage free."

Out of the sea

Shellfish are a good source of protein but don't provide all the essential amino acids. Different types of shellfish provide different amino acids, and I wouldn't recommend trying to cobble them together to get the essential amino acids you need. (It's much more efficient to get your amino acids from other meat or vegetable sources.)

Fish also don't have all the essential amino acids, but they do contain some and they can be a very healthy addition to your diet for other reasons.

Both fish and shellfish contain omega-3 fatty acids, which are wonderful for your health. However, as I mention several times in this book, mercury toxicity is a problem when it comes to eating fish, especially swordfish, shark, king mackerel, tile fish, and tuna. Be sure to read up and choose wisely.

Sticking with vegetarian varieties

Eating a vegetarian diet can be completely healthy, but it takes more effort and planning to eat no animal products and still bring key nutritional requirements into your body, particularly when it comes to essential amino acids. I do not recommend a vegetarian diet for most people because it's so difficult to do right. I have seen many patients who have tried to be vegetarians and ended up in very poor health. Most food plants simply don't contain all the essential amino acids. However, if you're willing to mix and match, you can definitely get the job done (and you can cut down on your toxin intake while you're at it).

Vegetarians fall into one of four broad categories:

- **Vegans** eat only plant-based foods. They don't eat dairy foods, poultry, eggs, or meat from any animal or fish.
- **Lacto-vegetarians** consume some dairy products as well as plant-based foods.
- **Lacto-ovo vegetarians** eat plant-based foods, dairy products, and eggs.
- **Flexitarians** eat mostly plants, dairy products, and eggs but occasionally have small amounts of fish or poultry.

If you're a vegetarian or if you're considering making the jump to a vegetarian diet, you need to make sure you're getting plenty of essential amino acids. Here, I tell you how to go about doing just that while still keeping an eye out for potential toxic influences.

Accumulating amino acids

To get all your essential amino acids from plant-based foods, you need to broaden your diet horizons and be open to the idea of mixing and matching.

If you're trying to cobble together the right plant-based foods in a vegetarian diet to make sure you're bringing in all your essential amino acids, start by including plenty of legumes in your meals. Legumes provide a range of amino acids, and they're readily available. What's more, you can very likely find legumes with that gold standard "100% Organic" label, so you can get your amino acids and stiff-arm the toxins that could otherwise be left over from the use of pesticides and fertilizers on your legumes. Here are a few examples of amino acid–heavy legumes and how you may incorporate them in your diet:

- **Adzuki beans:** Also known as *red oriental beans*. Try them in rice dishes.

- **Anasazi beans:** Make good refried beans, or you can use them in soups.

- **Black beans:** Go great with rice, soups, stews, and any Mexican dishes you prepare.

- **Black-eyed peas:** Good in salads, casseroles, and fritters, or served with ham and rice.

- **Chickpeas:** Also known as *garbanzo beans*. They're the key ingredient in hummus.

- **Edamame:** Green soybeans that work wonderfully as side dishes (particularly with Oriental cuisine).

- **Fava beans:** A nice side dish (and of course they go great with a nice Chianti).

- **Lentils:** Another extremely versatile legume. Use them in soups, salads, and stews.

- **Lima beans:** Also known as *butter beans*. They're a great addition to healthy casseroles, soups, and salads.

- **Red kidney beans:** One of the most dynamic legumes out there. What would chili or mixed bean salad be without red kidney beans?

- **Soy nuts:** Also called *soybean seeds*. They work well as a stand-alone snack or as a topper for salads.

In addition to providing essential amino acids, legumes also give you important nutritional musts like folic acid, potassium, iron, and magnesium. You can also count on them for a healthy dose of natural fiber!

Luckily, the vegetarian options for including protein in your diet don't end at legumes. There are also some notable and wonderful exceptions to the protein limitations of most grains. These make a terrific option for vegetarians and also represent a healthy protein source for non-vegetarians:

✔ **Buckwheat:** Despite its name, this grain-like crop isn't related to wheat and doesn't have anything to do with the Little Rascals. It also doesn't contain any gluten, which can be very helpful for people with gluten allergies. Buckwheat is great because it contains all the essential amino acids — even the ones that contain sulfur, which most plant sources of protein don't have.

✔ **Quinoa:** Pronounced *KEEN-wah,* this unique plant isn't a cereal, and it isn't a grass. However, it is gluten-free and contains all the essential amino acids and omega-3 fatty acids required for humans. A true nutritional powerhouse, quinoa is also loaded with other vitamins and nutrients.

✔ **Hemp seed:** Two basic types of hemp plants exist. One is the kind that produces the plant materials used to smoke marijuana. The other is an excellent food source, and it provides the healthful hemp seed. Hemp seed contains all the essential amino acids, as well as all the essential fatty acids and omega-3s. You can do all sorts of tasty things with the seeds, including grinding them into a meal (for use in baking), eating them whole, steeping them in a tea, and pressing them to create hemp seed oil. Just like buckwheat and quinoa, hemp seed is gluten-free and packed full of minerals and nutrients.

Hemp seed is as close to a perfect food as I have found. It contains a huge range of healthful components, and I think everyone should include it in their diet. (Look for a 100 percent organic variety, of course.)

Nailing down other nutrients

If you're a vegetarian, you have to make sure you're getting the right levels of amino acids in your diet, but you have to also keep an eye on several other types of nutrients. Here's a quick rundown of what you need and where you can get it:

✔ **Calcium:** You can get loads of calcium from dark green vegetables like broccoli, kale, collard and turnip greens, and spinach.

✔ **Vitamin B-12:** This vitamin is tough to find outside animal-based food, but you can definitely get some from eating yeast and seaweed. (You can always get additional B-12 from supplements, of course.)

✔ **Iron:** Introduce more iron in your diet by eating more dried beans and peas, lentils, and dark leafy vegetables. If you eat these foods in combination with foods that are high in vitamin C, you can increase your absorption rates.

✔ **Zinc:** Compared to some other important nutrients, zinc is relatively easy to find. You can get zinc in whole grains, soy products, nuts, and wheat germ.

✔ **Omega-3 fatty acids:** If you're a vegan, your only real dietary options for omega-3 fatty acids are micro algae and brown kelp (ask at your health food store for details), as well as walnuts. Non-vegans can find omega-3s in fish and fortified eggs.

Corraling Carbohydrates

Carbohydrates are substances that your body converts into *glucose,* which is the sugar that your cells use as fuel. Excess glucose that can't be used as fuel right away is stored as fat. Any successful detox diet will allow you to get just the right amount of carbohydrates and make sure that the carbohydrates you eat are the good kind.

Two different kinds of carbs exist — one unhealthy and one healthy:

✔ **Simple carbohydrates** include things like *fructose* (fruit sugar), *sucrose* (table sugar), and *lactose* (milk sugar). Simple carbohydrates are easily and rapidly absorbed into your bloodstream, and they don't offer much in the way of vitamins, minerals, or fiber. You can consume a lot of simple carbohydrates before your brain tells you to stop eating, and simple carbohydrates usually make food taste good. (Who doesn't like sugar?) Therefore, it's probably very easy for you to consume more than your body needs for energy in the short term. When that happens, the extra is stored as fat.

✔ **Complex carbohydrates** are the good kind. They're broken down slowly, and your body absorbs them at a slower rate than simple carbohydrates. That may not seem like a big deal, but it means that when you're eating a meal heavy on complex carbohydrates, your brain has time to respond and send you the message that you're full and it's time to quit eating before you've consumed excessive amounts. Even better, complex carbohydrates have vitamins, minerals, antioxidants, and fiber that your body really needs. You can find complex carbohydrates in foods like vegetables, whole grains, peas, and beans.

As a general rule, try to maintain complex carbohydrates as the primary carbohydrate source in your diet. Too many simple carbohydrates can cause a lot of health problems.

Not only are complex carbohydrates better for you from a strictly dietary perspective, but they're also healthier when it comes to detoxification. The fiber in complex carbohydrates can absorb toxins that are present in broken-down food in your intestine and remove those toxins with your stool. (Two kinds of fiber exist: soluble and insoluble. *Insoluble fiber* increases the bulk of your stool and helps it to move through your intestines. You find it in foods like bran, nuts, and many vegetables. *Soluble fiber* retains water and helps to control your levels of bad cholesterol and sugar. Good sources include apples, beans, peas, and oats.)

And here's yet another reason to focus on complex rather than simple carbohydrates: The carbohydrates that you find in almost all unhealthy processed foods are simple. Remember that processed foods offer very little in the way of nutritional value and very often contain toxins.

The battle between simple and complex carbs has become a popular way to evaluate carbohydrates in your diet, but there's another and often better way to slice it: the glycemic index and the glucose load. Check out Chapter 9 for more about this method for evaluating your diet.

Getting Some Good Fats

People are generally concerned about fats for two reasons:

- ✔ Fat has twice the amount of calories as carbohydrates and protein.
- ✔ Animal fat contains cholesterol.

For years the topic of dietary fat has consumed the minds of healthcare providers and the general public. The big issue about fat is cholesterol and its role in causing cardiovascular disease. If you ask most people (even physicians) what causes heart disease, most of them would say cholesterol. But more and more evidence suggests that's not the case at all, and I want you to be aware of that trend.

First, let's look at a few facts about cholesterol:

- ✔ Cholesterol is essential for many of your body's normal functions. For example, your body uses it to make many different kinds of hormones.
- ✔ Most of the cholesterol in your body is made by your body. It doesn't make a whole lot of sense that your body would manufacture something that will kill you.
- ✔ Fifty percent of heart attack victims have healthy cholesterol levels at the time of their heart attacks.
- ✔ In 1900, heart disease wasn't a top-ten cause of death, and back then people cooked with lard — lots of it.

Do these facts begin to make you think that cholesterol may not play such a big role in heart disease? They should. And there's more.

In his book *Hidden Truth About Cholesterol-Lowering Drugs* (Health Myths Exposed Publishing), Shane Ellison offers further insight into the cholesterol issue. He reports studies that refute the idea that lower cholesterol is better. Here's a little taste of what he discovered:

- ✔ Low cholesterol is associated with heart arrhythmias.

- ✔ The American Geriatric Society reported that people over 65 years old with elevated cholesterol levels had decreased mortality. People with cholesterol levels as high as 417 had a better survival rate than people under 189.

- ✔ The *Journal of Cardiac Failure* published an analysis of 1,134 patients with heart disease that showed lower survival rates among those with low cholesterol than among those with high cholesterol.

These stats should raise your eyebrows. You can read much more about the relationship between fat, cholesterol, and heart disease in Chapter 13, but I wanted to give you some context before jumping into my explanation on fats and how you should treat them in your diet.

You can put all fats in one of two broad categories: animal fats and vegetable fats. I cover each here.

Animal fats

Animal fats are usually saturated (unhealthy) fats and considered by some people to contribute to the clogging of the arteries. Animal fats can be found in meat and dairy products, including butter.

Unless you're eating 100 percent organic animal fat, you should try to limit the amounts of animal fat that you include in your diet — not because of the cholesterol, but because the fat is a storehouse of toxins that the animal received. Simply put, non-organic animal fats have a lot of toxicity and do very little to contribute to your overall health, and you should dodge them whenever possible.

In addition, strike these items off your shopping list immediately: anything that contains *trans fat, hydrogenated fat,* or *partially hydrogenated fat.* These substances are awful for you and have no place in a healthy diet!

Although fish oil is technically an animal fat, it's really in a class of its own and is a healthy oil to consume if it is free of toxins.

Vegetable fats

Vegetable fats are easier to think of as vegetable oils. They include oils like almond, canola, corn, flaxseed, grapeseed, hempseed, olive, peanut, safflower, soybean, sunflower, walnut, and motor oil. (Okay, that last one isn't true. Just wanted to make sure you're paying attention.)

Vegetable oils are usually considered to be healthier than animal fats, but that isn't always the case. Cottonseed oil, for instance, is usually very saturated and quite unhealthy. On the flip side, some vegetable oils have been unfairly given a bum rap. Take coconut oil, for example. Some studies have shown coconut oil to be harmful, but those studies were conducted with hydrogenated coconut oil, which is different from more natural versions of the oil. Natural coconut oil isn't nearly as bad for you as you may have heard, especially when you get 100 percent organic virgin coconut oil. In fact, I think coconut is one of the best oils you can use when cooking. It's also worth noting that coconut oil contains a substance called *lauric acid,* which has been shown to have antibacterial, antiviral, and antifungal properties. (Some indications exist that it works as an immune system booster, too!)

You can also feel good about using flaxseed oil, olive oil, and hempseed oil for cooking or for putting directly on your food.

Venturing beyond Your Grocery Store

Earlier in this chapter I clue you in on how to sort through the various organic food options you find at your local grocery store, and in Chapter 6 I give you advice on how to avoid nasty processed foods when you're in the grocery store. But what if you want to set your sights beyond the grocery in your quest to find healthy, non-toxic food options?

If that's the case, let me first commend you on making the decision to step beyond the easy and obvious sources for food that so many people limit themselves to. You don't have to buy all your food from one store, and in many cases it can pay off to shop around both in terms of the variety of healthy food on offer and also in terms of price. In this section, I cover three options to consider for food shopping: health food stores, farmers' markets, and Web or catalog suppliers.

Going to a health food store

More and more health food stores have been popping up lately, and I think that's a wonderful thing. Not every health food store offers a huge variety of healthy, organic, and toxin-free foods, but you're still likely to find options that don't often pop up on conventional grocery store shelves.

Picking low-toxin food at a health food store is easier than at the grocery store because you won't be bombarded with unhealthy and processed alternatives. However, you still need to pay attention to the labels and make sure you're getting the right level of organic. (Remember that 100 percent organic is the best.)

If you plan to do a lot of shopping in a health food store, take the time to get to know some members of the store staff. It's always useful to make friends with the person who's most informed about where the food is sourced. He or she can help you figure out which food options are the most healthful and which ones fit in best with your particular diet. As a rule, you should also be able to find someone who is borderline militant about the purity of the organic foods in the store, and that's a good person to know, too.

Some health food stores have co-op arrangements that allow you to pay a set amount of money and get a certain amount of organic food each week. These arrangements can be very cost efficient and much easier than handpicking the food at a conventional grocery store. The co-op practice is also a good one because it limits the amount of food that the stores have to throw away due to spoilage. However, you lose some flexibility because you essentially get whatever the store gives you during a given week. If you're interested in a co-op arrangement, be sure to ask someone at your local health food store.

Capitalizing on farmers' markets

Farmers' markets and roadside stands are great places to buy food, but you really *must* get to know the growers to make sure they're dedicated to organic farming practices. Otherwise, you run the risk of buying food that has been grown using conventional methods involving pesticides, chemical fertilizers, and more. If you develop a relationship with a grower at a local stand or farmers' market, you should be able to find out pretty quickly whether or not he is indeed committed to growing his crops in a non-toxic way. You can always ask about the farm's organic certification status, too.

Turning to the Web and catalogs

It's becoming more common for people to turn to the Internet and to catalogs for their food needs, and that's both a good thing and a bad thing. It's good because those options — particularly the Internet — can put a huge amount of possibilities at your fingertips. You can find a tremendous range of foods available online, and because many of the companies have very low overhead you can sometimes find great prices.

The problem with ordering food over the Internet or through a catalog is that you can be faced with a more difficult challenge when it comes time to confirm the quality of the food. If you're considering ordering food products from one of these sources, be sure to study up on the organic labeling standards I describe earlier in this chapter and do your homework before ordering. (Ask for referrals, read reviews, and get all the details on how long the site or catalog has been in business before you lay down that credit card information.)

Chapter 8

How Toxic Are You? The Detoxification Quiz

No matter how hard you try, you're bound to end up with toxins in your body. That doesn't mean you shouldn't strive to keep toxins out and detoxify your body after they're already in, but in truth you can never completely win the battle against toxins. Toxins are inescapable, especially now that the presence of heavy metal, chemical, and biologic toxins in the environment is greater than ever before.

This chapter is short but important. In the next few pages, I offer a series of quizzes that you can take to figure out just how toxic your body has become. Take the time to evaluate any symptoms of these toxin-related ailments, and you can get a good feel for how much toxins are causing problems for your body's many systems.

The quizzes in this chapter aren't meant to diagnose an ailment or disease. Rather, they can alert you if you have frequent symptoms that are an indicator of toxicity. If you have significant symptoms, you should consult a physician — preferably an open-minded one who is willing to consider toxicity as a real threat to your health (see Chapter 5).

Here's how this chapter works: For each of the quizzes, score the frequency with which you experience each symptom. Then total your score and compare that number to the severity rating scale that corresponds with that quiz.

Note that if your score is low, that doesn't necessarily mean you're in the clear if some of your symptoms are severe. Also note that some symptoms are involved in several different types of toxicity.

Here's the frequency rating scale that you can use throughout the chapter:

0 = Never

1 = Infrequently

2 = Occasionally

3 = Frequently

4 = Constantly

Yeast Toxicity

____Chronic sore throat

____Chronic ear infection

____Infertility

____Itchy ears

____Low stomach acid

____Diabetes

____Flatulence (gas)

____Belching

____Reflux (heartburn)

____Bloating

____Constipation (hard stools)

____Obstipation (less than one stool/day)

____Irritable bowel syndrome

____Crohn's disease

____Ulcerative colitis

____Abdominal cramping

____Vaginal yeast infections

____Anal puritis (itching)

____Chronic fatigue

____Fatigue

____Depression

____Irritability

____Decreased concentration

____Headaches

____Brain fog

____Sinus problems

____Bladder infections

____Rashes

____Allergies

____Difficulty losing weight

____Craving sweets

____Craving breads

____Sensitivity to chemicals

____Feeling intoxicated without drinking

____Delusions

____Insomnia

____General itching

____Fibromyalgia

Total Score____

36–54: Mild toxicity
55–72: Moderate toxicity
Above 72: Probable severe toxicity

If your score is in the moderate to severe range, you may also want to consider the following:

✔ Do you use antibiotics frequently?

✔ Do you use stomach acid–reducing medications frequently?

✔ Do you use medicinal steroids frequently?

✔ Do you receive radiation or chemotherapy treatments?

✔ Have you been diagnosed with elevated mercury toxicity in the past?

If your score on the quiz puts you in the moderate or severe categories and you answered "yes" to any of the above questions, your risk of yeast toxicity is that much higher. If your score causes you some concern, flip back to Chapter 5 for some information on how to lower your yeast levels. You also want to consult with a physician who is well versed in yeast toxicity.

Gastrointestinal Toxicity

____Food allergies

____Offensive breath

____Body odor

____Recurring acne

____Dermatitis

____Eczema

____Psoriasis

____Gum disease

____Ulcers

____Low-fiber diet

____High-sugar diet

____Hiatal hernia

____Crohn's disease

____Ulcerative colitis

____Use of acid-reducing medication

____Frequent headaches

____Depression

____ADD/ADHD

____Less than one stool per day

____Hard stool

____Daily loose stools

____More than five stools per day

____Indigestion

____Heartburn (reflux)

____Burning anus

____Low back pain

____Hemorrhoids

____Excessive gas

____Very foul gas

____Very foul stools

____Abdominal bloating

____Excessive belching

____Skin boils   ____Mouth ulcers

____Coated tongue   ____Autism Spectrum Disorders

Total Score_____

25–40: Mild toxicity
41–67: Moderate toxicity
Above 67: Probable severe toxicity

How did your scores add up? If you're in the moderate or severe toxicity range, take another minute and think about the following questions:

- Do you use laxatives frequently?

- Do you often travel internationally?

If you answer either or both questions in the affirmative and your scores are high, you could very well have a problem with gastrointestinal toxicity. If that's the case, consider talking to your doctor, and be sure to flip back to Chapter 5 for details on bowel toxins and Chapter 4 for information on how your body works to detoxify your digestive system.

Allergic Toxicity

____Depression   ____ADD/ADHD

____Ill after eating   ____Frequent illness

____Weakness   ____Chronic fatigue syndrome

____Severe fatigue   ____Irritable bowel syndrome

____Poor concentration   ____Crohn's disease

____Headaches   ____Colitis

____Insomnia   ____Indigestion

____Frequent ear, sinus, or bronchial   ____Obesity
infection
                                     ____Allergic shiners (circles under eyes)
____Hyperactivity
                                     ____Asthma
____Learning disability
                                     ____Chronic cough
____Brain fog
                                     ____Recurrent hives or rash
____Poor memory
                                     ____Genital itch
____Diarrhea
                                     ____Bed wetting
____Constipation
                                     ____Frequent urination

____Arthritis   ____Eczema, psoriasis

____Autism Spectrum Disorders   ____Fibromyalgia

Total Score____

25–37: Mild toxicity
38–62: Moderate toxicity
Above 62: Possible severe toxicity

Did you end up with a score in the moderate or severe range? If so, you may want to visit your physician to talk about your symptoms. You can also flip ahead to Chapter 12 to read up on how toxins can affect allergies.

Chemical Toxicity

____Depression   ____Low basal body temperature

____Behavioral change   ____Persistent hoarseness

____Headaches   ____Rashes, hives

____Insomnia   ____Persistent cough

____Tremors   ____Anemia

____Seizures   ____Loss of sense of smell

____Body pains   ____Infertility

____Change in bowel frequency   ____Numb or tingling extremities

____Abdominal cramps   ____History of miscarriage

____Flu-like symptoms   ____Unexplained nausea

____Decreased coordination   ____Multiple sclerosis

____Muscle pain   ____Parkinson's Disease

____Arthritis   ____Amyotrophic lateral sclerosis

____Reaction to chemical fumes   ____Fibromyalgia

____Difficulty with memory   ____Chronic Fatigue Syndrome

____ADD/ADHD   ____Autism Spectrum Disorders

Total Score____

25–38: Mild toxicity
39–64: Moderate toxicity
Above 64: Possible severe toxicity

Chemical toxicity — an overwhelming level of toxins like pesticides, fertilizers, phthalates, and food additives to name just a few — can result in many different kinds of symptoms and ailments. It's a general problem that is best solved with a wide-ranging detoxification effort. Check out Chapter 3 for some information on where those toxins may be coming from, and go to Chapter 18 for some basic information on a few detoxification methods that may work for you. Of course, a visit to a physician who is familiar with toxicity may also be in order if your symptoms are severe.

Heavy Metal Toxicity

____Depression

____Psychosis

____Confusion

____Decreased short-term memory

____Numbness or tingling

____Drowsiness

____Brain fog

____Restlessness

____Irritability

____Neuropathy

____Infertility

____Impotence

____Decreased libido

____Miscarriage

____Menstrual irregularities

____Tremors

____Low body temperature

____Low thyroid function

____Alzheimer's disease

____Multiple sclerosis

____Nausea

____Vomiting

____Abdominal pain

____Constipation

____Metallic taste

____Anemia

____Atherosclerosis

____Angina

____Peripheral vascular disease

____Kidney failure

____Joint pain or swelling

____Lymph node swelling

____Decreased vision

____Low adrenal function

____Increased skin pigmentation

____Seizures

____Autism Spectrum Disorders

____ADD/ADHD

____Parkinson's disease

____Amyotrophic lateral sclerosis

Total Score_____

32–49: Mild toxicity
50–80: Moderate toxicity
Above 80: Possible severe toxicity

This quiz includes symptoms of toxicity that are caused by mercury, lead, arsenic, and aluminum. The symptoms from different metals often overlap, and multiple metal toxicities can be as much as 100 times more toxic than the individual toxins.

If you register moderate or severe toxicity according to this quiz, ask yourself these questions to continue the process:

✔ Have you received multiple influenza vaccinations?

✔ Do you have amalgam dental fillings?

✔ Do you often use antacids that contain aluminum?

✔ Did you receive childhood vaccines before 2001?

✔ Do you eat fish frequently?

If you answer yes to these questions and you also have a high level of toxicity according to the quiz, you could very well be suffering the effects of having too many heavy metals in your body. Check out Chapter 18 for some useful detox guidance so you can start detoxing immediately, and be sure to read Chapter 3 so you understand how you're being exposed to harmful materials. You should also consider going to the doctor to get tested for mercury, lead, arsenic, or aluminum.

Liver Toxicity

____Decreased memory

____Decreased concentration

____Headaches

____Dizziness

____Autoimmune disease

____Greasy stools

____Fibrocystic breast

____Easy bruising

____Gallbladder problems

____Excessive chemical sensitivity

____Generalized itching

____Overweight

____Constipation

____Fatigue

____Frequent urination

____Food allergies

____Abdominal bloating or pain

____Excessive gas

____Fat intolerance

____Light-colored stools

____High calorie intake

____Slow healing

____Acne

____Jaundice

____Diarrhea

Total Score____

20–31: Mild toxicity
32–52: Moderate toxicity
Above 52: Possible severe toxicity

How did you do? If your score puts you in the moderate or severe toxicity range, please think about the questions that follow.

✔ Do you have a history of chemical exposure?

✔ Do you consume excess amounts of fat and protein?

✔ Do you consume a lot of alcohol or use drugs?

✔ Have you contracted hepatitis at any point in the past?

Answering yes to one or more of these questions can mean that you have an increased risk for liver toxicity. Your liver is a completely essential organ, and you want to make sure it's healthy. If you think your liver may be suffering, flip back to Chapter 4 to get some details on liver detoxification and think hard about scheduling an appointment with your physician to discuss the problem.

Part III
Enhancing Wellness through Detoxification

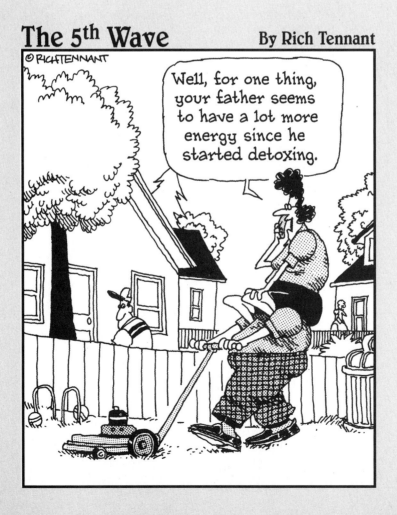

In this part . . .

You can think of this part as a menu of choices. Want to improve your immune system? Go to Chapter 10. Want to beat your allergies so you're not suffering from them all the time? Have a look at Chapter 12. Or maybe you want to be able to stop smoking and put down the bottle, once and for all. If so, read all about these topics in Chapters 14 and 15, respectively. That's just the beginning, too — I include plenty of information in this part about how you can make improvements to specific areas of your health using the techniques that make up detoxification and detox dieting.

As if that weren't enough, this part contains the most delicious material of all: recipes to help you eat right and accomplish specific health goals.

Chapter 9

Reaching Your Ideal Weight (And Staying There!) with Detox Dieting

In This Chapter

▶ Rethinking what it means to go on a diet

▶ Identifying destructive eating behaviors

▶ Focusing on the right eating habits

▶ Putting some thought and planning into your eating

As you've no doubt seen, read, and heard on the news, obesity is more of a problem now than it ever has been before. The unhealthy, toxin-filled foods that people consume on a massive scale have caused many to become overweight, and the trend doesn't seem to be letting up anytime soon.

If you're interested in losing weight or staying at a healthy weight, the best way to do so is to choose and eat healthy, toxin-free foods. Doing so isn't always easy, but it's certainly something that you can accomplish, and I'm happy to provide you with the basics in this chapter.

I start out by asking you to rethink what it means to go on a diet, and then I set out a number of ways that you can change the way you think about food and the way you eat. A successful detox diet really starts with a particular mindset. If you can begin to think about food and eating in a certain way, you've already won half the battle.

Changing the Way You Think about Dieting

What does it mean to go on a diet? For most people, dieting means committing to eating in some unusual and bizarre way for as short a period of time as possible to achieve significant weight loss. People who go on diets want to shed pounds until they reach some magical weight. (For most, that means getting down to what they weighed several years ago, when they could eat whatever they wanted without gaining any weight.)

This concept of dieting is pretty strange when you really think about it, and dieting very rarely works. Most diets fail spectacularly even though we spend outrageous sums of money on them. The amount spent on diets in the United States each year — upward of $50 billion — is higher than the entire gross domestic product of Costa Rica! Combine that staggering figure with the fact that we're still one of the fattest countries in the history of the world, and you can clearly see that we're going about dieting in the wrong way.

Identifying the problem with diet pills

Diet pills are a popular choice for people who struggle with their weight. Most people think that if they use diet pills for a period of time, they can simply get used to eating less and watch in amazement as the weight drops (and stays) off. Nothing could be further from the truth.

Diet pills reduce your appetite so you can eat all you want and lose weight — you just want less. But when you stop the diet pills, you continue the same behavior. You still eat all you want, but because you're not taking the pills anymore, your body wants a lot more. The end result: You gain weight.

Research has shown that almost all people who use diet pills to lose weight end up weighing more than they did before they started the pills. In the end they would've been better off not buying the pills at all.

Realizing why limiting your consumption doesn't work

Many other diets focus on reducing the amount or types of food you can eat to the point that you're miserable all the time. Maybe you're allowed to have only a mug of hot water for breakfast and lunch (followed by "a sensible dinner"!), or maybe you can eat all the beef and cheese you want but not much else.

On many such diets, people will lose 5 pounds in the first week and think that means they'll reach their goal of losing 20 pounds in just a month. The problem? That first 5 pounds is mostly water weight. After the second week of dieting, the pounds stop coming off and the feeling of failure starts setting in. Then the dieter gives up, saying that hormones must be causing the weight gain and she can't do anything about it. So she goes on an eating binge to reward herself for making such a valiant effort and ends up gaining 10 pounds.

Does this pattern sound familiar?

Seeking the big picture

As a country, the United States has a weight problem. But the true problem is not the weight itself; it's the way we think about eating.

If you want to lose weight, you have to look at the process not as an isolated diet but rather as a change in the way you eat for the rest of your life. If you look at dieting in any other way, you're dooming yourself to fail. That's the bad news. The good news is that if you approach dieting in the right frame of mind, you can make the kind of long-term changes that will help you to lose weight, detoxify your body, and enjoy better all-around health. The rest of this chapter shows you how.

Doing Away with Dysfunctional Eating Behaviors

The first step you can take toward establishing a healthy, sustainable diet for you and your family is to cut out key dysfunctional eating behaviors that you've developed over the years. Please don't feel bad if you've fallen into one of the traps I describe in this section; our culture makes it very easy to start down the wrong path and very challenging to keep your guard up all the time.

Here are the biggest behavioral pitfalls:

- **Eating whatever is quickest and easiest to procure:** When you're really hungry, what could be easier than driving through a fast food restaurant? You pay just a few bucks for a big bag full of greasy, toxin-filled food and maybe another buck or two to get a 64-ounce cup of an equally unhealthy soft drink. No planning or preparation is required. You get hungry, and you hammer back some grub — that's the end of it.

✔ **Failing to plan your at-home meals:** Even when you're at home, the fastest and easiest meals are often the first choice. That's especially true when everyone in the house is eating at different times. Why take the time to chop up some vegetables or run some produce through a juicer when you can microwave a frozen dinner, pop open a couple cans of processed side dishes, and sit down to eat?

✔ **Racing through meals:** After you've spent mere minutes microwaving your dinner, you may sit down in front of the TV to eat. Then, after you've gulped down your food (very likely in mere minutes as well), you're right back to the TV, videogames, or the Internet. I know some families who have a little game to see who can finish their food the fastest! That's a very bad habit to encourage (as I explain later in this chapter).

Sometimes family members save arguments or stressful conversations for dinner time. Not a good idea! You should be relaxed when you eat so your body is ready to turn its attention toward effective digestion.

If you're intent on detoxifying your body and losing weight, you have to make a long-term commitment to putting a stop to harmful eating behaviors you've developed over the years. It's not easy, and if you have a family you may face resistance on the home front. But you simply won't succeed if you try to approach the process with anything other than the long view.

Going Back to the Basics

To better understand how you should be approaching food, think about what life was like generations ago, when many people were farmers and focused almost exclusively on growing food for their families. Everyone in the family worked extremely hard (especially compared to today's standards), and people were outside for much of the year. They cared for crops grown organically without chemical fertilizers or harsh pesticides. The food they grew, and the food they caught or killed in the form of wild game, was relatively hard to procure and was overwhelmingly toxin-free. Families ate together, taking time to slowly enjoy the food that they had worked so hard to produce. Then they relaxed for the rest of the evening before getting up early to do it all over again.

Obviously, people back then faced their share of problems and hardships. But as far as food quality and toxicity, they had it pretty good. People didn't suffer from the effects of widespread toxins in their air, water, and food. Health problems like Alzheimer's, multiple sclerosis, autism, and ADHD weren't an issue, and the population wasn't enslaved by heart disease, cancer, arthritis, and hypertension.

I know that you're not going to go back to living the way people lived back then. I can't ask you to quit your job and start working out in the fields with hand tools and a mule-driven plow to grow your own food, which you could enjoy eating over the course of a couple of hours with your family in front of the fireplace. However, when it comes to food and eating, you can certainly incorporate certain aspects of that lifestyle into your routine. The effects on your health (and weight) can be tremendous.

Chewing the right way

Chewing is extremely important to your health. You can do your body a lot of good just by chewing the right way. Chewing is the first step in the digestive process, and if it's not done correctly, your digestion can really suffer.

One of the most important aspects of the chewing process is the act of physically breaking down your food into smaller pieces. If the food pieces are too big when they get to your stomach, the next part of the digestive process doesn't work properly. The result is that you won't absorb the nutrients in your food nearly as well.

To make sure you get the most out of the nutrients in your food, take the time to chew your food into smaller and smaller pieces until it's essentially a liquid before swallowing.

The interaction that your saliva has with your food is also very important. Your goal should be to make sure that saliva touches every last surface of your food. If you can accomplish that, you can be confident that you're starting your digestion off right because your saliva contains digestive enzymes. You can also feel good about reducing your risks for irritating or damaging your esophagus. If you don't take the time to mix plenty of saliva in with your food when you chew, you can harm the surface tissue of your esophagus when you swallow.

When you're eating, take your time and chew slowly. Taking plenty of time to chew is a great way to ensure that you're breaking your food down into small enough bits and also saturating it with adequate amounts of saliva.

Slowing down your eating

So many aspects of our modern culture lead to eating much too fast. Fast-paced lives include fast-paced meals, and that trend is flat-out unhealthy. The slower you can eat your food, the better. Why? Here are two key reasons:

> ✔ **The physical reason:** Your stomach has a limited amount of acid and enzymes available to break down your food. If you eat extremely quickly and throw a lot of food at your stomach at once, your stomach has a hard time soaking all the food with the right amount of acid. That means your stomach isn't able to do its job, and lousy nutrient absorption is often the result.

✔ **The mental reason:** The mental aspect of eating is often overlooked. Your stomach and intestines respond to your emotional state. If you're anxious, nervous, hurried, or physically active when you eat, there's a discernable decrease in blood flow to your stomach and intestines. Digesting your food properly is a blood-intensive process, so eating at a frenzied pace when you're not relaxed can put your digestion at risk. Also, you eat a lot more if you are multitasking while you eat rather than paying attention to your food.

Resisting the urge to wash it down

The standard American diet includes a drink with every meal. How many meals have you had recently that weren't accompanied by a glass, can, or bottle of something to drink? Some people have a hard time believing this, but having a drink with your meal can actually cause a problem when it comes to healthy nutrition.

When you're eating and you take a drink, the food and saliva combination in your mouth is immediately diluted, and the digestive enzymes in your saliva are compromised. Then, when you swallow the mix of food, drink, and saliva, the slippery texture of your saliva is cut by the drink, and swallowing becomes more likely to irritate your esophagus.

Drinking with meals can also create problems for your stomach. Your stomach is about the same size as both of your hands cupped together. When you drink a big beverage while eating, you can really fill up your stomach and drastically dilute your stomach acid, which throws a wrench in digestion. If your stomach can't thoroughly soak the food you put in it with powerful acid, it can't properly prepare the food to enter the intestines, where much of digestion — particularly nutrient absorption — takes place. And the effect trickles down: Drinks can also dilute enzymes from other sources, like the pancreas.

Drinking lots of water is a good thing for dieting and for detoxification, but don't drink anything with your meals. Wait at least one hour after eating before having a big glass of water, and your digestion will improve as a result.

Less is more, more often

Most people have experienced the ravages of indigestion from eating a really big meal. It's an uncomfortable, unnatural feeling, and it contributes to weight gain and general damage to your health.

A large meal — especially one that you eat quickly — challenges your stomach's ability to produce the acid and *pepsin* (an important digestive enzyme) necessary to break down your food. A lack of acid is a problem, and the problem is further compounded by the fact that it triggers your pancreas to produce less of its important digestive enzymes. That leaves you with some pretty poorly digested food that starts heading into the intestines where it can wreak all sorts of havoc and cause you plenty of discomfort.

Like many of the problems I describe earlier in this chapter, big meals also decrease your chances of properly absorbing the nutrients in your food. Finally, eating a huge amount of food at one time can cause your blood sugar to rise and fall dramatically, which makes your energy levels go haywire and can even contribute to diabetes over time.

How can you avoid these complications? It's pretty easy, really. The best way to get the most out of your digestive system is to eat small meals on a more frequent basis. This eating pattern allows all the digestive processes to do their work without being overwhelmed, and it helps to ensure that your blood sugar stays at steady, pleasant levels (no big peaks and troughs in your energy levels). Smaller and more frequent meals also allow for more absorption of nutrients.

The best eating pattern for a detoxification diet is to eat smaller meals more often throughout the day. One good plan is to eat three small meals a day — breakfast, lunch, and dinner work fine — and also eat a small snack between each meal.

Taking a break

How often have you heard the term "eat and run"? You've probably heard it a lot, and if you're like a lot of Americans, you've probably done it far more than you should. To get the most out of your food, you need to take a break after eating a meal. It doesn't have to be a long break, so please don't think I'm suggesting that you need to lie down on the couch for 60 minutes after a mid-afternoon snack. But it does help the digestive process if you can avoid any vigorous activity for a short period of time — 30 minutes is a good rule — right after you eat.

Why is this break important? A natural process occurs right after you eat that involves an increased level of blood flow to your stomach and intestines and a decreased blood flow to your muscles. Healthy digestion depends on an ample supply of available blood for your digestive organs and other tissues. If you engage in physical activity soon after eating, you allow your muscles to place a demand for your blood at the expense of your stomach and intestines. The shift of blood flow that occurs directly after you eat allows all the digestive processes to function at a high level, and it also allows for better absorption of nutrients. Don't jeopardize those benefits by shifting into high gear right after you have a meal.

Taking time for a BM

Let's face it: What goes in has to come out. Nobody likes to talk about having a bowel movement, but I would be remiss if I didn't touch on the importance of normal, healthy BMs as a part of any successful detox diet.

The gastrointestinal tract produces quite a lot of trash, and the trash has to be emptied on a regular basis. If your stool sits too long in your colon, too much water is removed from it and it becomes dry and hard to pass. That's very uncomfortable and even harmful when the situation is extreme. It can also contribute to toxicity because when higher-than-normal amounts of water are absorbed from your stool into your intestines, the chances increase that toxins will be absorbed at the same time.

From the time we are born, a natural reflex called the *gastro-colic reflex* is present. This reflex stimulates you to have a bowel movement shortly after a meal. For many people, it can be a subtle reflex that is relatively easy to override. That's unfortunate. Many people resist the natural urge to have a BM after a meal, waiting instead until they can take care of it at a more convenient time and in a more convenient location.

If at all possible, don't fight your body's natural reflex to have a bowel movement after a meal. A healthy BM schedule is vital for good health and detoxification, and you need to make sure you're making your body's needs #1 when it comes to #2.

Practicing Essential (And Realistic) Eating Habits

I can go on and on about the specific steps you should take to detoxify your body and improve your health, but none of it amounts to much if you can't make those practices part of your everyday life, and fast.

When it comes to detox dieting, you need to do as much as you can to put your diet in proper perspective and make eating properly a major priority in your life. The food you choose to eat has a big impact on your health, as does the food you choose *not* to eat. Some of the steps are easy, and some can be quite difficult if you've been stuck in an unhealthy food rut for a long period of time. But you have to commit to making the changes or you'll never see any success with your detox diet. Proper non-toxic eating habits will provide you with good health, whereas most prescriptions treat only the symptoms of disease.

The practices I describe next are not suggestions; they're rules. Thinking of them as rules is the only way you'll make the kinds of long-term adjustments to your eating habits that will allow you to rid your body of toxins and reach your ideal weight through detox dieting.

Dodging food served through a window

Fast food is designed to be prepared rapidly (hence the name) and to appeal to the taste buds of the majority of the population. It's cheap to prepare and sell. Providing good nutrition and avoiding toxins have never been part of the formula when it comes to fast food.

If I started writing now and promised that I wouldn't stop until I had covered all the various unhealthy qualities of fast food, I'd still be writing when the last Styrofoam cup from the last fast food restaurant finally biodegraded. Fast food is truly awful for you. Here are just a few tidbits for you to consider.

- ✔ A recent study found that 100 percent of chicken from fast food restaurants contains at least some amount of arsenic, which is an extremely harmful toxin.

- ✔ The vast majority of beef used in fast food is raised on massive commercial feed lots where the cows are pumped full of hormones, antibiotics, and steroids.

- ✔ Cooking — if you can call it that — in fast food restaurants is done almost exclusively with trans fats, which are the most unhealthy, toxin-laden fats you can consume.

The worst part of the fast food picture is that fast food restaurant chains spend billions of dollars each year on marketing tricks, which are designed to make you feel better about eating their food. One chain offers a large packet of salad dressing that has only 70 calories per serving. The problem is that in very small print at the bottom of the package it says the package contains 5 servings. That's 350 calories in one packet alone, which is as many calories as the standard cheeseburger.

It's not impossible to make food choices at fast food restaurants that aren't completely horrible for your body — salads come to mind. But you always need to remember that the ingredients you find even in those somewhat healthy alternatives were chosen because they were the cheapest (not because they were the healthiest, and certainly not because they contained the fewest toxins).

Don't eat fast food. The convenience and the price simply aren't worth the damaging effects that fast food has on your health.

Avoiding white foods

If you're looking for a simple rule that can go quite a long way toward making your detox diet a success, this is the one for you. It seems like such a simple thing, but by avoiding white foods you automatically miss out on the things that are loaded with calories, short on nutrients, and often jam-packed with toxins. Avoiding white foods is a fantastic rule to live by for diabetics and anyone who wants to be healthy and maintain a decent weight. Avoid anything white and anything that started out white.

A few exceptions to the "Don't eat white foods" rule exist, the most notable being cauliflower. Feel free to make that vegetable a part of your diet, and of course try to use a 100 percent organic option if you can!

Getting out the gluten

Gluten is a substance found in barley, rye, wheat, and oats. It's used as a major protein source in many cultures and is common in the United States. Gluten is present in all wheat products and is used as an additive to make food thicker or stick foods together. You find it in breads, wheat pastas, pastries, cookies, cakes, and literally anything made from flour (which is typically white). If you're reading your food labels like you should be, you'll see that gluten pops up in an incredible array of food products.

Dodging gluten in wheat and grains is hard enough, but food manufacturers make avoiding gluten even trickier because they add it to a dizzying variety of foods. You can find it in soups, casseroles, pastes, cereals, and even beef jerky. Forms of gluten can be included in ingredients lists with many names, including *starch, binders,* and *natural flavorings.*

The steps necessary to cut gluten out of your diet are too complex for me to cover here. If you'd like to eliminate gluten from your diet, try reading *Living Gluten-Free For Dummies* by Danna Korn (Wiley).

Increasing numbers of people have a gluten allergy, and many others suffer from an ailment called *celiac disease.* That's an autoimmune disorder where the presence of gluten in the diet causes multiple, extremely unpleasant effects. Some estimates indicate that as many as one out of every eight people has some form of celiac disease. The small intestines of people who suffer from celiac disease are damaged when the diet includes gluten, and over time the damage can cause the intestine to leak substances that aren't intended to get into the bloodstream, like harmful bacteria and toxins. It's not a pretty picture, but it's one that many people live with.

Common symptoms of celiac disease include diarrhea, vomiting, and abdominal pain. It can also contribute to growth retardation and psychosocial problems in children. If you think you may be suffering from celiac disease, consult your doctor. Keep in mind, though, that if your doctor is firmly rooted in conventional medicine, she may be prone to look for every other possible cause for your symptoms before considering celiac disease or a similar form of gluten sensitivity. Common misdiagnoses include irritable bowel syndrome, Crohn's disease, regional enteritis, gastroenteritis, nervous stomach, and stomach flu.

Your doctor can order blood tests to determine whether you have celiac disease, but the best way to confirm the problem is to go on a gluten-free diet because it's possible that gluten is giving you fits but not at the level that would be confirmed with a blood test. A gluten-free diet isn't an easy thing to do, but if your body is sensitive to gluten, the rewards are enormous.

Here's one other note on gluten for you to consider: After it's in the body, gluten can be transformed into a compound called *glutomorphine*. That compound is commonly identified in autistic children, and some experts think that it causes additional complications within the autism spectrum. If someone you know is affected by autism, you may want to consider trying to limit his gluten intake to see if doing so has a positive effect on his symptoms.

Removing milk and milk products

Milk is processed in some very strange and unnatural ways these days, and the result can be a product that has questionable health benefits and could, in fact, contribute to some ailments. Quite a lot of the milk available today also contains hormones and antibiotics because those substances are frequently given to dairy cows.

About 20 percent of the U.S. population is *lactose intolerant,* meaning that milk and products made from milk cause quite a few problems. For these people, caseins could be the culprit.

Caseins are proteins found in milk. Casein is structurally very similar to gluten, and it may cause some of the same effects. We don't yet fully understand how caseins could wreak havoc on the intestines and other parts of the body, and we also don't know how many people may be casein intolerant. But some experts believe that for some people, casein causes long-term disruption to the digestive system and can also have negative effects on mental and immune function.

Some interesting case studies suggest a connection between casein and the symptoms of autism in children. *Avoidance diets* — in which children don't eat or drink anything containing casein — have resulted in remarkable improvements in the behavior of some children with autism. As with gluten, if you are close to a child with autism, you may consider putting him on a diet that cuts out casein to see if there's a positive effect.

If you're suffering from a digestive system problem and your doctor isn't having much luck diagnosing or treating it successfully, consider cutting milk and milk products out of your diet for three months. An avoidance diet of that length will tell you whether milk is creating problems for your intestines. And don't worry about missing out on calcium: You can get all the calcium you need from vegetables, and you can get your vitamin D with supplements.

Keep in mind that most conventional physicians don't consider casein to be a real problem, so you may have to decide for yourself whether consuming milk or milk products is damaging to your health.

If you choose to eliminate milk from your diet, be on the lookout for milk products hidden in other foods. Milk or milk proteins are added to a wide variety of foods, particularly processed foods. Check labels for *sodium caseinate, calcium caseinate,* and *milk protein;* all three are milk-based materials.

Giving sweeteners the slip

Sweeteners are one of the biggest problem areas when it comes to detoxification and detox dieting. Sweeteners are present in a mind-boggling array of foods, and they can add up quickly to cause a bigger waistline and higher levels of toxins in your body.

As you begin your detox diet and general detoxification efforts, do your best to cut out foods and beverages that contain sweeteners. Sweeteners contribute to obesity (either directly or indirectly) and are often loaded with toxins. The one exception is *stevia,* a plant-based sweetener that doesn't contribute to weight gain, diabetes, or any other ailments that are common among people who consume excessive amounts of sweeteners.

The many faces of sugar

Sugar comes in many, many forms on ingredient lists, and you need to be sure you're checking for all of them when you're scanning ingredients to select healthy, toxin-free foods. Here are a few common forms of sugar you need to watch out for:

- Dextrin
- Fructose
- Galactose
- Glucose
- Lactose
- Maltose
- Sucrose

In addition to dodging the different kinds of sugar, you also need to make sure you cut out the artificial sweeteners. Here are the most common examples:

 ✔ Acesulfame

 ✔ Aspartame

 ✔ Neotame

 ✔ Saccharin

 ✔ Sucralose

High fructose corn syrup

High fructose corn syrup deserves its own section because it's used in all kinds of processed foods and food products. It's everywhere, and it's horrible for you! Not only is the substance itself really bad for your health, but it also often contains mercury. Do whatever you can to cut high fructose corn syrup out of your diet immediately!

Planning ahead

Unhealthy, toxic food has crept into the diets of most people because it's incredibly easy and often cheap to obtain. You can get nutritionally lousy, high-toxin food in a huge number of places these days.

If you want to eat healthy, lose weight, and cut out toxins, you have to commit to thinking about and planning your meals. Planning ahead is the key to success for detoxing and for weight loss. Here are a few useful tips that will help you adjust to the idea of putting some thought into the food you eat:

 ✔ Remember that you're changing the way you eat for the rest of your life. Even if it feels like a pain to read labels, shop for healthy ingredients, and make a concerted effort to dodge toxins, doing so will get easier over time as it becomes the norm.

 ✔ Go through your pantry and refrigerator and get rid of the unhealthy, toxic foods that I describe in Chapter 6. If a food is in your house, you'll probably eat it, so either trash it or donate it.

 ✔ If you're going to be away from home at a meal time, either pack a healthy meal or snack or figure out a healthy place to eat beforehand. Decisions made on the fly with limited choices rarely turn out well.

 ✔ Build a few more minutes into your meal schedule. Taking the time to eat your food slowly and giving your digestive system a few minutes to work its magic before you're off to the races again can pay dividends for any detoxification diet. Also consider taking digestive enzymes at meal-times; they can never hurt. And remember that having a bowel movement after a meal is a normal reflex, so don't fight it.

 ✔ Make sure you have a good source of clean water available at all times, but don't drink it during meal time!

Recipes for Detox Dieting Success

One important thing to bear in mind when starting out on a detox diet is that the food you eat doesn't have to be bland or boring. You can cook up some really fantastic dishes and stay safely within the tenets of detox dieting. Don't believe me? Check out the recipes in the next few pages.

Curried Chicken with Amaranth Pilaf

Curry powder is an excellent spice combination to add to your diet. It is flavorful and warm. One of the main ingredients of this delicious chicken recipe is *turmeric,* a root with powerful anti-inflammatory properties. It helps improve liver and cardiovascular function. And whole grains like amaranth contain lots of soluble fiber, which helps you feel full more quickly so you eat less.

Preparation time: *15 minutes*

Cooking time: *30 minutes*

Yield: *6 servings*

1 tablespoon olive oil	*1 tablespoon curry powder*
1 organic yellow onion, chopped	*1 teaspoon cinnamon*
3 cloves organic garlic, chopped	*1/8 teaspoon white pepper*
2 teaspoons curry powder	*1 tablespoon olive oil*
1 cup organic amaranth, rinsed	*1/2 cup fresh orange juice*
2/3 cup chopped organic dates	*2 tablespoons local organic honey*
2 cups filtered water	*2 tablespoons freshly squeezed lemon juice*
1 cup freshly squeezed orange juice	*1 cup sliced organic cherries or 1/2 cup dried organic cherries*
1 1/2 pounds organic, free-range, skinless chicken breasts, cut into strips	*2 tablespoons toasted sesame seeds*

1 In large saucepan, place 1 tablespoon olive oil. Add onion and garlic; cook over medium heat and stir 5–6 minutes until tender. Add 2 teaspoons curry powder; cook 1 minute. Stir in amaranth and cook 1 minute. Add dates, water, and orange juice. Bring to a simmer. Cover, reduce heat, and simmer 20 minutes.

2 Meanwhile, combine chicken with 1 tablespoon curry powder, cinnamon, and pepper; toss to coat. Heat 1 tablespoon olive oil over medium high heat in another saucepan; add chicken mixture. Brown chicken, stirring several times, until chicken is almost done, about 6 minutes.

3 Add 1/2 cup orange juice and 2 tablespoons honey to the chicken mixture; bring to a simmer. Simmer 3–5 minutes until chicken is cooked. Cover and remove from heat.

4 When amaranth is tender, stir in lemon juice and cherries, cover, and let stand 5 minutes. Then place on serving platter. Pour chicken mixture over, sprinkle with sesame seeds, and serve.

Per serving: Calories 422 (From Fat 102); Fat 11g (Saturated 2g); Cholesterol 63mg; Sodium 65mg; Carbohydrate 52g; Dietary Fiber 8g ; Protein 30g.

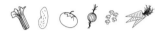

☞ *Chopped Veggie Salad*

Raw vegetables are important to a detox diet, especially when focusing on weight loss. They're rich in fiber, vitamins, and minerals, and they contain enzymes that help your liver focus on converting stored fat into energy. That helps the pounds come off!

One of the nicest things about salads is that it's so easy to change them, adding foods you love or deleting foods you don't like. Just about anything goes — as long as it's 100 percent organic. Other vegetables that would be good in this salad include shredded raw parsnips, sliced fresh mushrooms, and chopped tomatoes, fennel, or celery.

Preparation time: *10 minutes*

Cooking time: *0 minutes*

Yield: *4–6 servings*

2/3 cup plain low fat yogurt	*2 cups cauliflower florets, chopped*
2 tablespoons flaxseed oil	*1 pound organic asparagus, chopped*
3 tablespoons Dijon mustard	*2 small beets, peeled and shredded*
2 tablespoons freshly squeezed lemon juice	*3 organic carrots, peeled and shredded*
1/4 cup chopped organic flat-leaf parsley	*2 avocados, peeled and chopped*
1/8 teaspoon freshly ground pepper	*1/2 cup sliced toasted almonds*
2 cups chopped organic red cabbage	

1 In large bowl, combine yogurt, flaxseed oil, mustard, lemon juice, parsley, and pepper; mix well. Add cabbage, cauliflower, asparagus, beets, and carrots and stir to coat. Refrigerate until ready to serve.

2 Just before serving, add avocados and toss gently. Sprinkle with almonds and serve.

You can also serve this salad on a bed of mixed organic greens or cooked brown rice mixed with chopped nuts and a mustard vinaigrette.

Per serving: Calories 387 (From Fat 246); Fat 27g (Saturated 0g); Cholesterol 3mg; Sodium 400mg; Carbohydrate 32g; Dietary Fiber 15g ; Protein 12g.

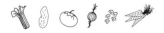

⟡ Root Vegetable Lentil Soup

Root vegetables are hearty and filling, and they contain lots of antioxidants and fiber. Cooking these vegetables makes their nutrients more available, and it concentrates their flavor. Lentils are an excellent diet food: nutty, creamy, and a wonderful source of protein. This soup is warming and satisfying on a cold day.

Preparation time: *20 minutes*

Cooking time: *70 minutes*

Yield: *6 servings*

2 tablespoons organic olive oil	*5 cups filtered water*
2 organic onions, peeled and chopped	*1 1/2 cups organic apple juice*
5 cloves garlic, peeled and minced	*1 cup organic Puy lentils*
2 tablespoons grated organic ginger root	*2 tablespoons freshly squeezed lemon juice*
2 organic sweet potatoes, peeled and chopped	*1/4 teaspoon freshly ground pepper*
1 parsnip, peeled and chopped	*1/2 cup chopped organic flat-leaf parsley*
4 organic carrots, chopped	*1 cup plain yogurt, drained in cheesecloth*
1 teaspoon turmeric	*1/2 cup toasted pumpkin seeds*
2 sprigs fresh organic rosemary	

1 In a large pot, place olive oil; add onions, garlic, and ginger root. Cook over medium high heat, stirring occasionally, until vegetables are tender, about 6–7 minutes. Add sweet potatoes and parsnip; cook and stir until vegetables start to soften.

2 Add carrots, turmeric, rosemary, water, apple juice, and lentils; bring to a simmer. Reduce heat to low, cover, and simmer 40–50 minutes until vegetables and lentils are tender.

3 Remove rosemary stems. Stir in lemon juice, pepper, and parsley. Correct seasonings if necessary, and serve dolloped with yogurt and topped with pumpkin seeds.

Per serving: *Calories 353 (From Fat 70); Fat 8g (Saturated 2g); Cholesterol 5mg; Sodium 65mg; Carbohydrate 60g; Dietary Fiber 12g ; Protein 14g.*

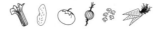

⟡ *Quinoa Fruit Breakfast Cereal*

Quinoa (pronounced *keen-wah*) is a super-crop, containing all the amino acids necessary for the human body to stay healthy. It's an ancient grain, eaten by pre-Columbian peoples.

Make sure that you rinse quinoa well before using because it's coated with a substance called *saponin,* which is a bitter chemical that prevents birds from eating the seeds.

The berries add a fresh finish to this hearty breakfast, providing you with antioxidants, vitamin C, flavonoids, and phytochemicals. And raspberries have *anthocyanins,* a compound that stabilizes blood sugar to keep hunger pangs away.

Preparation time: *25 minutes*

Cooking time: *25 minutes*

Yield: *4–6 servings*

1 1/3 cups quinoa, well rinsed	*1 cup chopped organic strawberries*
1 cup filtered water	*1 cup organic blueberries*
1 cup freshly squeezed orange juice	*1 cup organic raspberries*
1 cup organic apple juice	*1 tablespoon freshly squeezed lemon juice*
1/4 teaspoon stevia	*2 tablespoons organic honey*
1 teaspoon cinnamon	*1 tablespoon organic fresh thyme leaves*
1/2 cup toasted slivered almonds	

1 Spread the rinsed quinoa on a paper towel and let dry 10–15 minutes. (Note: It will still be somewhat wet after 15 minutes, which is fine.)

2 Place quinoa in a skillet over medium heat and toast it, stirring frequently, until it begins to pop. Remove from heat; place quinoa in heavy saucepan.

3 Add filtered water, orange juice, apple juice, stevia, and cinnamon and bring to a simmer. Reduce heat to low, cover, and simmer 20–25 minutes until quinoa is tender.

4 Stir in almonds, remove from heat, cover, and let stand 5 minutes. Meanwhile, combine berries with lemon juice, honey, and thyme in small bowl. Serve the quinoa and top with the berry mixture.

Per serving: *Calories 430 (From Fat 97); Fat 11g (Saturated 1g); Cholesterol 0mg; Sodium 18mg; Carbohydrate 77g; Dietary Fiber 10g; Protein 12g.*

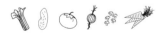

Crunchy Curried Salmon Wraps

One of the secrets of eating well with fewer calories is to add interest and flavor to your food. Curry powder adds no calories but is full of flavor and nutrients. Nuts are an important part of any diet; they provide good fats and lots of protein. And using whole grain organic tortillas as wraps satisfies your need for carbohydrates in a healthy way.

Preparation time: *15 minutes*

Cooking time: *8 minutes*

Yield: *8 servings*

1 pound wild Alaskan salmon fillets

1/2 cup freshly squeezed orange juice

1 tablespoon grated fresh organic ginger root

1 cup sliced organic celery

1/2 cup diced organic dried apricots

1/2 cup diced organic prunes

1/4 cup diced unsalted cashews

2/3 cup organic low fat yogurt

1–2 tablespoons curry powder

1/8 teaspoon white pepper

1 1/2 cups organic arugula

1 1/2 cups organic broccoli sprouts or mung bean sprouts

8 organic 10-inch whole-grain tortillas

1 Place salmon fillets in large skillet; pour juice over; sprinkle with ginger root. Bring to a simmer over medium heat. Reduce heat to low, cover, and poach salmon for 7–8 minutes until done. Remove salmon from pan; reserve 2 tablespoons poaching liquid.

2 Flake salmon and place in medium bowl. Add celery, apricots, prunes, and cashews.

3 In small bowl, combine yogurt, curry powder, poaching liquid, and pepper; mix. Add to salmon mixture and stir gently.

4 Divide arugula and sprouts among the tortillas; add salmon mixture. Roll up and cut each roll in half. Serve immediately.

Per serving: Calories 362 (From Fat 84); Fat 9g (Saturated 2g); Cholesterol 37mg; Sodium 249mg; Carbohydrate 46g; Dietary Fiber 5g; Protein 23g.

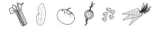

☜ Nutty Hummus Dip

Hummus is a puree of chickpeas (also called *garbanzo beans*), garlic, sesame, and lemon. It's high in folate, manganese, fiber, and protein and very low in fat, making it the perfect diet snack. Hummus is also delicious as a sandwich spread or topping for grilled salmon or chicken. Serve it with lots of fresh vegetables for dipping, and if you can find whole grain organic pita bread, cut it into triangles and toast it for another great dipper. For this recipe keep in mind that you can substitute a 15-ounce can of organic chickpeas for the cooked chickpeas, but the result will be higher in sodium.

Preparation time: 25 minutes (plus overnight soaking time)

Cooking time: 2 hours

Yield: 6–8 servings

1 cup dried organic chickpeas or garbanzo beans	*1/2 cup toasted slivered almonds*
6 cups filtered water	*3 tablespoons toasted sesame seeds*
1 head organic garlic	*5 tablespoons freshly squeezed lemon juice*
2 teaspoons toasted sesame oil	*1/2 teaspoon ground cumin*
2 tablespoons flaxseed oil	*1/8 teaspoon red pepper flakes*
1/4 cup organic tahini (sesame paste), like Artisana	

1 Pick over the chickpeas and rinse well. Cover with filtered water and soak overnight.

2 In the morning, drain and rinse the chickpeas. Place in heavy saucepan, cover with 6 cups filtered water, and bring to a boil. Reduce heat, cover pan, and simmer 70–120 minutes until they are tender. (Check after 1 hour to see if they are soft.) Drain well, reserving 1/3 cup cooking liquid.

3 Preheat oven to 400 degrees F. Cut garlic head in half crosswise and place, cut side up, on small baking sheet. Drizzle each half with a teaspoon of sesame oil. Bake for 35–45 minutes until garlic is very soft. Let cool 15 minutes, then remove cloves from skin; set aside.

4 In food processor, combine roasted garlic, cooked and drained chickpeas, and remaining ingredients. Process until desired consistency, adding reserved cooking liquid as desired. Hummus can be very smooth or it can be chunky. You may need to add more water, lemon juice, or flaxseed oil until the hummus is creamy. Serve with vegetable dippers.

Per serving: Calories 321 (From Fat 179); Fat 20g (Saturated 2g); Cholesterol 0mg; Sodium 10mg; Carbohydrate 27g; Dietary Fiber 7g; Protein 11g.

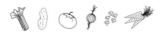

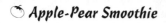

Apple-Pear Smoothie

Apples and pears are available year-round, so they're perfect for this easy breakfast smoothie. Each packs a lot of soluble and insoluble fiber. Pectin in apples can lead to a reduction in the body's need for insulin. Apples are also rich in *quercetin*, a flavonoid that fights inflammation and oxidation in the body.

Preparation time: *5 minutes*

Cooking time: *0 min*

Yield: *4 servings*

2 organic apples, unpeeled, chopped

2 organic pears, unpeeled, chopped

1 frozen organic banana, peeled

1 cup freshly squeezed orange juice

1/2 cup nonfat organic yogurt

2 tablespoons organic honey

1/2 teaspoon stevia

3 tablespoons freshly squeezed lemon juice

1 teaspoon cinnamon

2 tablespoons ground flaxseed

1 cup ice made from filtered water

1 Combine all ingredients in a heavy-duty blender or food processor. Process or blend until mixture is smooth. Immediately pour into chilled glasses and serve.

Per serving: *Calories 211 (From Fat 29); Fat 3g (Saturated 0g); Cholesterol 1mg; Sodium 23mg; Carbohydrate 46g; Dietary Fiber 7g; Protein 4g.*

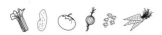

☕ Butternut Squash and Rice Stew

Any root vegetable or squash that's brightly colored, like pumpkin, sweet potatoes, carrots, or butternut squash, is packed with carotenoids and beta-carotenes, as well as fiber. These nutrients help protect your body from disease. The slow cooker is a healthy cooking method. When cooked at low temperatures, foods do not develop *advanced glycation end products,* or AGEs. These compounds are formed when sugars, protein, and fat are combined at high heat. They irritate cells in your body and may increase your risk for heart disease and diabetes.

Preparation time: *10 minutes*

Cooking time: *9 hours 45 minutes*

Yield: *6 servings*

2 organic onions, peeled and chopped	*1 cup freshly squeezed orange juice*
4 cloves organic garlic, peeled and minced	*2 tablespoons organic mustard*
2 pounds butternut squash, peeled, seeded, and cubed	*1 teaspoon dried basil leaves*
2 organic carrots, sliced	*3 sprigs fresh rosemary*
1 organic Granny Smith apple, peeled, cored, and cubed	*3/4 cup long grain organic brown rice*
3 cups filtered water	*2 tablespoons freshly squeezed lemon juice*
2 cups organic pear juice	*1/8 teaspoon cayenne pepper*
	1/8 teaspoon black pepper

1 In 5-quart slow cooker, place onions, garlic, squash, and carrots. Place apple on top. Add water and pear juice.

2 In small bowl, combine orange juice with mustard and basil; whisk until smooth and stir into slow cooker.

3 Add rosemary, and then cover and cook on low for 8–9 hours until vegetables are tender.

4 Add rice, lemon juice, and peppers; remove rosemary stems. Cover and cook on high 55–65 minutes until rice is tender.

Per serving: Calories 248 (From Fat 14); Fat 2g (Saturated 0g); Cholesterol 0mg; Sodium 151mg; Carbohydrate 57g; Dietary Fiber 8g; Protein 5g.

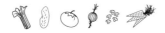

Chapter 10

Boosting Your Immune System

*Y*our immune system is truly a wonder. It's a vast, complex system with all kinds of unique, specialized parts that work together to keep your body from being overrun with foreign invaders like bacteria, viruses, parasites, toxins, and cancer. When it's healthy, your immune system can do some mind-boggling things. When it's not healthy, however, it can break down easily and allow you to fall victim to the harmful things that are around us all the time.

With that in mind, you should be very happy to know that you have quite a lot of control over the health of your immune system. Most people don't give their immunity much thought until they get sick, but we all should be mindful of our immune systems and do whatever is possible to keep things running at a high level. The best way to avoid illness is to stay healthy.

In this chapter, I fill you in on many of the toxic threats that bombard your immune system and can make it difficult for your body to effectively prevent and fight disease. I also lead you through the ways that you can avoid these toxins and detoxify your body if some of the nasty substances have already found their way inside you. A top-notch immune system isn't possible without good nutrition, so I clue you in on the foods and supplements you can select to keep your immune function at its best. Finally, I wrap up the chapter with some tasty, easy recipes for dishes you can make to provide your immune system with the healthy fuel it needs to perform its critical job.

Avoiding Toxins that Challenge Your Immune System

Like so many other things in life, your immune system will eventually break down if it's overworked for a long period of time. If your body is exposed to harmful, foreign influences like organisms or chemicals in amounts that exceed what your immune system can handle, disease will be the result.

As I mention many times throughout this book, the environment around you has reached an unprecedented level of toxicity in the last few decades. The vast amounts of toxic threats that come at you from all sides are more than enough to overwhelm your immune system. Some people would disagree, of course, but in my opinion the toxic threat has become the most significant health hazard of our time.

In this section, I give you a concise but rounded view of the various types of toxins that can give your immune system fits. Just like the toxins I describe in other chapters, these will do the least amount of damage to your body's systems if you're aware of them and able to avoid them in your daily life.

Biologic toxins

On an average day, you're exposed to millions of microscopic organisms that can potentially do your body harm. Many of these tiny creatures could have a seriously negative effect on your health if they ended up in your body in large quantities, so you should consider yourself lucky to have some lines of defense set up that stop most of the onslaught before it gets into your bloodstream or internal tissues. These defenses include your skin, which repels quite a lot of microorganisms, and also your stomach acid, which kills off many of the living things that enter your body when you eat, drink, or breathe.

Some microscopic cells are able to penetrate those first lines of defense, however, and that's when your immune system saves the day. If you can keep your immune system healthy and make sure it isn't completely overwhelmed by the critters I describe in the next couple pages, it will prevent those organisms from congregating and multiplying in your body. If your immune system persists, you continue to live a healthy life. If it breaks down and the organisms get a foothold in your body, they will soon begin to invade your tissues, reproduce in large quantities, and produce chemical toxins that keep overloading your immune system to cause infection and disease.

We all know that in order to avoid coming into contact with dangerous micro-organisms, we should stay away from sick people and avoid eating or drinking foods and liquids that have clearly gone rancid. But you can also take many other steps to prevent yeast, bacteria, and parasites from invading your body.

Yucky yeast

Yeast cells are on and in your body all the time, and you can't do much about that. They're simply too tiny, numerous, and common in your environment for you to keep every last cell away from you. And that's okay. A few yeast cells here and there both inside and outside your body are just fine. If you can keep them in check, they won't give you any problems.

The real trouble starts when yeast cells are able to increase their numbers to the point that as a group they're big enough to negatively affect you. Yeast and the byproducts that yeast cells create can cause all manner of nasty effects in your body; check out Chapter 2 for details.

How can you avoid giving yeast cells room to run in your body? You want to dodge several scenarios:

- **Too much sugar in your diet:** Yeast cells thrive on sugars and simple carbohydrates, so keep those to a minimum in order to keep yeasts under control.

- **Excessive use of antibiotics:** Just one round of antibiotics is enough to kill 80 percent of the good bacteria in your intestines, which creates all kinds of room for yeast cells to flourish. Make sure you use antibiotics only when necessary.

- **Anything that slows down or speeds up your bowels:** If the food your intestines are trying to digest moves through too slowly or too quickly, the normal bacteria in there can be disrupted, and yeast cells are given the chance to multiply rapidly. Staying regular with a healthy detox diet helps you avoid the problem.

- **Use of certain medications:** Any medication or over-the-counter product that can cause harm to the lining of your stomach or your intestines can do enough damage to give yeast a foothold in your body. Chemotherapy, radiation, and long-term use of steroids can have the same effect. Even common anti-inflammatory drugs like ibuprofen or aspirin can cause enough disruption to allow yeast overgrowth.

If you want to discourage the overgrowth of harmful yeast cells in your body, you can take *Saccharomyces* probiotics. Saccharomyces is actually a type of yeast, but it's a good yeast that behaves itself in your body, and it can help to keep the harmful yeasts under control. You can find Saccharomyces in capsule form at your health food store, likely for less than $20 per bottle. Try to take Saccharomyces anytime you have an infection that requires you to take antibiotics.

Bad bacteria

Like yeasts, bacteria are on and in us all the time, including the kinds of bacteria that can cause infections. The trick is that they're present in extremely small numbers, and they don't start being harmful unless they're given the chance to multiply. You want to keep several things in mind to make sure the bacteria around you don't get enough momentum to grow in number and challenge your immune system on a dangerous level. Here goes:

- ✔ **Wash your hands and bathe regularly.** I know this is some pretty basic advice, but I can't stress enough the importance of washing your hands — especially before you eat anything — and bathing on a regular basis. If you do these two things, you'll greatly reduce the bacterial threat without much effort at all.

- ✔ **Wash your food.** Of course, it doesn't do you much good to wash your hands if bacteria are on your food. Fruits and vegetables should be washed thoroughly as soon as you get them home. Most people wait to wash until they're going to eat their produce, but it's better to wash it as soon as you get home from the store. Don't let fruits and vegetables sit unwashed in the fridge or on the counter because that situation encourages bacterial growth and also allows any toxins on the produce to continue to penetrate into the interior of the food.

- ✔ **Cook meat thoroughly.** If you eat meat, be sure it's cooked all the way through. And don't allow meat to sit at room temperature for any extended period of time.

- ✔ **Maintain a healthy level of stomach acid.** You need the right amount and strength of stomach acid to kill off the bacteria that could otherwise enter your body through your digestive system. To assure that your stomach acid is at the right levels, don't take acid reducers unless you have documented high acid levels.

If you have problems with acid reflux or ulcers, you need to see a doctor and be tested for *H. pylori,* a bacterium that causes many of these types of ailments. You also need to have your stomach acid level tested with the Heidelberg gastric analysis. Go to `www.phcapsule.com/drref.htm` to find a physician who has this equipment and can do the testing.

- ✔ **Avoid contaminated water.** If your main source of water is a well, make sure you have it tested for the presence of dangerous bacteria. (Flip back to Chapter 3 for more information on how to get your water tested.) If you travel internationally, be sure to drink water that you know has been treated to kill bacteria and other microorganisms. (Bottled water may be your only option in these situations.)

When you travel to another country, don't assume that you can drink from a water source just because you see the locals drinking from it. People adapt to the bacteria where they live, and what is commonplace and not detrimental to the health of one person in one area could cause disease in another person.

Pushy parasites

Parasites are nasty little critters that use you as a home, help themselves to your resources, and don't offer anything helpful in return. Most of them aren't so bad that they will kill you — after all, they'd sort of be shooting themselves in the foot because they'd be ruining their home. However, they can make you very sick, and they can push your immune system to its limits. Humans have always been exposed to parasites, and we still are today. People just don't want to talk or think about it, and parasites are often one of the last things a doctor considers unless you really push the issue.

With international travel and immigration, people are exposed to a wider variety of parasites than ever before. If you travel abroad, be sure that the water you drink and ice you eat has been purified. Don't eat raw vegetables or fruit unless you're sure that they have been peeled, washed with purified water, or thoroughly cooked.

Natural bodies of water are often loaded with parasites, and you don't have to drink the water to catch them; swimming in the water can be enough to catch the bug. Having pets that spend time both inside and outside the house can also increase your exposure to parasites; you can contract several parasites just as easily as your cat or dog would. Getting tested for parasites is extremely uncommon, but most people wouldn't dream of not getting their pets wormed every year. What's wrong with this picture?

Because testing for parasites is uncommon, patients often figure out they're harboring some sort of critter only after the symptoms have set in for a while. Parasites cause many different types of illnesses, and if you catch one, you can count on it being a constant drain on your immune system. I recommend that you do a parasite cleanse every year. See the upcoming section "Destroying parasites" for details.

Environmental elements

The range and amount of environmental toxins that people are faced with today have exceeded the capability of many people's bodies to carry out detoxification without any help. The result? Widespread disease. Environmental toxins like heavy metals and chemicals can be disastrous for your immune system, and you need to prioritize limiting your exposure to these substances and acting quickly to detoxify your body if you need to.

Heavy metals

Avoiding heavy metals is a long-term, difficult challenge, but it's one that you should take on with enthusiasm if you're committed to good health. Check out Chapter 2 for all the details on heavy metals, from the kinds that are increasingly prevalent (like mercury and lead) to the many problems they can cause in your system. Everyone needs to avoid heavy metals whenever possible, but it's absolutely imperative that children, pregnant women, and women who plan on getting pregnant do whatever they can to avoid and remove heavy metals.

Which metals are the hardest on your immune system? Here's a helpful list of the most harmful heavy metals, along with the places you can encounter them if you're not careful:

- **Aluminum:** A common metal found in some vaccines, antacids, cookware, and antiperspirant.
- **Antimony:** Found in fire-retardant textiles like bedding.
- **Arsenic:** Present in some foods (chicken is a top offender), wood preservatives, fuel oils, fertilizers, and weed killer.
- **Barium:** Often present in some ceramics, plastics, textiles, and fuel.
- **Beryllium:** Found in neon signs, bicycle wheels, and fishing rods.
- **Bisthmuth:** Present in many medicines used to treat stomach aches.
- **Bromine:** Often used as a disinfectant for swimming pools and hot tubs.
- **Cadmium:** Present in cigarettes, batteries, and refined foods.
- **Lead:** Found in old paint, tin cans, pewter, dust, ceramics, and insecticides.
- **Manganese:** Sources include welding equipment and supplies.
- **Mercury:** Sources include amalgam fillings, fish and other types of seafood, flu vaccines, and high fructose corn syrup.
- **Nickel:** Present in tobacco, auto exhaust, fertilizer, and baking powder.
- **Thallium:** Found in metal alloys, rodenticides, and fireworks.

For a thorough discussion on how you can avoid these heavy metals, flip back to Chapter 3.

Chemicals

Avoiding toxic chemicals is no easy task, but if you make a concerted effort, your immune system will be much better off. Chemical toxins harm and kill many of our bodies' cells, and the dynamic cells that make up your immune system are especially fragile and prone to being killed or rendered useless by chemical toxins. Here are a few tips for cutting toxic chemicals out of your life:

- **Don't use toxic cleaning products in your home.** Plenty of non-toxic options are available online and at your local health food store, and they will get your house just as clean as their harsh chemical counterparts. Vodka in a spray bottle is a good option (one spray for the countertop and one for the tonsils!).

✔ **Avoid using products with fragrances.** These include room sprays, dryer sheets, carpet deodorizing powders, and even some candles.

   Many candles have wicks that contain lead. If you use candles in your home, be sure to choose lead-free options when buying.

✔ **Reduce your exposure to fumes.** If you're working with substances that produce fumes, make sure you're doing so for only short periods of time and in a well-ventilated space. This includes paint!

✔ **Wash all your fruits and vegetables thoroughly.** Your best bet is to do so as soon as you bring them home from the store.

✔ **Purify your air.** Invest in a good HEPA air purifier to cut down on the airborne toxins that you inhale while indoors.

Removing Toxins for Better Immune Response

The previous section is all about how to identify and avoid the toxins that can damage your immune system. Unfortunately, no matter how vigilant you are about dodging toxins, you'll likely still end up with them in your system just because those materials are now so abundant. That's why this section focuses on the detoxification of immune-damaging materials from your system.

Different methods of detoxification work best for different toxins, so you may have to take a multi-pronged attack. But the good news is that almost all toxins can be removed, so even if your toxicity is pretty high you can start now to correct the situation. (If you need help figuring out how toxic you are, check out the quiz in Chapter 8.)

You may have a hard time getting motivated to change your routine and diet or to take supplements to treat a problem that isn't always blatantly obvious. Finding motivation is even more difficult because traditional medicine doesn't focus much on toxicity. (In many cases doctors don't even test for toxicity when trying to diagnose an illness.) The challenge for you is to recognize the toxins that are in your body now and to take an active role in your detoxification. No one else is going to do it for you.

Saying goodbye to living toxins

Earlier in this chapter I explain how you can avoid letting yeast, bacteria, and parasites enter your body and put a strain on your immune system. But chances are you already have some of these living toxins in your body, and you need to get rid of them if you want your immune function to be tip-top.

Killing yeasts

Yeasts are very aggressive in the body when they have a steady stream of simple carbohydrates and sugar to feast on, so the first thing you should do to limit yeast growth is to cut out as many of those materials from your diet as possible. Taking out most of the sugar from your diet will starve the yeast cells, which can go a long way toward slashing their numbers down to manageable levels. You can also take a variety of natural products that kill yeast, including grapefruit seed, black walnut hull extract, slippery elm bark, goldenseal root extract, and bearberry leaf. I also recommend trying the antifungal drugs Nystatin or Diflucan and using them for about three weeks. (You'll need a doctor's prescription.) That usually does the trick.

Eliminating bacteria

High levels of harmful bacteria in your colon can produce a lot of toxins, and these toxins can strain your immune system in some pretty heinous ways and have direct effects on other organs like the brain. To remedy that kind of problem, try a colon cleanse followed by a concerted effort to repopulate your gut with good bacteria. (Have a look at Chapter 5 for details on how to carry out that process.) If that method fails, sometimes it may be necessary to use antibiotics. If that's the case, ask your doctor to prescribe oral antibiotics that don't get absorbed into your bloodstream but instead do all their killing right in the intestines.

Destroying parasites

Parasites can be extremely pesky, but natural solutions can take care of the problem. Ask at your health food store for natural products that contain black walnut husks, wormwood, Pau D'Arco, garlic, pumpkin seed, ginger root, clove, and gentian root. Keep in mind that if natural alternatives don't do the trick, you can always fall back on a few old and very safe prescription drugs like Vermox and Biltricide for killing parasites.

Giving chemicals and heavy metals the heave-ho

Toxic chemicals and heavy metals are bound to damage your immune system, so you should take action to remove these substances from your body. A range of helpful detox methods is available, and they are treatments available to everyone — nothing too exotic or expensive.

Everyone should be interested in removing from their bodies toxins that compromise immune health. But at the very top of the list are children and women who are trying to get pregnant.

If you are in good health and you're just getting started on a detoxification regimen to rid your body of the toxins that affect the immune system, consider doing a two-day water fast, meaning that you eat nothing and drink only water for two full days. Doing so is easier than you think, and it's useful for cleaning out your body and giving your natural detoxification mechanisms a little bit of a rest before you shift them into high gear for your detox push. Just make sure you have a reliably clean, toxin-free water source before you get started.

Getting help from herbs and foods

You can eat a variety of herbs and foods to help your body fight and get rid of the toxins that are harmful to your immune system. Many of these options are excellent for general health, too, so you certainly won't be giving anything up in terms of nutrition if you work to include a range of them in your diet.

One of the most important dietary considerations for detoxifying your body against toxic threats to your immune system is your daily intake of fiber. If you get plenty of fiber in your diet, your body has an easier time eliminating the toxins in your digestive system that have been broken down or removed from your blood by your liver. Do your best to incorporate fiber into your diet whenever possible.

Here are some of the best herbs and foods for detoxification of the heavy metals and chemicals that can harm your immune system:

- **Sulfur-containing foods:** These include eggs, garlic, and onions.
- **Fresh vegetables juices:** Beet, carrot, and celery juices are three of the top varieties.
- **Cruciferous vegetables:** Focus on broccoli, Brussels sprouts, kale, and cabbage.
- **Dandelion greens:** These should be available at your grocery store, and you can probably even find a 100 percent organic variety. If not, try a health food store.
- **Green tea:** I mention this one in several other chapters as well. It's a detoxification powerhouse!
- **Other types of tea:** You can see benefits from tea made from cinnamon bark, licorice root, ginger root, and burdock root.
- **Rosemary:** This excellent herb helps increase your body's natural detoxification enzymes.
- **Cilantro:** It actually works to pull heavy metals from your tissues. Eat it fresh or buy a tincture from your health food store and follow the directions on the label.

✔ **Chlorella:** Like cilantro, this green algae acts to flush heavy metals from your body. Find it at your local health food store or online.

✔ **Fruits:** Some of the best options include grapes, berries, and citrus fruits.

If you're trying to eat certain herbs and foods to detoxify your body, you'd really be wasting your time if you were choosing options that contain toxins. To make sure that doesn't happen, get 100 percent organic foods and supplements whenever possible.

Seeking out suitable supplements

You can also use several different kinds of supplements to help you rid your body of chemical and heavy metal toxins. First, make sure that you're taking a high potency, high quality multivitamin to cover all the basic vitamins and minerals. (Check out Chapter 5 for a general discussion of how to pick out your supplements.) After you have that important step taken care of, you can focus on selecting some other supplements to help you clear out the toxins that can bombard your immune system. Here are some of the top examples, along with the dosages you need to achieve the desired effect:

✔ **Alpha-lipoic acid:** 100–600 mg per day

✔ **Amino acids:** 1,000 mg of both glycine and taurine per day

✔ **Carnitine:** 1–3 grams per day

✔ **Mixed carotenoids:** 15,000–25,000 units per day

✔ **Molybdenum:** 50–200 micrograms per day

✔ **N-acetylcysteine:** 500–1,000 mg per day

✔ **Omega-3 essential fatty acids:** 1–4 grams per day

✔ **Resveratrol:** 30 mg per day

✔ **Selenium:** 200 micrograms per day

✔ **Silymarin:** 50–200 mg per day

✔ **Vitamin C:** 2–4 grams per day

✔ **Zinc:** 30–50 mg per day

I know this may seem like a long list, but remember that you're trying to change the way your body functions on a very basic level to enhance toxin removal. Doing so takes a lot of effort, but the result — a robust immune system — is worth it!

Catching toxins with chelation

If you have a heavy load of heavy metals in your system and they're damaging your immune system, you may need to step up your detoxification efforts beyond food, herbs, and supplements. The next step is chelation, and it can really save the day.

Chelation involves taking a medication that's designed to attract and attach to heavy metals and then remove them through your urine. Chelating agents have been used for over 60 years and are extremely safe and efficient in removing heavy metals. I won't get into the chelation details here, but you can flip to Chapter 18 for a full rundown if you're interested.

Sweating out the heavy metals

Sweating is one of the most important ways to detox the body, and you can actually accomplish a useful amount of heavy metal detoxification by simply sweating through everyday activity and exercise. Sweating removes one-third as many toxins as your kidneys, and many of the toxins that sweating eliminates aren't removed effectively by any other means of detoxification. If you sweat out some of the heavy metals that plague your immune system, you can improve the health of your entire body. I encourage you to embrace that kind of sweating and make it part of your normal routine.

If you want to really increase the amount of heavy metals you eliminate from your system through sweating, you can always take advantage of saunas. You can use several types of saunas year-round to bolster your heavy metal detoxification. The most common types are wet, dry, and infrared. I cover all the details in Chapter 18, so if you're interested, grab a towel and a tall glass of clean water and get ready to sweat it out!

Using Nutrition to Bolster Immunity

Your immune system is a complex machine, and if you want to keep it healthy you need to get a range of important nutritional elements. But you can also go the extra mile and tweak your diet in a few key ways to ensure that your immunity is at its very best. That's what I encourage you to do in this section: Go beyond the basic requirements and shoot for the type of diet that can really make your immune system shine.

Picking foods to help thwart disease

I put a lot of emphasis on the importance of the food you choose to eat, and I'm certainly not changing my tune when it comes to keeping your immune system healthy. Eating the right foods can give you a leg up on robust immunity, and avoiding a few lousy foods can go just as far.

What you need to eat

First off, see to it that you're getting the following minerals and amino acids, which are very important in maintaining a high performance immune system:

- ✔ **Iron:** Low iron levels cause increased retention of the harmful heavy metal toxins aluminum, lead, and cadmium. You can get iron in beef, turkey, sardines, oysters, clams, shrimp, beans, lentils, and pumpkin seeds.

- ✔ **L-cysteine:** This amino acid is a key player in boosting your body's ability to detoxify itself. Make sure you get plenty of it in your diet! You'll find it in chicken, turkey, eggs, yogurt, garlic, onions, red peppers, broccoli, and Brussels sprouts.

- ✔ **Selenium:** If you don't get enough selenium, your body is more likely to retain mercury, which is one of the worst toxins known to man. Selenium is found in garlic, grains, shellfish, salmon, sunflower seeds, walnuts, ginseng, onions, and chives.

- ✔ **Zinc:** Don't skimp on the zinc or you'll make it harder for your body's natural detoxification efforts to clear out a range of heavy metals. Look for zinc in beef, lamb, turkey, chicken, and shellfish.

Also keep in mind that virtually any deficiency of vitamins or essential fatty acids has a negative impact on your immune system. Make sure you're getting what you need on those fronts — you can read more in Chapters 5 and 17 — and you'll give your body the firm foundation it needs to maintain health and fight disease.

Be sure to eat plenty of antioxidant-rich foods. Strive to include foods that are loaded with alpha-lipoic acid, beta-carotene, omega-3 fatty acids, resveratrol, sulforaphane, vitamin C, and vitamin E. These are essential substances for a bombastic immune system, and you can get them from the following food sources:

- ✔ **Alpha-lipoic acid:** This antioxidant supports the liver's detoxification function. Find it in nuts, seeds, broccoli, leafy green vegetables, grains, hempseed oil, flaxseed oil, and virgin unhydrogenated coconut oil.

- ✔ **Beta-carotene:** Eat fruits and vegetables that are orange in color, such as sweet potatoes, carrots, mangoes, apricots, and spinach. (Okay, I know that last one isn't orange, but it can't all be color-coded, can it?)

- ✔ **Omega-3 fatty acids:** Fish and grass-fed beef are good sources.

- ✔ **Resveratrol:** This substance is one of many reasons to eat your broccoli.

- ✔ **Sulforaphane:** This is one of the best antioxidants ever found. You get sulforaphane from broccoli and broccoli sprouts, but 90 percent is destroyed if you cook it.

✔ **Vitamin C:** Citrus fruits, green and red peppers, Brussels sprouts, and broccoli are great sources.

✔ **Vitamin E:** Find it in safflower, corn, and canola oils, as well as wheat germ and sunflower seeds.

Healthy immunity also depends on a good, steady source of protein in your diet. Two of the most beneficial amino acids for giving your immune system a boost and fighting disease are glutamine and arginine. Find them in eggs, lean beef, chicken, and turkey.

What you need to avoid eating

Trans fats are inflammatory, and saturated fats are loaded with toxins. They decrease the effectiveness of your immune system. You should be making every effort to cut them out of your diet anyway, but you can feel extra good about waving goodbye to them when you realize that in addition to increasing your cardiovascular health and decreasing your toxin intake, you're also helping your body to fight disease. All that, and you only have to give up a couple of nasty types of fat? Not a bad deal at all.

Figuring out what to eat if you're already sick

You could eat the best foods and maintain the healthiest lifestyle and still get sick. There's no escaping the fact that we live in a world full of viruses, bacteria, and toxins that can make us ill, and eventually your immune system is going to get overwhelmed and you'll get sick. When that happens, you should maintain your healthy lifestyle and continue to eat the wholesome, natural foods that I describe throughout this chapter (and elsewhere in the book). But you can also do a few other things to help your immune system fight off the intruders that are causing your ailment:

✔ **Ramp up the antioxidants:** Antioxidants are great at helping your immune system fight illness, and if you eat them when you're sick you should get well faster. (If you take them all the time, you may not get sick at all.) Flip to Chapter 5 for lots of information on how to select foods that are packed with antioxidants.

✔ **Load up on vitamin C:** When you're sick, you should take vitamin C up to *bowel tolerance.* That's the level at which the vitamin C causes loose stool, and of course you don't want to do that to yourself, especially when you're sick. Bowel tolerance for adults is about 8,000 to 10,000 mg per day. (The amounts are lower for children, of course.) To get that much vitamin C in your diet when you're sick, try to eat as many vitamin C–rich foods as you can (I list a few in this chapter) and take supplements to make up the difference.

✔ **Get lots of vitamin E and selenium:** These substances can also be extremely beneficial when you're sick, especially for viral and upper respiratory infections.

✔ **Drink water — and lots of it:** When you're sick, it's hugely important that you drink lots and lots of water. In Chapter 5 I explain your lymph system, which is almost like a second circulatory system that helps to flush toxins, bacteria, and viruses from your body. If you're extremely well hydrated, your lymph system has what it needs to flush out those harmful materials faster and more efficiently than if you're not drinking enough water.

Your immune and lymph systems desperately need lots of water to work properly and make you well, so make sure you're giving those important systems what they require. Drink up! (And make sure the water is purified and toxin-free, of course.)

Choosing Supplements that Boost Your Immunity

Boosting the immune system's function with vitamin and herbal supplements is a practice that has been going on for thousands of years. If you choose your supplements wisely, you can really enhance your body's ability to keep itself healthy and running smoothly, which in turn makes it much more adept at fighting off illnesses. In today's toxic world, I believe that everyone should supplement to maintain a robust immune system. With just a little extra effort, you can defeat disease before it gets started. You know what they say about an ounce of prevention.

How to deal with diarrhea

When some people get diarrhea, they immediately reach for some over-the-counter or prescription drug that is designed to patch up the problem and allow them to have solid stools again. That's not the healthiest move. When you get diarrhea, it's a crystal clear sign that your body is trying to get rid of something. Your colon is essentially stealing water from the rest of your body to liquefy the contents of your bowels and move them out as quickly as possible. When you get diarrhea, don't reach for a bottle of medicine right away. Let your colon do its job!

The best treatment for most types of diarrhea is to drink lots and lots of water and let the diarrhea run its course. If you work hard to stay hydrated, your colon will eventually clear out the harmful substances that are making you sick. After the toxic contents are out of your body, the diarrhea should stop. One caveat: If your diarrhea lasts for several days, the problem could be something that your colon isn't able to handle on its own, so you may need to consult your doctor.

One quick note: Don't confuse this information on immune system–boosting supplements with the information I provide earlier in the chapter on supplements that you can take to help your body detoxify itself when you've taken in toxins that threaten your immune system. The suggestions overlap somewhat, but there are key differences, as well.

Vitamins and minerals

If you're on a good daily multivitamin regimen, you're more than likely giving your immune system much of what it needs to flourish.

Be wary of a multivitamin that purports to provide you with all the vitamins and minerals you need in one capsule or tablet a day; if it really had everything you need in one dose, the pill would be as big as a golf ball. Most comprehensive multivitamins require several capsules a day. Four is a very common number and a good one for you to start with. Ask the experts at your local health food or vitamin store for a recommendation.

In addition to your multivitamin, you can take the following to boost your immune system's function. The abbreviation IU stands for *international units:* a measurement of biological activity that is established for each substance so that different products can be compared.

- ✔ **Beta-carotene or vitamin A:** 25,000 IU per day
- ✔ **Magnesium:** 600–1,200 mg per day
- ✔ **Vitamin C:** 2,000–4,000 mg per day
- ✔ **Vitamin D3:** 2,000–5,000 IU per day
- ✔ **Vitamin E:** 400–800 IU per day
- ✔ **Zinc:** 20–40 mg per day

Herbs and other supplements

Quality herbal supplements can greatly enhance your immune function. The quality and potency of the supplement is very important, so be sure to read the section in Chapter 5 that discusses how you can select high-quality supplements.

One immune-boosting supplement that has recently shown quite a bit of promise is *sulforaphane,* which is an extract of broccoli seeds. It enhances your immune system and has even shown some interesting results in fighting and preventing cancer.

You should also consider taking a supplement that contains concentrated antioxidants, which are extracted from multiple vegetables. These supplements are sold under different names but are usually called *greens.* You'll probably find them in powder form; check the shelves of your favorite health food shop or vitamin store.

When you're buying the supplements called *greens,* pay special attention to the ORAC number. You don't need to know the technical details of what that number means or how it's calculated, but just make sure the product you choose has an ORAC of at least 20,000 per scoop. That's the same as the antioxidant capacity of 15 servings of vegetables!

Here are a few other supplements you can take to gear up your immune system:

- ✔ **Arginine:** 3,000 mg per day
- ✔ **Garlic:** 600–1,000 mg per day
- ✔ **Glutamate:** 3,000 mg per day
- ✔ **Selenium:** 200 micrograms per day

Recipes for Improving Your Immune Function

Foods that contain the nutrients and other substances that help to keep you healthy and maintain your immune system just happen to be delicious and versatile in the kitchen. Try some of these recipes to help keep your immunity up to snuff or to give your body a boost when you start to feel a sniffle coming on.

Gingered Roasted Salmon with Berry Salsa

Berries are some of the best foods you can eat. They're very high in antioxidants, especially anthocyanins and flavonoids, and vitamin C, which helps support the immune system. In a recent study, blueberries were at the top of the list for best foods to eat for detoxification. Paired with smooth and nutty roasted salmon, this is a dish you'll want to eat again and again.

Wheat germ is very high in vitamin E, which helps the body defend against oxidation. Vitamin E may also reduce the risk of some kinds of cancers. Wheat germ is crunchy, nutty, and delicious. Store wheat germ in the refrigerator because the oils are delicate and perishable.

Preparation time: *15 minutes*

Cooking time: *25 minutes*

Yield: *4 servings*

1 cup organic blueberries	*1/2 teaspoon crushed red pepper flakes*
1/2 cup dried organic cranberries	*1 pound wild Alaska salmon fillets*
1 cup organic blackberries	*2 tablespoons organic honey*
2 tablespoons organic honey	*White pepper, to taste*
1 tablespoon grated fresh ginger root	*1/4 cup grated fresh ginger root*
1/2 teaspoon anise seeds	*3 cloves organic garlic, peeled and minced*
1 teaspoon apple cider vinegar	*1/3 cup organic wheat germ*

1 In medium bowl, combine blueberries, cranberries, and blackberries. In small bowl, combine 2 tablespoons honey, 1 tablespoon ginger root, anise seeds, vinegar, and red pepper flakes. Combine this mixture with the berries; mix well and set aside.

2 Preheat oven to 400 degrees F. Place salmon fillets on baking sheet, brush with 2 tablespoons honey and sprinkle with some white pepper. Combine 1/4 cup ginger root and minced garlic with wheat germ and pat on top of the salmon.

3 Roast salmon for 18–24 minutes until just barely done in center. Salmon should flake easily when tested with a fork. Serve with the berry salsa on the side.

Per serving: *Calories 330 (From Fat 51); Fat 6g (Saturated 1g); Cholesterol 53mg; Sodium 61mg; Carbohydrate 47g; Dietary Fiber 5g; Protein 26g.*

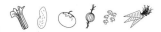

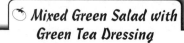

Mixed Green Salad with Green Tea Dressing

When you buy leafy greens, look for the darkest you can find. Darker greens (and vegetables, too) have more vitamins A, C, and K. These nutritious foods may help prevent some kinds of cancers, and they're a boon for your immune system. Green tea is full of antioxidants, too, including *catechin,* a compound that increases liver function.

You may find that this delicious recipe becomes part of your regular rotation.

Preparation time: *35 minutes*

Cooking time: *0 minutes*

Yield: *6 servings*

1/4 cup green tea leaves	2 cups organic arugula
1/4 cup freshly squeezed lemon juice	2 cups chopped organic mustard greens or organic microgreens
1 tablespoon apple cider vinegar	
1 tablespoon filtered water	2 cups organic baby spinach
2 tablespoons flaxseed oil	1/2 cup chopped organic flat-leaf parsley
1 organic garlic clove, peeled and minced	1 cup chopped organic fresh basil leaves
1 teaspoon turmeric	1 cup organic broccoli sprouts
1/4 teaspoon stevia	2 cups sliced organic mushrooms
1 cup organic plain yogurt	3 organic tomatoes, chopped

1 In small saucepan, combine tea leaves, lemon juice, and vinegar. Add filtered water and bring just to a simmer; remove pan from heat, cover, and let steep 20–30 minutes. Strain well; discard tea leaves. Stir in flaxseed oil, garlic, turmeric, stevia, and yogurt; blend well and refrigerate.

2 In serving bowl, combine arugula, mustard greens, spinach, parsley, basil, and broccoli sprouts; toss gently. Add mushrooms and tomatoes; pour yogurt dressing over all. Toss gently and serve immediately.

Per serving: *Calories 108 (From Fat 57); Fat 6g (Saturated 1g); Cholesterol 5mg; Sodium 50mg; Carbohydrate 11g; Dietary Fiber 3g; Protein 4g.*

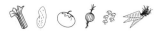

Berry Currant Chicken Salad

Chicken salad is a true comfort food. The combination of tender chicken with sweet and tart fruits is so good you won't believe it's good for you, too!

Black currants are very rich in vitamin C. It may be difficult to find them in regular grocery stores; look for them in organic and health food stores or order online. If you can't find them, the juice made from the black currant is a good substitute.

Borage seed oil is concentrated in GLA (*gamma-linolenic acid*), which your body converts into prostaglandins, increasing your immune strength. The oil can also ensure you have the right amounts of omega-3 and omega-6 fatty acids in your body.

Preparation time: *30 minutes*

Cooking time: *20 minutes*

Yield: *4 servings*

1/2 cup organic black currant juice	*4 organic boneless, skinless chicken breasts*
1/4 teaspoon stevia	*1 cup filtered water*
1 teaspoon organic borage seed oil	*1 cup organic black currants or red currants, rinsed*
2 tablespoons flaxseed oil	
3 tablespoons organic vegetable oil	*1/2 cup organic dried cranberries*
1 tablespoon apple cider vinegar	*1 cup organic raspberries*
1/8 teaspoon cayenne pepper	*3 cups mixed organic dark leafy greens*

1 In small bowl, combine juice, stevia, borage seed oil, flaxseed oil, vegetable oil, vinegar, and cayenne pepper; mix well and refrigerate.

2 Place chicken in skillet; pour water over. Bring to a simmer over medium heat. Reduce heat to low, cover, and poach chicken 12–17 minutes until just done. Place chicken in bowl; pour half of the poaching liquid over and let cool 20 minutes.

3 Remove chicken from liquid and cut into large chunks. Mix with currant dressing and place in serving bowl. Add currants, cranberries, and raspberries and toss gently. Serve on the dark leafy greens.

Per serving: *Calories 405 (From Fat 197); Fat 22g (Saturated 3g); Cholesterol 73mg; Sodium 77mg; Carbohydrate 25g; Dietary Fiber 6g; Protein 28g.*

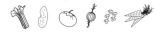

↻ *Cinnamon Granola*

Granola is the perfect choice for breakfast or snacks. Two classic ingredients, oats and wheat germ, help boost your immune system with high levels of fiber and vitamin E. And it's easy to make your own granola. Plus you get to control what goes into the granola! Top it with some plain yogurt with a bit of vanilla stirred in, and lots of fresh berries.

Preparation time: *15 minutes*

Cooking time: *40 minutes*

Yield: *10 1/2-cup servings*

3 cups organic rolled regular oats	*1/3 cup organic vegetable oil*
1 cup organic wheat germ	*1/2 cup organic local honey*
1/2 cup chopped walnuts	*2 tablespoons organic apple juice*
1/2 cup pumpkin seeds	*1 teaspoon cinnamon*
1/3 cup sesame seeds	*1 teaspoon vanilla extract*
1/4 cup organic flaxseed	

1 Preheat oven to 325 degrees F. In large bowl, combine oats, wheat germ, walnuts, pumpkin seeds, sesame seeds, and flaxseed. Set aside.

2 In saucepan, combine oil, honey, and apple juice; heat through until mixture is smooth. Remove from heat and add cinnamon and vanilla.

3 Pour sauce over oat mixture and stir gently. Spread evenly onto a baking sheet. Bake 30–40 minutes, stirring every 7 minutes, until granola is golden. Let cool completely, and then stir to break up clumps. Store in airtight container at room temperature.

Per serving: *Calories 345 (From Fat 156); Fat 17g (Saturated 2g); Cholesterol 0mg; Sodium 5mg; Carbohydrate 41g; Dietary Fiber 6g; Protein 10g.*

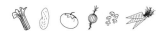

Chapter 11

Increasing Your Energy Level

*O*ne of the most common health complaints is a lack of energy. So many people are tired, and they just don't feel like they have the get-up-and-go that's necessary to keep up with their busy lives. If you're suffering from a lack of energy, take heart in the fact that you're not alone, and rest assured that you *can* take steps to improve your energy level and put that much needed pep in your step.

Many complicated biologic states can cause a lack of energy, but a few issues are really common and can be fixed with conventional medicine, natural therapies that involve detoxification, or a combination of both. Two of the top issues are thyroid problems and blood sugar problems, both of which I cover in this chapter.

Amazingly enough, the bacteria that you carry around in your gastrointestinal tract can also contribute to a lack of energy. You have more bacterial cells in your gut than in all other parts of your body combined. When the delicate balance of that bacteria is disturbed, several of your organ systems can be affected, and profound fatigue is a common result. The good news is that you can take steps to make sure that the balance of the bacteria in your intestines is right where it needs to be, and you may be surprised how much of a positive effect that change can have on your energy level. The bad news is that you'll have to put some thought into what's living in your belly, which can rank pretty high on the gross-out scale.

So if you've been feeling low on energy, hang in there and summon the zeal to flip through the pages of this chapter. You'll be doing back flips in no time! (Okay, maybe you'll just be energized and ready to get up and go each day — you'll have to find another book for the back flip instructions.)

Taking a Look at Your Thyroid

Your energy level is determined by your metabolism, which is controlled by hormones that your thyroid gland produces. If your thyroid is acting up, chances are you're seeing some pretty dramatic effects in your energy level.

If you're incredibly tired or wired all the time, you could very well have a thyroid problem and you should make an appointment to see your doctor. (If you're in need of a doctor or in the market for a new one, flip back to Chapter 5 for some tips on how to find and work with good doctors who are well versed in natural treatments like detoxification.) If you've already been diagnosed with a thyroid ailment and you're weighing your options for treatment (or already receiving conventional treatment), you may want to consider augmenting your progress with detoxification.

In this section, I dig into the details of the toxins that can affect your thyroid gland and what you can do to rid your body of those toxins (and keep them out). I also offer a quick look at some of the things that your thyroid gland has to have in order to function correctly, and I let you know where to find those things in foods that fit in with a detoxification diet.

While I focus on the dangers of mercury and aspartame in this section, you should know that fluoride also affects your thyroid in a negative way. Fluoride can attach to thyroid hormone molecules and prevent them from working in your tissues, but the hormones will still be counted in the standard blood test for thyroid function. In other words, the thyroid test will show that you have plenty of thyroid hormone, but the hormone doesn't work.

If your thyroid's function is just a little out of whack, you can probably make quite a bit of progress toward remedying the problem with natural means (diet and supplements are a couple examples). But if your thyroid is seriously misbehaving, you need medical treatment. You need to consult with your doctor to determine whether your thyroid problem is a minor or major one.

Mastering mercury

When it comes to thyroid-damaging toxins, nothing is more harmful than mercury. Mercury basically makes it impossible for your thyroid gland to successfully produce good hormones, and without hormones from your thyroid, your metabolism is terribly slow and your energy level goes crashing through the floor.

Considering an alternative thyroid test

Sometimes people suffering from low energy levels get a blood test — the standard test used to screen for thyroid problems — and the results indicate that their thyroid is normal. If that happens to you but your symptoms persist and you're still not convinced that your thyroid is working like it should, you may want to check your thyroid's function using the _basal body temperature method_. It's a relatively easy process that you can begin at home on your own.

1. **Get a basal thermometer.** A _basal thermometer_ is a specialty thermometer used to measure human body temperature. You can buy one at your local drug store or through many online retailers.

2. **Measure your body temperature in your armpit as soon as you wake up — before you get out of bed — every day for ten days.** Record the temperature measurement for each day.

3. **Average the temperatures.** If your temperature is where it should be, you'll get an average of 97.2 to 98.2 degrees Fahrenheit.

4. **If your average temperature is below the range specified in step 3, consult a physician.** You'll need to make sure you find a physician who is willing to treat you for a thyroid problem based on symptoms and basal body temperature. A good source for these types of physicians is the American College for Advancement in Medicine (ACAM). You'll also find that ACAM members are more likely to treat you with natural methods and products.

You can find a listing of physician members of the American College for Advancement in Medicine at the organization's Web site (www. acamnet.org). You may also want to check out the Web site of the International College of Integrative Medicine (www.icimed.com).

In addition to being extremely damaging to your thyroid, mercury is also a particularly problematic toxin because it's extremely powerful — the second most toxic substance on the planet, after plutonium — and it's found all over the place in our environment. (I fill you in on the details shortly when I explain how you can work toward limiting your mercury exposure.) To give you an idea of how toxic mercury is, consider that the amount of mercury in an old glass thermometer is enough to poison a 26-acre lake.

If you want to enjoy healthy energy levels, you need a fully functioning thyroid. And if you want your thyroid to perform at its best, you need to rid your body of mercury.

Getting rid of the mercury in your body

You can choose among several good ways to get rid of the mercury in your body. At the top of the list is a process called _chelation_. Chelation is a detoxification method that involves introducing a substance into your body and allowing that substance to attach itself to toxins, which are then carried out of your body in urine or feces. Chelation is a precise procedure that must be performed by a doctor. (I cover plenty of chelation details in Chapter 18.) For eliminating mercury, the best chelating agent is DMPS, which is administered using an IV.

In addition to DMPS, DMSA is also used as a chelating agent for mercury. DMSA is administered orally, but there's some debate among experts on whether or not DMSA can carry mercury into the brain.

If you're not too keen on chelation, don't dismay: You can use other methods to help eliminate mercury from your system on your own, at home. You can get started with a tincture of cilantro (also known as Chinese parsley), which is a solution made from the normal kitchen herb that you often find in salsa and pesto. You can buy tincture of cilantro at most vitamin stores. Tincture of cilantro mobilizes mercury, moving it to your liver where it's deposited in your bile and then moved to the intestines.

That's the first step, but if you stop there, your intestines will simply reabsorb the mercury and you'll be back at square one. To prevent that from happening, you need a *binding agent* that will bond to the mercury and hold it in the intestines until it eventually works its way down your digestive system and out of the body in your feces. For mercury detoxification, the best binding agent is a green algae called *chlorella* that you can buy in powder form.

Here are the details for using tincture of cilantro and chlorella to help clear the mercury out of your body:

1. **Take two drops of tincture of cilantro two times a day, and gradually increase the dosage over a period of days until you reach the point where you're taking ten drops, three times each day.** You can do this easily by making a simple tea with ten drops of the tincture mixed up in a cup of hot water. Take this dosage for a week, take a two-week break, and then do it for another week.

2. **While you're taking the tincture of cilantro, make sure you're also using your chlorella.** Start with one gram of powder four times a day and increase that amount to three grams, four times a day.

3. **Continue taking the tincture of cilantro and chlorella on the alternating schedule (on for one week, off for two weeks) for six months.**

If you get an upset stomach during the process of detoxifying with tincture of cilantro and chlorella, your first reaction may be to take less chlorella. Don't do that! Instead, increase your dose of chlorella to three grams five times a day or more. Your upset stomach is a sign that you're removing a lot of mercury from your system, and you need more chlorella to keep that process moving in the right direction.

Steering clear of mercury exposure

After you've made an effort to get rid of the mercury in your body, what can you do to keep it out? Unfortunately, it's not an easy task.

Despite the fact that mercury is one of the most toxic substances known to man, it's surprisingly ubiquitous in the world today. If you're striving to limit your mercury exposure — and you should be — you need to be aware of the following sources of mercury:

✓ **Fish:** If you include fish in your diet, chances are you're also including mercury. Fish and the waters they inhabit are extremely susceptible to mercury contamination, and when fish are caught and eventually end up on your dinner table, the mercury is transferred to you. Because fish are native to and farm-raised in a variety of environments, the mercury levels in fish can vary widely. If you want to add fish to your dinner table but you're not interested in also adding a dangerous toxin like mercury, try using Alaskan salmon, which generally contains less mercury than many other types of fish. You can also buy fish that has been analyzed and certified safe by independent lab testing.

If you're pregnant, be extremely cautious about eating fish. The mercury risk is high: The U.S. Food and Drug Administration (FDA) recently issued a warning for pregnant women that even one 3-ounce portion of swordfish, shark, king mackerel, or tilefish during the entire pregnancy can contain enough mercury to cause fetal brain damage.

✓ **Flu vaccines:** Vaccines for influenza have become increasingly popular in the past decade, but most doses of flu vaccine still contain mercury. A mercury-containing chemical called *thiomersal* (commonly called *thimerosal*) is used in vaccines as a preservative.

Mercury-free flu vaccines are available in limited amounts each year, so if you're planning to get vaccinated, ask your doctor about obtaining a vaccine that doesn't contain mercury.

✓ **Dental fillings:** The amalgam fillings (commonly referred to incorrectly as *silver* fillings) used by dentists can contain up to 50 percent mercury. Many people in the dentistry community suggest that amalgam fillings are harmless, but in my opinion that's hard to believe when you consider that the Environmental Protection Agency (EPA) requires that when dentists remove amalgam fillings they treat the material as toxic waste.

If you need a filling, ask your dentist about alternatives to amalgam that don't contain mercury. Several options are available, and the choice is yours!

✓ **Coal:** Coal contains mercury, but chances are you don't often come in contact with coal. The problem arises when trillions of tons of coal are burned in coal-burning power plants across the globe each year, and the mercury that was contained in the coal is released into our atmosphere. The further you live from a coal-burning power plant the better, but if you're like most people and you can't let proximity to a power plant be the deciding factor when choosing where you live, consider using some of the air detoxification techniques I describe in Chapter 3.

✔ **Compact fluorescent light bulbs:** In an effort to conserve energy, many people are now installing efficient compact fluorescent light bulbs in their homes and businesses. The bulbs are extremely energy efficient, but unfortunately they contain mercury. When you dispose of compact fluorescent bulbs, place them in a plastic bag with a tight seal and take them to a nearby household hazardous waste collection site.

If a compact fluorescent bulb breaks, take special care to limit your mercury exposure. The EPA suggests that you immediately open all nearby windows and carefully sweep up the pieces without touching them with your hands. Then use a paper towel to remove all of the broken glass — do not use a vacuum — and place everything in a sealed plastic bag for disposal at a household hazardous waste collection site. You can read more at www.epa.gov.

Assessing the risks of aspartame

The sugar substitute aspartame is used in a wide range of processed food products, from diet sodas to chewing gum, and unfortunately there have been numerous implications that aspartame can have some harmful effects on the human body.

It's important to note here that aspartame was approved by the U.S. Food and Drug Administration (FDA) for use in food products. But anecdotal evidence and some clinical studies have suggested that for at least a portion of the population, aspartame could be responsible for negative health effects. Some of the anecdotal evidence points to the fact that aspartame can cause or contribute to thyroid problems, so if you're suffering from a thyroid ailment you should consider taking action to reduce the amount of aspartame you're introducing into your body. At the worst, you're looking at a "can't hurt, might help" scenario.

Detoxifying for aspartame

At this point, no detoxification methods focus specifically on removing aspartame from your body. But you can see some related benefits by adding lots of high antioxidant foods to your diet. The following are just a few of the many kinds of foods that are loaded with antioxidants:

✔ Artichokes

✔ Blackberries

✔ Cranberries

✔ Pecans

✔ Russet potatoes

✔ Walnuts

Avoiding aspartame

You can dodge this substance by paying attention to what you're eating. It's simple: Just read the ingredient lists on food labels!

If you're keen on sugar substitutes, I recommend trying stevia, which is a natural sweetener partly derived from a shrub that's native to South America. It has been used as a sweetener in Japan for more than 30 years. You can find stevia at almost all heath food stores, and it comes in many forms.

Giving your thyroid what it needs to succeed

Your thyroid needs a few minerals in order do its important work. The list below shows you the minerals that are critical to healthy thyroid function and includes suggestions on the types of foods you can eat to make sure you're getting enough of the important minerals.

- ✔ **Iodine:** Get iodine from sources like seafood (fish and shellfish) and sea vegetables (such as kelp, dulse, bladderwrack, and alaria).

  Many people get their iodine from iodized salt or from tap water. Be wary of both sources. Iodized salt usually has sugar added (dextrose) and can contain the toxin aluminum. And tap water has many toxic drawbacks, as you can read about in Chapter 3.

- ✔ **Copper:** Your thyroid needs copper, and you can make sure you're getting enough copper in your diet by eating plenty of eggs, legumes, nuts, and raisins. And no, you can't just toss in a handful of pennies with your garden salad.

- ✔ **Zinc:** Zinc is important for maintain healthy thyroid function. You can boost the amount of zinc in your diet by eating more oysters, dried beans, spinach, seeds, and nuts.

- ✔ **Selenium:** This mineral is particularly helpful in taming overactive thyroid glands. You can get more selenium by eating raw Brussels sprouts, cabbage, broccoli, and cauliflower.

Grasping Glucose Control

Maintaining healthy glucose (also known as *blood sugar*) levels in your body is a great way to ensure that you'll have the kind of energy that makes you feel like jumping out of bed in the morning, ready to take on the day. The amount of sugar that you bring into your body is almost entirely dependent upon your diet. If you make smart choices about the sugar you consume, you'll take an important step toward feeling good and staying healthy.

The problem, of course, is that sugar is delicious! And in a world full of sugar-filled, processed foods, it can be all too easy to let sugar creep into your diet in unhealthy and dangerous amounts. To help keep your hand out of the cookie jar, remember that in high enough amounts, sugar actually has a toxic effect on your body. In this section, I explain how sugar can act as a toxin, and I clue you in on how you can take steps to make sure your blood sugar stays at a level that makes you feel energetic but doesn't take you down a path that leads to diabetes and other sugar-related ailments.

Recognizing sugar as a toxin

When you look at a piece of candy, a soft drink, or a jelly donut, do you immediately think *toxin*? I know you may find it hard to believe, but the sugar that makes up a huge part of those types of sweet treats can have a toxic effect on your body's systems. A spoonful of sugar may help the medicine go down, but keep in mind that the reason you may need medicine in the first place is because you've had way too much sugar over the years.

High levels of blood sugar in your body have an inflammatory effect on your blood vessels. When you have high blood sugar, your body produces additional *insulin* (a hormone that helps your body move sugar into the tissue where it can be converted into energy). But if you have too much insulin in your system, the result is also inflamed blood vessels. In that respect, sugar and insulin can act just like many other toxins because the inflammation of your blood vessels is the start of a long, nasty process that includes the buildup of plaque, a decrease in blood flow, and damage to your organs. And I haven't even mentioned the many dangers of diabetes, which affects more than 20 million Americans. (If you'd like more information on diabetes, check out *Diabetes For Dummies,* 3rd Edition, by Dr. Alan Rubin [Wiley].)

But you do have to keep your blood sugar levels high enough to provide the fuel you need to keep your body working properly and leave you feeling energized. The brain does not keep any stored sugar reserves and operates directly off of the blood sugar, so maintaining constant blood sugar levels is extremely important. How can you tell when you've got the right amount of sugar in your system, and when you need to cut back on your sugar intake or risk damaging your health? For a few simple ways to keep tabs on your blood sugar; keep reading.

Keeping an eye on your sugar

A blood sugar level of 70–100 mg/dl (milligrams per deciliter of blood) is considered normal and healthy. If you keep an eye on the amount of sugar in your diet, you should have no problem staying within that range. Unfortunately, it's virtually impossible to accurately gauge your blood sugar levels based on how you feel. Luckily, though, you can use some very common tests to measure your blood sugar, including tests you can do yourself and tests that a doctor should administer.

Doing it yourself

If you'd like to monitor your blood sugar levels at home on your own, you can do so very easily with a blood glucose meter. You can buy a meter at your local drug store or from a wide variety of online retailers. Although each meter includes slightly different instructions for use, the basic steps are usually the same.

These instructions give you a general idea of what to expect if you choose to use a do-it-yourself blood glucose meter. But please be sure to read all the instructions for your meter because differences exist between devices that you'll need to take into account to ensure safety and an accurate reading.

1. **Turn on your meter.**

2. **Wash your hands with soap and warm water, and be sure to thoroughly clean the finger you plan to prick with the *lancet* (needle).**

3. **Insert a test strip in the meter and prick your finger with the lancet.**

4. **Put a drop of blood on the test strip and wait for the meter to display your results.**

If your blood sugar level falls in that ideal 70–100 mg/dl range, you can rest assured that you're doing a nice job of eating the right amount of sugar, and your energy levels should be good. If your blood sugar is in that range and you're still pooped all the time, be sure to read about the other possible causes for a lack of energy that I detail in this chapter.

If you're overweight, sedentary, or have a family history of diabetes, you should buy a blood glucose meter and check your levels periodically. If you don't eat anything for eight hours and your blood sugar is over 126 mg/dl, or if your blood sugar is over 200 mg/dl when you test two hours after a meal, you could have diabetes and you should make an appointment with your doctor immediately.

Getting tested by your doctor

In addition to the blood glucose meters that make it easy to keep an eye on your blood sugar levels by yourself, you can also visit your doctor for an even more accurate, comprehensive test. Scheduling a yearly hemoglobin A1c (HgbA1c) test is a good idea. This test shows you what your average blood sugar level has been for the previous three months. Your doctor should be happy to discuss the results with you, but keep in mind that you want your measurement to be less than 6.1. If you make that cut, you shouldn't be experiencing a lack of energy because of blood sugar concerns. However, keep in mind that a good test result doesn't guarantee you're not at risk for diabetes in the future.

If you visit your doctor for a blood glucose test, ask her to give you both a *fasting* and a *two-hour postprandial* blood sugar and insulin test. (The former is a test that is administered after you haven't eaten for eight hours, and the latter is administered exactly two hours after you eat a meal.) This combination of tests will give you a nice, full indication of your blood glucose and insulin levels and whether you have diabetes. Believe it or not, the fasting and two-hour postprandial insulin tests can detect sugar problems up to ten years before you become diabetic!

Solving your sugar problem

If your blood sugar levels are causing a health problem, you can use a variety of effective ways to get the problem under control. Luckily, these types of fixes will have a positive effect on your health in general, and they're quite easy to do.

Eating smaller portions more frequently

If you eat a small number of large meals (three or fewer) each day, you're probably forcing your body to accommodate sudden, sizable increases in sugar and carbohydrates. That situation creates a very unstable pattern for blood sugar levels, and the result can be big increases of energy followed by crashes. That's a blood sugar roller coaster that you don't want to be on if you're interested in keeping up a healthy, pleasant energy level throughout the day.

Fixing the problem is pretty simple: Eat more meals per day, and make sure they're smaller than the meals you were eating before. If you eat, say, five small meals a day instead of three big ones, you end up consuming about the same amount of food but your body has a much more constant supply of fuel, and the exhausting variations won't be nearly as much of an issue.

Avoiding unhealthy amounts of sugar

There's no better way to head sugar-related problems off at the pass than by curbing the amount of sugar and simple carbohydrates you include in your diet. Why do I include simple carbohydrates here? Consider this: Bread turns to sugar as soon as it hits the stomach; in terms of blood sugar levels, a slice of bread is no different than a spoonful of sugar. (Note that whole wheat bread, while healthier for you than white bread, is no different in terms of raising your blood sugar.) Limiting your sugar and simple carbohydrate intake can help give you healthy, steady energy throughout the day, and doing so also helps you avoid a lot of the common health problems that many Americans face. (Obesity and diabetes are prime examples.)

Dodging sugar can be harder than you think. Sugar is added to the majority of processed foods, and sugar can be listed lots of different ways in ingredients lists. If you see any of the following words listed as an ingredient, you're really just seeing another term for sugar:

- ✔ Dextrose
- ✔ Fructose
- ✔ Glucose
- ✔ High fructose corn syrup
- ✔ Sucrose

High fructose corn syrup can be particularly nasty, so do your best to avoid eating it. A recent U.S. Department of Agriculture study showed that 80 percent of high fructose corn syrup samples revealed the presence of mercury, which is one of the worst toxins out there.

You never know where a form of sugar is going to pop up. If you want a real shock, have a look at the ingredients on a container of iodized salt. You're almost guaranteed to see *dextrose* — a form of sugar — listed as one of the ingredients!

Seeking out the right foods

This may come as a surprise, but a diabetic diet is a good diet for anyone. Sugar is kept to a minimum in diabetic diets, and the basic food types that form the diet's foundation are vegetables (especially those with color), a variety of protein, and regular (but small) amounts of fruit. If you're faced with an overabundance of blood sugar, make sure those types of foods are the focus of your diet.

Several nutrients, minerals, spices, and herbs have also been shown to help regulate blood sugar levels. The following are just a few of many examples:

- ✔ **American ginseng:** This herb has shown promise for people interested in a very natural way to control blood sugar. You can buy American ginseng at vitamin or health food stores.

- ✔ **Chromium:** People who don't get enough chromium in their diets have been known to suffer from elevated glucose levels, and when their chromium levels are increased their blood sugar returns to normal. Make sure you're getting plenty of chromium by eating eggs, organic beef, cheese, and wine.

- ✔ **Cinnamon:** Recent studies have shown that 1 to 8 grams per day of cinnamon have helped to reduce blood sugar in diabetics. You can add cinnamon to many different kinds of foods, but don't even think about using cinnamon rolls as a source of cinnamon in your diet! To get enough, you need to supplement.

> ✔ **Vitamin E:** To up your vitamin E intake, eat more nuts, vegetable oils, and leafy vegetables. You'll help to control your blood sugar and, at the same time, boost your antioxidant levels. It's a win-win!

Getting plenty of exercise

I can't say enough good things about the tremendous health benefits you can enjoy if you exercise regularly. Exercising is critical for a healthy life, and it can even help lower your blood sugar levels. During exercise, muscles take sugar directly out of the bloodstream without insulin, which can go a long way toward limiting your glucose levels.

You don't have to do a triathlon or carry a log up the side of a mountain to help reduce your blood sugar levels with exercise. You can make quite a bit of positive progress by simply walking for 30 minutes at a fast pace every day.

Considering the Effects of Abnormal Bowel Flora

Your intestines are about 26 feet long and contain more than a trillion bacterial cells, called *bowel flora.* You have more bacterial cells inside you than you have human cells in your body. Most of these bacteria are *probiotics* (good bacteria), which help you break down food so you can absorb the nutrients. This bowel flora plays a major role in keeping you healthy, and if it gets disrupted by an increase in *abnormal bowel flora* (bacteria and other organisms in your gut that don't really belong there), the result can be all sorts of health problems, including severe fatigue.

Over the next few pages, I fill you in on abnormal bowel flora: the different types, the tests that can discover them, and how you can get rid of and avoid them. Your goal should be to eradicate the vast majority of abnormal bowel flora in your intestine because doing so will go a long way toward boosting your energy level.

Peeking at what's hiding in your gut

Even when you consider the jungles, deep forests, and coral reefs spread across the globe, very few places contain as wide a variety of living things as your intestines. The three major types of problem-causing abnormal bowel flora are yeast, parasites, and bad bacteria, and I give you the rundown on all three in this section. I also provide you with some ways to get rid of these critters.

As with many ailments, prevention is the best cure for abnormal bowel flora, so if you'd rather just find out how to avoid the problem, feel free to skip ahead to the "Avoiding abnormal bowel flora" section later in this chapter.

Yeast

Yeasts are microscopic organisms that are almost always present in your intestines. A certain type called *Candida* is extremely common, and if you have only small amounts of it among all the good bacteria in your intestines, it doesn't cause any trouble. But if you accidentally clear out a lot of your good bacteria, Candida suddenly has less competition and begins to multiply and grow. When that happens, Candida can hurt you in a lot of different ways, because it releases toxins that affect most of your body's systems. The following are just a few of the problems that can occur:

- ✔ Brain fog
- ✔ Constipation
- ✔ Irritable bowel syndrome
- ✔ Mouth and gum soreness
- ✔ Severe fatigue
- ✔ Urinary pain or itching

You can keep Candida and other yeasts in their place by using antibiotics only when really necessary and using probiotics when you do. Antibiotics don't just kill the bacteria that make you sick; they also kill the good bacteria in your intestines. After the good bacteria are gone, the yeasts suddenly have a lot more freedom, so they begin multiplying almost immediately.

If you've recently finished a round of antibiotics and you're suffering from some of the symptoms of a yeast problem, you can take steps to get the yeasts back under control. Cut your sugar and carbohydrate levels down to a minimum, and help support your good bacteria by eating yogurt or taking supplements that contain probiotics. One of the best supplements to take when taking antibiotics is Saccharomyces boulardii. If these steps don't help and you're still suffering from symptoms after a week, see a physician.

Sometimes the symptoms of a yeast problem can be severe and prolonged, and if that's the case it's time to schedule an appointment with your doctor. He can give you the tests I explain in the "Getting tested for abnormal bowel flora" section later in this chapter, and he can also prescribe medications that will help clear out the excess yeast.

Parasites

Parasites are organisms that can live in your body, feeding on the materials that your body uses to make energy. They rob you of your body's nutrients and cause all sorts of problems — including fatigue — but parasites usually don't kill you. They come in all shapes and varieties, including worms. (These worms are closer to the types that dogs and cats often suffer from than the worms that live in your garden and make good fishing bait.) Two of the most common types of human parasite worms are

- ✔ **Roundworms:** Also known as *Ascaris worms,* this parasite thrives in your intestine and is transmitted through fecal-oral contact (when people don't wash their hands thoroughly after coming in contact with human or animal feces, for example).

- ✔ **Tapeworms:** Several kinds of these nasty worms exist, and they're transmitted through undercooked beef, pork, and fish. They can grow to dozens of feet in length within your intestines.

But worms are only part of the picture. There are hundreds of different types of parasites and almost as many ways to contract them. Don't be surprised if you end up with a parasite at some point in your life. (Don't be embarrassed, either, because most people get at least one parasite and plenty of people suffer from several.) Parasites can be treated with prescription medications, which are generally very effective but can also be harsh and hard on the body. If you'd rather pursue a more natural solution, you can try adding wormwood, black walnut hulls, garlic, grapefruit seed extract, and pumpkin seeds to your diet. Talk to someone at your local health food store for more information on how to buy and use these materials.

Bad bacteria

As I mention at the start of this section, quite a lot of good, beneficial bacteria live in your intestine, and you need them to survive. Good bacteria help you to break down your food and make your digestive system more dynamic and versatile. But bad, abnormal types of intestinal bacteria exist, too, and if they end up in your intestine and multiply rapidly, you can easily suffer from energy levels that go crashing through the floor.

There are too many different types of abnormal bacteria to cover here, and several of these varieties are probably living in your intestine even as you read this. As with the yeasts I explain earlier in this chapter, the bad bacteria don't cause problems unless the good bacteria in your intestines are killed off. In that situation, the bad bacteria are suddenly left with less competition and can multiply. This situation can happen when you take antibiotics (because 80 percent of your good bacteria can be wiped out with a single round of antibiotics), and it can also be made worse when you consume contaminated food that contains relatively large amounts of bad bacteria.

Excessive amounts of bad bacteria in your intestine often cause gas that has a particularly foul smell. If you're suffering from extremely foul-smelling gas, please consider that you may have an overabundance of bad bacteria, and take some of the steps I describe in this section to correct the problem. You (and anyone you spend time with) will be happy you did.

The best way to rid yourself of bad bacteria is to overwhelm it with good bacteria. You can actually ingest good bacteria that will multiply and thrive when they reach your intestines. A couple examples of good bacteria are *lactobacillus acidophilus* and *lactobacillus bifidus.* You can add them to your diet by drinking acidophilus milk or by taking supplements that contain the bacteria, both of which are available at any health food store.

Getting tested for abnormal bowel flora

If you're experiencing the symptoms of a yeast, parasite, or bad bacteria problem, your doctor can test your urine and feces to help you figure out if you have a problem with abnormal bowel flora. Any general physician could do this type of testing, but most aren't familiar with the tests. Your best bet is to find a doctor who practices natural medicine. Go online and visit the Web sites for the American College for Advancement in Medicine (www.acamnet.org) or the International College of Integrative Medicine (www.icimed.com) to find a list of doctors who can help.

Stool sample tests

Stool samples can be analyzed for parasites, yeast, and abnormal bacteria. The process is simple: You provide a sample, and a lab examines the sample to determine if you have healthy or unusually high levels of abnormal bowel flora.

Urine tests

Abnormal bacteria and yeasts in your intestines produce chemicals that are absorbed into your bloodstream and eventually make their way out of your body through your urine. Lab tests can analyze your urine to detect these chemicals. If the chemicals are present in high enough quantities, you have a solid indication that you could be suffering from an overabundance of abnormal bowel flora. Unfortunately, these types of urine tests (and the stool tests I describe in the previous paragraph) aren't usually covered by health insurance plans.

Avoiding abnormal bowel flora

Hands down, the best way to deal with an abnormal bowel flora problem is to never get a problem in the first place. If you can prevent yeasts, parasites, and bad bacteria from getting out of control, you've taken an important step to fight off fatigue. Keep in mind that you must have a very acidic stomach to keep normal bowel flora. (See Chapter 4 for a complete discussion of the importance of stomach acid.)

Washing and cooking your food

Your food is by no means sterile, and although your stomach acid kills a lot of potentially problematic bowel flora, you need to make sure you're washing and cooking your food. All fruits and vegetables should be washed thoroughly. All meats should be cooked through, and be sure to wash any utensil used on uncooked meat before using it on other foods.

Finding foods that can help

You can make some simple food choices that will help to limit growth of abnormal bowel flora and promote the health of probiotics. Include plenty of vegetables in your diet, and focus on greens, tomatoes, celery, broccoli, cauliflower, asparagus, and beans.

To get the maximum health benefit from your vegetables, eat fresh, 100 percent organic products whenever you can. If you're not able to eat fresh vegetables, the next best option is frozen, followed by canned (a distant third).

Any meat you consume should be well cooked, or you risk introducing a whole host of parasites into your system. If you can, buy free-range meat and check to see that it was produced without antibiotics or growth hormones.

Seeking the right supplements

Supplements can be a good way for you to boost the amount of probiotics in your intestine, which can thwart unhealthy increases in abnormal bowel flora. These supplements are taken orally, and you can find them at health food stores or at reputable online retailers. You can try one or a combination of the following:

- ✔ Acidophilus
- ✔ Bifidus
- ✔ Saccharomyces

All three have technical-sounding names, but they're common supplements and pretty easy to find.

Recipes for Boosting Your Energy Level

Following are some easy recipes that can help you increase and maintain your energy level.

⟁ Mixed Green Salad with Cinnamon Almonds

Almonds, vegetable oil, and dark leafy greens are high in Vitamin E, a crucial component of the detox diet and an important nutrient. The nuts are toasted and tossed with cinnamon and stevia to glaze. They make a perfect finishing touch to a simple salad with a slightly spicy dressing.

Preparation time: *15 minutes*

Cooking time: *5–7 minutes*

Yield: *4–6 servings*

3/4 cup sliced almonds	*1 teaspoon minced ginger root*
1 tablespoon vegetable oil	*Pinch organic sea salt*
1 teaspoon cinnamon	*Pinch cayenne pepper*
1/4 teaspoon stevia	*2 cups organic baby beet greens*
1/3 cup olive oil	*2 cups organic baby spinach leaves*
3 tablespoons apple cider vinegar	*1 cup organic arugula*
1/4 teaspoon stevia	*1 cup torn organic romaine lettuce*
1/2 teaspoon cinnamon	

1 In small saucepan, combine almonds with oil. Toast over medium-low heat until almonds are fragrant, 5–7 minutes. Remove to small bowl; sprinkle with 1 teaspoon cinnamon and 1/4 teaspoon stevia; toss to mix and let cool.

2 In serving bowl, beat together 1/3 cup oil, vinegar, 1/4 teaspoon stevia, 1/2 teaspoon cinnamon, ginger root, salt, and cayenne pepper until blended. Add greens; toss to coat. Sprinkle with almonds and serve immediately.

Per serving: *Calories 308 (From Fat 274); Fat 31g (Saturated 3g); Cholesterol 0mg; Sodium 133mg; Carbohydrate 8g; Dietary Fiber 4g; Protein 5g.*

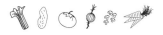

☞ Herbed Greek Yogurt Omelet

Your body needs chromium to regulate metabolism and blood sugar levels. This nutrient is found in eggs and cheese. This easy and flavorful omelet is a great way to start your day, or you can serve it for a late-night dinner with the mixed green salad.

Preparation time: *7 minutes*

Cooking time: *7 minutes*

Yield: *4 servings*

2 ripe organic tomatoes, chopped	*1 teaspoon minced fresh rosemary*
2 tablespoons lemon juice	*2 tablespoons minced parsley*
1/2 cucumber, peeled, seeded, and chopped	*1/4 teaspoon organic sea salt*
2 green onions, sliced	*1/8 teaspoon pepper*
1 minced jalapeno pepper, if desired	*1 tablespoon vegetable oil*
8 organic eggs	*2 cloves garlic, minced*
1/2 cup plain organic yogurt	*1/2 cup crumbled organic feta cheese (or 1 cup shredded kasseri cheese)*
1 tablespoon minced fresh fennel fronds	

1 In small bowl, combine tomatoes, lemon juice, cucumber, green onions, and jalapeno; mix well and set aside.

2 Combine eggs, yogurt, fennel, rosemary, parsley, salt, and pepper in medium bowl; beat until combined.

3 In 10" to 12" saucepan, heat oil over medium heat. Add garlic; cook and stir for 1 minute until fragrant. Add egg mixture to saucepan and let cook without stirring for 1 minute.

4 Shake pan gently and as the omelet sets, lift the edges so uncooked portion of eggs can flow underneath. When the omelet is almost set but still moist, sprinkle cheese evenly on surface.

5 Remove pan from heat and cover for 1 minute, then fold omelet in half and slide onto serving plate. Garnish with more parsley and fennel fronds, if desired, and serve with tomato mixture.

Per serving: *Calories 275 (From Fat 170); Fat 19g (Saturated 7g); Cholesterol 446mg; Sodium 504mg; Carbohydrate 10g; Dietary Fiber 1g; Protein 17g.*

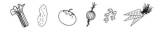

Ginseng Wine Punch

The fleshy root of the American Ginseng plant can be used in many ways. The root itself can be simmered to make tea, or it can be dried and ground into a powder that can be added to many foods. Ginseng can boost your immune system and helps eliminate fatigue due to the body's reaction to stress.

Preparation time: *20 minutes*

Cooking time: *15 minutes*

Chilling time: *3–5 hours*

Yield: *8–10 servings*

2 quarts purified water	1 organic orange, washed and thinly sliced
10 (1/8-inch thick) slices American ginseng root	1/2 organic lemon, washed and thinly sliced
1 bottle rose wine	3 cups sparkling water
1/2 teaspoon stevia	

1 Place purified water in a stainless steel or glass saucepan and bring to a boil. Add the ginseng slices, reduce the heat to low, cover, and simmer for 15 minutes. Strain the liquid, discarding the ginseng, and let cool for 1 hour.

2 Add the wine and stevia to taste. Pour into a pitcher, add sliced oranges and lemons, cover, and chill for 2–4 hours until cold. Just before serving, add the sparkling water and serve.

Per serving: *Calories 75 (From Fat 0); Fat 0g (Saturated 0g); Cholesterol 0mg; Sodium 5mg; Carbohydrate 4g; Dietary Fiber 1g; Protein 0g.*

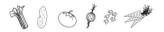

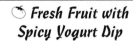

Fresh Fruit with Spicy Yogurt Dip

Kids love any type of dip; it turns ordinary fruit and vegetables into party food. This method of straining yogurt makes "yogurt cheese" that can be used as a substitute for cream cheese in recipes. Yogurt contains *probiotics:* good bacteria that can help boost your immune system.

Preparation time: *8 hours (for straining the yogurt)*

Chilling time: *2–3 hours*

Yield: *6 servings*

2 cups plain organic yogurt	1/4 teaspoon stevia
2 tablespoons orange juice	Fresh pineapple slices
1/2 teaspoon turmeric	Sliced, peeled kiwi fruit
1/2 teaspoon cinnamon	Fresh pear slices

1 Line a fine sieve with cheesecloth and add yogurt. Place in medium bowl, cover, and refrigerate overnight. Reserve the thin liquid, or whey, for use in soups or baking. Alternatively, you can substitute thick Greek organic yogurt for the plain yogurt and omit the straining step.

2 Place the thick yogurt in a small bowl. Add orange juice, turmeric, cinnamon, and stevia; mix well. Cover and chill the dip for 2–3 hours to blend flavors. Serve dip with fresh fruit.

Per serving: Calories 54 (From Fat 24); Fat 3g (Saturated 2g); Cholesterol 11mg; Sodium 38mg; Carbohydrate 5g; Dietary Fiber 0g; Protein 3g.

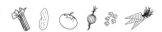

Chapter 12

Fighting Allergies

Allergies are an extremely common health problem. About 55 percent of all Americans have a reaction to at least one allergen, and about $18 billion per year is spent on diagnosing, treating, and preventing allergies. What's worse is that hundreds of deaths occur each year because of extreme allergies to certain foods, stinging insects, and medicines like penicillin. Maybe the most worrying statistic of all is that allergies are becoming more common: The presence of allergies in the U.S. population has increased by 300 percent since 1960.

Allergies are a result of the immune system reacting in an unusual way to some substance — an *allergen* — that has entered the body. The unpleasant and in some cases dangerous symptoms that come along with allergies all start with your immune system, so keeping that critical part of your body healthy is terrifically important when it comes to reining in allergy problems. (I talk all about the immune system in Chapter 10, and all the rules I explain there certainly apply here.)

Toxins wreak havoc on every part of your body, and your immune system is no exception. An increased amount of toxins in your body can throw a wrench in your immune function, which can make you more prone to the ravages of allergies. If you have allergies, you need to focus on cutting out toxins and taking steps to improve your immune system now. You also want to embrace a few allergy-fighting techniques. I cover all these bases in this chapter.

To figure out just how much of an allergy problem you may have, take a few minutes to go through the allergy quiz included in Chapter 8.

Covering Allergy Basics

Allergies are caused when your immune system has a response to an allergen. I won't go into all the nitty gritty details of an allergic reaction because it involves more technical information than you really want to know. Here's the short version: You end up with a reaction when your immune system identifies and responds to an allergen in a way that, through a series of steps, gives you elevated levels of certain chemicals — *histamine* is the main one — in your bloodstream, and these chemicals cause allergy symptoms. The symptoms are wide ranging and can affect many areas of your body, including the following:

- **Eyes:** Itching, burning, redness, watering, *allergic shiners* (a dark or blue hue under the eyes), blurred or double vision

- **Mouth:** Sores, constant bad taste, trouble swallowing

- **Sinuses:** Itching or runny/stuffy nose, recurrent infections, pain, sneezing, decreased smell

- **Ears:** Recurrent infections, sensitivity to sound, ringing, pain, clogged feeling, itching

- **Lungs:** Shortness of breath, tight chest, cough, excessive phlegm — and even complete swelling of the throat that stops breathing

- **Cardiovascular system:** Heart pain, palpitations or irregular beat, high or low blood pressure, inflammation of arteries or veins

- **Stomach and intestines:** Bloating, gas, heartburn, nausea, constipation or diarrhea, ulcers, irritable bowel, spasms, Crohn's disease, ulcerative colitis

- **Muscles:** Inflammation, tremors, weakness, stiffness, pain

- **Joints:** Stiffness, swelling, pain, arthritis

- **Skin:** Rash, itching, swelling, redness, perspiration, eczema

The vast number of symptoms caused by allergic reactions is matched only by the hundreds of different kinds of allergens that are commonly found in the world around you. I don't have room to list all the allergens out there, but here are some of the most common offenders:

- **Pollen:** Many different kinds are released by a variety of plants, from weeds to trees.

- **Mold:** Lots of different types of molds cause allergic reactions.

- **Drugs:** Some drugs can cause an allergic response in humans; antibiotics like penicillin are among the most common drug allergens.

Itching to control the poison ivy allergy

One of the most common allergies of all is an allergy to poison ivy. The resin on the poison ivy plant causes an itchy, burning rash on the skin of most people, and a prevalent misconception only makes the problem worse. Let me clear things up: Poison ivy does not spread. If you're exposed to it and you get an allergic reaction, the resulting rash can't spread to other parts of your body (or to other people). After you shower with hot soapy water, all the poison ivy resin is gone from your body.

So how does poison ivy get from one place to another? The problem is usually large amounts of poison ivy resin that remain on clothes, shoes, and other items after the exposure has taken place. If you get the resin on your shoes,

the next morning you can put your shoes on and get the resin on your hands, which you can then rub on your neck, arms, or even your eyes. That action spreads the resin all over, and the rash spreads with it. The resin off the plant can stay active for three weeks.

It's easy to beat this common allergic reaction. If you find that you've gotten into some poison ivy, take off your clothes and wash them with lots of detergent and hot water. Then take a long, hot, soapy shower and don't miss any spots when you're washing. After the shower, put on fresh gloves and wash everything that may have come in contact with the resin, including shoes, belts, hats, watches, glasses, tools, and even pets.

 ✔ **Animal dander:** *Dander* is made up of scales of old animal skin, which slough off and are inhaled through breathing. Many people assume that pet hair or fur causes allergies to animals like cats or dogs, but dander is the real culprit.

 ✔ **Latex rubber:** Sources include gloves, balloons, and condoms.

 ✔ **Foods:** Allergic reactions to certain foods are a concern for millions of people. Common food allergens include shellfish, peanuts, dairy products, eggs, and gluten.

If you think you're having an allergic reaction to a food, don't immediately focus on a food that you've just eaten or one that you've had for the first time. Reactions because of food allergens can be delayed, so think about what you've eaten over the course of the last two or three days. And you can't be allergic to something the first time you're exposed to it; your immune system has to be exposed at least one previous time before it goes haywire and causes an allergy. Instead, focus on foods that you have had a limited number of times in the past and eaten again recently.

Many people assume that allergies are inherited, but that's only partly true. Research has shown that the tendency to develop allergies is influenced by heredity, but being allergic to a specific allergen isn't inherited. So if one or both of your parents had allergies, you're more likely to have them. But if your mom or dad is allergic to ragweed, that doesn't mean you will be allergic to ragweed — just that the chances are greater you'll develop an allergy to something.

If you have a new baby or you're expecting one, you can limit the baby's chances of developing allergies by breastfeeding. Infants often develop food allergies because they're exposed to food too early in life. Infants don't start making digestive enzymes to break down food other than breast milk until they're about 1 year old, and introducing those foods can contribute to the development of allergies.

Maintaining a healthy digestive tract can help you to avoid allergies. When your intestines are irritated or inflamed by toxins, they can malfunction and leak allergens into your bloodstream. Read up about how to keep your intestines healthy and toxin-free in Chapters 4 and 5.

Nothing to Sneeze At: Supplements for Beating Allergies

Years ago, the wholesome, natural foods that people ate were high-quality and nutrient-rich enough to provide the substances necessary to keep their immune systems healthy and less likely to get out of whack, so allergy problems were less common. In the last 100 years or so, however, the quality of our food has gone way down and the amount of toxins in the environment has shot through the roof. One of the results is a dramatic increase in the number of people who suffer from allergies.

If you have problems with allergies and you want to solve them the natural way, adjust your diet accordingly — that's the focus of the next section — and consider taking some supplements to expedite the process. In this section, I present two different categories of supplements that can help tame your allergies: supplements that give your immune system the kind of kick in the pants it needs to perform efficiently and not create allergy issues, and supplements that help you to keep existing allergy problems under control.

Energizing immunity

Because your immune system's response is the root of your allergies, it pays to take supplements that keep your immune system from getting out of whack. A range of products is on the market, but I'm a fan of the following options, which are widely available both at health food stores and online. (For some basic information on how to pick out safe, high-quality supplements, be sure to visit Chapter 5.)

- **American skullcap:** 1–2 grams per day

- **Astragalus:** 250–500 mg per day

- **Devils claw:** 600–1,200 mg per day

- **Evening primrose:** 2–8 grams daily

- **Folic acid:** 800 micrograms per day

- **Gamma-linolenic acid:** 2,800 mg per day in several divided doses

- **Licorice:** 250–500 mg three times per day

- **Omega-3 fatty acids:** 1–4 grams per day

- **Quercetin:** 50–200 mg three times a day

- **Spirulina:** 2,000–3,000 mg per day

In Chapter 10, I sing the praises of concentrated antioxidant supplement powders, which are commonly called *greens.* They're terrific for your immune system and can therefore help you to get your allergy problems under control. Make sure you look for products that have an ORAC of at least 20,000 per scoop in powder form.

Helping to keep allergies under control

In addition to the supplements listed in the previous section, which will keep your immune system humming along as it should, you can also try taking some supplements that have been shown to help nip allergy problems in the bud. I list some of the most promising options here. These supplements are good for sinus-type problems but also help with any allergic reaction:

- **Butterbur:** Recent studies have shown that tablets made from this herb can treat allergy symptoms as well as some of the common prescription allergy drugs that have become increasingly popular in recent years.

- **Goldenseal:** Natural compounds in the root of the goldenseal plant can help with your allergies. Look for capsules containing goldenseal, and take the supplement according to the dosage recommendations on the product label.

- **Stinging nettle:** As you can tell by its name, the stinging nettle plant isn't something you want to encounter when you're walking through the woods or on a creek bank. But when its leaves and roots are freeze-dried and packaged in capsule form, the plant can help you fight seasonal allergies. You should be able to find several varieties at your favorite health food store or at a shop that specializes in vitamins or supplements.

Controlling Allergies with Smart Food Decisions

The food choices you make can have a tremendous impact on your allergies. Of course, when it comes to food allergies, the choices you make about what you eat can be a matter of life or death (in extreme cases). But even with more common allergies, like pet or seasonal allergies, you can make a lot of headway just by picking out the right food options.

As always, the general rules for food apply: Avoid toxins by cutting out processed foods, skip on foods that contain additives, and eat organic whenever possible (remembering that 100 percent organic is the best). Just taking these steps can do you a world of good because you'll eliminate the toxic load from your diet and greatly reduce the stress you put on your immune system. Here are a few examples of healthful foods that will help you keep your body in tip-top shape and less likely to fall prey to uncomfortable and dangerous allergies:

- **Fish and fish oil:** Be sure to keep in mind — and avoid — the types of fish that commonly contain mercury. (See Chapter 2 for details.)
- **Fruits:** Apples, blueberries, and papaya are a great place to start.
- **Green vegetables:** Try broccoli, spinach, Brussels sprouts, and asparagus.
- **Orange or yellow vegetables:** Carrots, squash, peppers, and pumpkin are just a few examples.

Choosing locally grown or produced foods is another way to lessen your allergy troubles. One of the top choices is local honey, made by bees that live in your area. This may sound a little farfetched, but local honey can help you with your allergies. All honey contains very small amounts of pollen, which bees constantly bring back to their hives after visiting hundreds and thousands of plants to collect the nectar that provides their food source. Local honey contains trace amounts of the types of pollen that are most common in your area — the pollens that cause your seasonal allergies to flare up twice a year (or more for some people). When you eat the honey, you expose your body to just a little bit of the pollen — not too much. Over time, your immune system figures out how to deal with these allergens in a healthy, normal way, instead of going haywire and causing dreadful allergy symptoms like sneezing, wheezing, and itchy eyes.

Even if you haven't had problems with food allergies in the past, it always helps to be alert when you're eating top offenders like milk, wheat (gluten), eggs, peanuts, shellfish, soy, and tree nuts. If you experience troubling allergy symptoms after consuming these types of foods, consult your doctor. You can also read up with *Food Allergies For Dummies* by Robert A. Wood, MD and Joe Kraynak (Wiley).

Recipes for Getting Your Allergies under Control

Fighting allergies with food can be effective and also extremely enjoyable. The recipes in this section will please your palate and also help to keep your allergy troubles at bay.

◌ *Sweet Apple Dip*

Everyone loves apples, and they're easy to use in recipes. They provide a good amount of soluble and insoluble fiber, as well as pectin, which helps lower LDL cholesterol. Apples also contain quercetin, an antioxidant that fights free radicals that lead to disease and aging. Children with asthma who eat apples and drink apple juice have less wheezing.

Serve this dip with more apples and other fruits and vegetables, like carrots, pear slices, and kiwifruit.

Preparation time: *5 minutes*

Chilling time: *2–3 hours*

Yield: *4–6 servings*

2 large organic apples, grated

2 tablespoons freshly squeezed lemon juice

1 tablespoon honey

1/2 teaspoon cinnamon

1/4 teaspoon turmeric

1/4 teaspoon stevia

1 cup organic or homemade applesauce

1 Toss grated apples with lemon juice, then mix with all other ingredients in a medium bowl. Serve immediately with other fruits and vegetables, or cover and chill for 2–3 hours.

Per serving: *Calories 108 (From Fat 4); Fat 0g (Saturated 0g); Cholesterol 0mg; Sodium 2mg; Carbohydrate 29g; Dietary Fiber 4g; Protein 0g.*

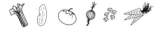

Garlic Salmon Vegetable Salad

If you have food allergies, you need to avoid certain foods. Never eat the specific food you are allergic to, of course, but also make sure to avoid caffeine, sugar, and alcohol. The most allergenic foods include eggs, soy, wheat, tree nuts, peanuts, milk, and shellfish. Luckily, there are many foods you can eat!

Vegetables and fruits, along with salmon, local honey, and tea, are all excellent sources of nutrients, especially omega-3 fatty acids. You'll start feeling better when eating to detox your body.

Preparation time: *20 minutes*

Cooking time: *7 minutes*

Yield: *4 servings*

5 tablespoons extra virgin olive oil	*5 cloves organic garlic, peeled and minced*
2 tablespoons flaxseed oil	*1 pound wild Alaskan salmon*
1/3 cup freshly squeezed orange juice	*1 organic red bell pepper, chopped*
2 tablespoons freshly squeezed lemon juice	*1 organic yellow bell pepper, chopped*
1 tablespoon mustard	*8 ounces organic button mushrooms, sliced*
1/8 teaspoon cayenne pepper	*4 cups dark leafy organic greens*
1 tablespoon fresh thyme leaves	*1 cup mung bean sprouts*
2 tablespoons olive oil	

1 In small bowl, combine extra virgin olive oil, flaxseed oil, orange juice, lemon juice, mustard, cayenne pepper, and thyme; mix well and set aside.

2 Heat 2 tablespoons olive oil in skillet over medium heat. Add garlic; cook 1 minute. Then add salmon; sauté 4 minutes, then turn. Sauté 2–3 minutes longer until just cooked. Remove salmon and garlic from heat; let cool 10 minutes. Break salmon into chunks.

3 Combine salmon with bell peppers and mushrooms in large bowl; pour dressing over all. Toss to mix. Serve on greens; garnish with sprouts.

Per serving: *Calories 469 (From Fat 319); Fat 35g (Saturated 5g); Cholesterol 53mg; Sodium 180mg; Carbohydrate 13g; Dietary Fiber 3g; Protein 27g.*

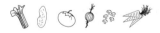

☙ Stir-Fried Vegetables on Quinoa

Stir-frying is a very quick and healthy way of cooking. Before you start to stir-fry, make sure all the ingredients are prepped and ready to use. There's no time to stop and prepare an ingredient while things are hopping in the wok!

In this recipe you can substitute long grain brown organic rice for the quinoa if you'd like, but do try the quinoa. It's nutty and mild and contains all the amino acids your body needs.

Preparation time: *20 minutes*

Cooking time: *35 minutes*

Yield: *4 servings*

1 cup quinoa, rinsed	*2 organic carrots, sliced*
2 cups filtered water	*1 cup organic green beans, cut into 1/2-inch pieces*
2 tablespoons olive oil	*1/2 cup filtered water*
1 organic yellow onion, peeled and chopped	*2 tablespoons apple cider vinegar*
3 cloves organic garlic, peeled and minced	*2 tablespoons honey*
2 tablespoons grated fresh ginger root	*1/8 teaspoon cayenne pepper*
2 cups organic Brussels sprouts, quartered	*1 cup organic broccoli or mung bean sprouts*
1 head organic broccoli, cut into florets	

1 In saucepan, combine quinoa and 2 cups filtered water; bring to a boil. Reduce heat, cover pan, and simmer 15–18 minutes until quinoa is tender; set aside.

2 Meanwhile, prepare all the vegetables. In large skillet or wok, heat olive oil over medium-high heat. Add onion and garlic; stir-fry 2 minutes. Add ginger root, Brussels sprouts, broccoli, carrots, and beans; stir-fry 5–6 minutes until crisp-tender.

3 Combine 1/2 cup water, vinegar, honey, and cayenne pepper in small bowl; stir well and add to skillet with sprouts. Stir-fry 3–4 minutes until liquid thickens slightly. Serve over quinoa.

Per serving: *Calories 342 (From Fat 89); Fat 10g (Saturated 1g); Cholesterol 0mg; Sodium 61mg; Carbohydrate 57g; Dietary Fiber 9g; Protein 11g.*

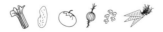

☝ Honeyed Pineapple Rice Pudding

Rice pudding is a creamy, rich, and comforting dessert that almost anyone with allergies can eat. You can omit the pineapple if you are allergic to it, or you can simply substitute another fruit. Rice milk is easily found in most grocery stores. Be sure to look for a 100 percent organic variety.

Eating locally produced honey may actually help relieve allergy symptoms. Honey is an immune system booster and may work like a vaccination, helping your body become accustomed to the allergens in the air and environment. Be sure you aren't allergic to honey before you eat it or use it in a health regimen.

Don't give honey to infants, as it can contain a certain kind of bacteria that is harmless to adults but can make infants extremely ill.

Preparation time: *10 minutes*

Cooking time: *1 hour 40 minutes*

Yield: *6 servings*

1 cup long grain organic brown rice	*1/3 cup local organic honey*
2 cups filtered water	*1 tablespoon grated fresh ginger root*
2 cups cubed fresh organic pineapple	*1 teaspoon cinnamon*
1 1/2 cups organic pineapple juice	*1/4 teaspoon stevia*
3 cups organic rice milk	*1 teaspoon vanilla*

1 In medium saucepan, combine rice with filtered water. Bring to a boil, reduce heat, cover, and simmer 45–60 minutes until rice is tender.

2 Combine cooked rice, pineapple, juice, rice milk, honey, ginger root, and cinnamon in a large saucepan. Cook over medium heat 30–40 minutes, stirring frequently, until very thick. Stir in stevia and vanilla, remove from heat, and serve warm or cold.

Per serving: *Calories 307 (From Fat 20); Fat 2g (Saturated 0g); Cholesterol 0mg; Sodium 50mg; Carbohydrate 69g; Dietary Fiber 4g; Protein 5g.*

Chapter 13

Improving Circulation

Cardiovascular disease is the number one cause of death in the United States. The numbers are staggering: Recent years have seen deaths from cardiovascular causes nearing the 1 million mark, and more than 16 million people alive today have had a heart attack or significant *angina* (heart pain). Almost 6 million of those have had heart failure.

All this suffering and death due to ailments of the heart and the rest of the circulatory system are even scarier when you consider that just over 100 years ago, heart disease wasn't even in the top ten causes of death. What is causing such a high rate of cardiovascular disease today that wasn't present in 1900? A lot of things have changed since then, of course, but one of the major changes in terms of health and our environment is an unprecedented influx of toxins in our food, air, and water.

In this chapter, I present some information that could very well conflict with what you've heard in the past about circulatory problems and cardiovascular disease. I urge you to keep an open mind and consider that conventional medicine may be going about this extremely important fight in the wrong way; we may be focusing too much on potential causes of these diseases that aren't as significant as we once thought. Keep reading to find out more and to discover what you can do to avoid this ubiquitous killer.

Focusing on Blood Vessel Inflammation

The major contributing factor in lousy circulation and cardiovascular disease is the development of plaque in the arteries. I'm not talking about the kind of plaque that can form on your teeth (and certainly not about the kind you receive onstage at an awards ceremony). The plaque that forms in your arteries is made up of cholesterol and calcium. Over time, it can grow and eventually get big enough to close off a blood vessel to the point where the tissue downstream doesn't get enough blood to function. Or, the plaque can break apart and cause a plug in an artery with a clot.

When people hear about arterial plaque, most of them immediately assume that cholesterol is the problem — after all, we've been conditioned by news reports and millions of drug company marketing dollars to think of cholesterol as the primary cause of cardiovascular disease and circulatory system problems. (I cover the cholesterol question in detail a little later in this chapter.) But here's a key question: Is the arterial plaque the root of the problem, or is it the result of another, underlying problem?

For some reason, the most popular line of reasoning in the medical field is that we shouldn't be looking at why plaque develops; instead, we should focus on how to get rid of the plaque or the basic materials your body uses to make the plaque (calcium and cholesterol). But that approach doesn't really solve the problem. We need to understand the reasons the body is trying to form plaque in the first place.

A growing body of evidence indicates that the initial cause for a plaque to develop is blood vessel inflammation. This inflammation can be caused by a lot of different things, and one of them is — you guessed it — toxins. Toxic materials, including heavy metals, chemicals, and biologic toxins (like bacteria and yeast), can all cause inflammation. In fact, all the toxins I cover in Chapters 2 and 3 can cause inflammation to some degree, which can lead to the buildup of plaque in the arteries and a slow-down in blood flow.

To make sure you're getting screened properly for cardiovascular disease and potential problems with circulation, ask your doctor to do a *c-reactive protein* (CRP) test when you schedule your next checkup. A highly sensitive cardiac CRP test measures inflammation in your blood vessels and is the best way to detect potential problems with your circulatory system. The test is common, and just about any medical lab can perform one. Multiple studies have shown CRP to be more predictive of who is going to have a heart attack than cholesterol.

Pinpointing Toxins That Hinder Circulation

In this section, I give you the rundown of how specific toxins can affect your blood vessels and your heart.

Feeling the strain from heavy metals

Heavy metals earn their name because their weight is at least five times the weight of water. A handful of heavy metals are required for normal health; zinc and copper are two examples. But most heavy metals are toxic in any amount. The most toxic heavy metals include mercury, lead, antimony, arsenic, cadmium, excessive iron, aluminum, and nickel, and they all wreak havoc on your cardiovascular system. Here are some of their effects:

- ✔ **Aluminum** and **iron** in high levels can cause damage to blood vessel linings.

- ✔ **Arsenic** causes major blood vessel inflammation.

- ✔ **Cadmium** causes high blood pressure and can enlarge the heart and inflame the blood vessels.

- ✔ **Lead** is also known to cause high blood pressure, which is a leading cause of cardiovascular damage.

- ✔ **Nickel** produces inflammation of the blood vessels and has been identified as being a cause of heart attacks.

The heavy metals in this list are very hard on your circulatory system, but they pale in comparison to mercury. For humans, mercury is the most toxic non-radioactive substance on the planet. I cover mercury's effects in several places throughout this book, but for the purposes of this chapter it's important that you know mercury is extremely toxic to the blood vessels and to the heart muscle itself.

One recent study looked at patients with a dangerous condition called *enlarged heart* and found that they had mercury levels in their heart muscles that were 22,000 times higher than patients with normal hearts.

Mercury can be extremely damaging to your heart. Studies of patients with elevated mercury levels have revealed increased heart attacks, abnormal electrocardiograms, rapid heartbeat, premature heartbeats, and inflammation of the heart muscle. Despite all this evidence, most cardiologists don't pay much attention to mercury.

If you or someone in your family is suffering from heart disease, be sure to talk with your cardiologist about getting tested for mercury toxicity. Just be sure that you get a proactive urine test instead of a blood test, because mercury stays in the blood for only a few days before it goes into your tissue.

In addition to its direct effects on the circulatory system, mercury can also cause loads of indirect negative effects. For instance, mercury can greatly damage the thyroid, and an out-of-whack thyroid is a huge strain on the heart. (Read all about the ways in which mercury can harm your thyroid in Chapter 11.) Mercury can also bond with insulin and contribute to diabetes, which is a major stressor on the heart and blood vessels. As if that weren't enough, mercury fouls up the function of your pituitary gland, which plays a critical role in regulating your blood pressure.

Here are a few other common diseases and conditions that mercury contributes to. All these ailments have either direct or indirect consequences for your heart and the rest of your circulatory system:

- Alzheimer's disease
- Amyotrophic lateral sclerosis (Lou Gehrig's disease)
- Autism
- Candida overgrowth syndrome
- Chronic fatigue syndrome
- Colitis of any type
- Crohn's disease
- Fibromyalgia
- Gastritis
- Graves' disease
- Multiple sclerosis
- Myasthenia gravis
- Obsessive compulsive disorder
- Panic disorder
- Parkinson's disease
- Rheumatoid arthritis
- Sjogren's disease
- Systemic lupus erythematosus

Mercury is a tremendous risk to your health, and you need to take an active role in limiting your exposure to it. Flip back to Chapter 2 to get the skinny on where mercury comes from, and read through Chapter 3 to begin your understanding of how you can avoid eating, drinking, and breathing it in.

Looking at reactive oxygen species

Many of the toxins that I cover throughout this book fall in the category of *reactive oxygen species* (ROS): a large group of chemicals that contain oxygen and can cause damaging effects to your body's cells and tissues. ROS can have a particularly nasty effect on the lining of your blood vessels. Inflammation occurs as a result, and when that happens your body starts building plaque in an effort to cope with the inflammation. Before you know it, you have cardiovascular disease. Clearly it's in your best interest to limit the amount of ROS in your system and to limit the negative impact of the ROS already present inside you.

You won't ever be able to cut out all the ROS because certain types are made by your body through its natural chemical processes. Even before the levels of toxins in our environment shot through the roof in the last century or so, people had some ROS in their bodies. That wasn't much of an issue, however, because humans are able to deal with a certain level of ROS with antioxidants, assuming that proper diet and nutrition are in place.

But we live in an era of extremely high toxicity, and the ROS levels that most people are exposed to are much too high for their bodies to handle. ROS can come from fertilizers, pesticides, food additives, food packaging, household cleaning products, and aerosols, just to name a few sources. Your body can get overwhelmed, and the problem can snowball if you're not eating the right kind of diet and getting loads of antioxidants to help your body fight the good fight. The results are often devastating, and some of your body's systems and tissues are more vulnerable than others. Your circulatory system is very sensitive to ROS.

An increasing amount of evidence points to the fact that the inflammation that leads to the buildup of plaque in the blood vessels, which causes cardiovascular disease, begins with toxic threats like those posed by reactive oxygen species. You need to start cutting down on the amount of toxins you're exposed to immediately (see Chapter 3) and do what you can to clear out the toxins that are already in your body (Chapter 5 offers plenty of good starting points).

Understanding the Many Levels of Toxic Damage to Your Circulatory System

In addition to directly damaging the major components of your circulatory system — your blood vessels and your heart — toxins can also contribute to problems in other areas of your body that cause indirect harm to your cardiovascular health. Three such problems are stress on your adrenal glands, changes to the way your body handles glucose, and dangerous fluctuations in your blood pressure. In this section, you get a feel for how toxins can cause indirect (but significant) damage to your body's delicate circulatory system.

Stressing the adrenal glands

You have a couple of adrenals glands — one on top of each kidney. Most people don't think much about their adrenal glands, but they do a lot of very important things for you. Your adrenal glands produce some hormones that you simply can't live without, and all these hormones have an effect on your circulatory system.

The adrenal glands are easily damaged by toxins, and damaged adrenal glands can have a negative impact on your cardiovascular health right away. Here are a few ways that can happen:

✔ Stress put on the adrenal glands by toxins can cause the glands to produce excess amounts of a hormone called *cortisol*. Higher-than-normal levels of cortisol can spike your blood sugar, which in turn causes inflammation in your blood vessels.

✔ Toxic damage to your adrenal glands can also result in unhealthy fluctuations in the amount of *aldosterone* (another hormone) your adrenals produce. The complications are serious and include a change in your blood volume (not good), elevated blood pressure (also not good), and damage to your circulatory system tissues (downright bad).

✔ Long-term stress on your adrenal glands from elevated toxicity can cause adrenal failure, which is nothing short of disastrous for your circulatory system.

Gauging glucose

The direct correlation between cardiovascular disease and diabetes is no secret. Most people understand that diabetics with higher blood sugar are more likely to suffer from diseases that affect the circulatory system, and they're more likely to die from these conditions. Recently, some studies have shown that even among non-diabetics, the frequency of cardiovascular problems is much higher among those who have consistently higher blood sugar. Clearly blood sugar (glucose) has an effect on the circulatory system, and when blood sugar is high that effect isn't good at all.

The ways in which elevated blood sugar levels challenge the circulatory system are many, and they're pretty complicated, so I won't get into the gory details here. The bottom line is that high blood sugar causes damage to blood vessels. High blood sugar also leads to high insulin levels, and it turns out that insulin also harms blood vessels.

A very clear connection exists between high blood sugar and cardiovascular problems, so if you're facing any kind of heart disease be sure you go into your fight knowing that you need to keep your blood sugar in check.

When you eat a large meal, especially one that's full of simple carbohydrates, your blood sugar spikes, and your insulin levels follow suit. Both things harm your blood vessels. This is another reason that it's best for you to eat small meals more frequently instead of eating a lower number of big meals. Obviously, it's also crucial to keep your sugar intake to a minimum. Even if you're not diabetic, don't push the envelope; you want to keep your blood sugar at safe, healthy levels.

Rapid rises in blood sugar are very hard on your circulatory system. To help keep this problem to a minimum, cut down on your intake of simple carbohydrates (which include sugars, high fructose corn syrup, potatoes, and anything made of flour.) A good rule is to avoid eating anything white, except cauliflower. You should also be sure to eat a breakfast that contains some sort of protein source. Doing so gets your blood sugar levels started off right in the morning so you don't have harmful blood sugar peaks and valleys throughout the day.

If you're worried about circulatory problems and heart disease, it's a good idea to go ahead and get your blood sugar and insulin tested. If your blood sugar or insulin levels are concerning, you could soon see an effect on your cardiovascular health, particularly if diabetes runs in your family.

Battling high blood pressure

When you visit any doctor's office or get a health checkup of any kind, what's one of the first things the nurse checks? Your blood pressure. That fact alone should tell you the importance of your blood pressure on your health.

High blood pressure (also called *hypertension*) is a problem that has grown quite a lot in recent years. Some estimates indicate that 30 percent of Americans suffer from high blood pressure, which is a pretty scary statistic considering how dangerous the condition can be for your health.

High blood pressure harms your circulatory system in two ways:

- ✔ It creates tension or stress in your blood vessels, which results in inflammation and damage to these important structures and leads to the formation of plaque.

- ✔ It makes your heart work harder than it should, which causes unnecessary cardiac strain that can lead to thicker and stiffer heart walls that don't function normally. Remember that your heart beats about 40 million times each year, so you really can't afford for it to be operating at anything less than its best.

Making sure your blood pressure problem is really a problem

Hypertension, or high blood pressure, is a condition in which your blood pressure is elevated at an unhealthy level all the time. Even if you have normal, healthy blood pressure, you're bound to see increases in your blood pressure when your body is subjected to different conditions. For example, if you take the blood pressure of a person while she's lifting a heavy box, her blood pressure is probably going to be very high because she's engaged in strenuous physical activity. By the same token, if you take someone's blood pressure when he's taking an important test at school or at his job, his blood pressure will inevitably be higher, and in many cases higher than what's considered a healthy level. There's also a very common condition often referred to as "white coat hypertension" that involves a temporary spike in blood pressure that results from people being nervous when they're in a doctor's office. That means their blood pressure could be at much higher than normal levels right when they're getting their blood pressure taken!

Because of these types of blood pressure variations, you should have your blood pressure tested multiple times in a few different settings before coming to the conclusion that you indeed have a constantly elevated blood pressure problem. You may consider investing in a blood pressure cuff, which is available at your local drug store or online, so you can take your blood pressure at home on a more frequent basis. You don't want to start taking blood pressure medication, which is very serious stuff, if your blood pressure really isn't a problem. Some researchers estimate that nearly half the people taking hypertension medication don't really have sustained high blood pressure!

Many factors contribute to high blood pressure, but one of the biggest is the formation of plaque in blood vessels, which is the result of inflammation caused by high levels of toxins in the body. All the toxins that end up in your body from food, air, and water can cause harmful changes to your blood vessels and dangerous, elevated blood pressure. It's just another reason why you need to put detoxification at the top of your health priority list.

Putting Cholesterol in Its Place

Very few natural substances are as vilified as cholesterol. You can't turn on a television or read a magazine today without seeing some sort of story about the dangers of cholesterol or an advertisement for a product — from prescription drugs to breakfast cereals — that will help to reduce your cholesterol.

The impact that cholesterol management has made in today's medicine is indeed remarkable. *Statin drugs,* which are used to lower cholesterol, produce sales of $27 billion dollars annually. That's a huge number!

But here's the problem with making cholesterol the boogeyman and spending billions of dollars a year on drugs to fight it: Cholesterol may not cause nearly as many health problems as the world thinks. Read on to find out what I mean.

Natural, normal, and necessary

Cholesterol is a natural product of your body. Your body manufactures cholesterol, and lots of it. In fact, cholesterol is the basic molecule that your body uses to make many of its most important hormones, including those that control blood sugar, mineral balance, blood pressure, and inflammation. Cholesterol is also the basic building block for sex hormones like estrogen and testosterone.

From a very simplistic point of view, it's difficult to imagine that your body would make a substance that would kill you. It seems even more of a stretch to think that a certain cholesterol level can be fine but a level just 1 or 2 percent higher is dangerous and requires medication.

As I mention at the start of this chapter, at the turn of the 20th century cardiovascular disease wasn't even in the top ten causes of death, and people didn't think a thing about their cholesterol levels. That's mind-boggling when you consider that in those days people commonly cooked with lard, bacon grease, and butter, and they ate many foods high in cholesterol. The genes of those people were almost exactly the same as the genes of people who walk the earth now. Why was cholesterol not more of a problem back then? Put simply, the people who lived just a few generations ago were more physically active, and they weren't exposed to nearly as many dangerous and deadly toxins as we are. They didn't eat, drink, and breathe toxic materials every day.

These observations support the idea that inflammation, not cholesterol, is the major culprit in causing cardiovascular disease and circulatory problems.

Looking at the facts about cholesterol

Understanding just how natural and important cholesterol is should make you think twice about the idea that cholesterol is behind the majority of cases of cardiovascular disease. Here's another tidbit that should raise your eyebrows: Fifty percent of people who have heart attacks don't have high cholesterol. Isn't that incredible? Doesn't that statistic alone make it difficult to say that cholesterol is the cause of heart disease?

Questioning the connections between cholesterol and cardiovascular disease

You can read study after study that makes the connection between high cholesterol and circulatory problems look weaker and weaker. Here are a few to consider:

- ✔ The *European Heart Journal* published a study of 11,500 patients over three years that showed that patients with low cholesterol had a death rate more than twice as high as patients with high cholesterol.

- ✔ The *Journal of Cardiac Failure* (really uplifting reading material, I know) published an analysis of more than a thousand patients with heart disease and found low cholesterol to be associated with higher death rates. Interestingly, higher cholesterol increased the chance of survival.

- ✔ A study reported in the *Archives of Gerontology and Geriatrics* looked at mortality and age, sex, body mass index, and total cholesterol. When it came to cholesterol, higher death rates were connected only with people who had extremely low cholesterol.

That's just the tip of the iceberg. You may be thinking, with all the evidence that flies in the face of those who say that cholesterol is the biggest cause of cardiovascular disease, who is continuing to insist that's the case? Well, consider this. A few years back a meeting of the National Cholesterol Education Program (NCEP) took place, and during that meeting the decision was made to lower the acceptable levels of cholesterol. As a result, 20 million Americans who didn't have high cholesterol levels before the meeting suddenly had them after the meeting. That's pretty shocking, but it's even more of a worry when you find out who sat on the committee that made the decision. Of the nine members on the committee, eight had financial connections to the manufacturers of statin drugs (drugs that are purported to lower cholesterol), and at the time they didn't disclose those relationships. Sort of seems like a case of the fox guarding the hen house, does it not?

Realizing that statin drugs aren't the answer

Conventional medicine's biggest weapons in the fight against cholesterol are statin drugs. These are the drugs that can reduce cholesterol levels in your body. You may have seen commercials that say statin drugs will reduce cardiovascular events (things like heart attacks) by about 33 percent. Sounds promising, right? Not so fast. Consider what the number means.

Let's say that a drug company monitors 100 people who aren't taking statin drugs, and three of those people have a heart attack. The company also monitors another 100 people who are taking statin drugs, and only two of them have a heart attack. Two versus three is a 33 percent decrease in heart attacks in the group taking statin drugs. Most people would look at that same data and say there there's really a reduction of only 1 in 100, but of course the folks selling the statin drugs are interested in finessing the data in a slightly different way.

Here are a couple other reasons that you may want to think hard before turning to statin drugs as your primary means of fighting heart disease:

✔ Statin drugs slow down enzymes that the body uses to make cholesterol. However, some of these enzymes help to make other enzymes that are used in every cell in your body in the generation of energy. This is why people who take statins often have leg cramps and aches; their muscles basically run out of energy and start contracting in weird ways.

You have an enzyme in your body called *coenzyme Q10,* which plays a key role in generating energy for your cells. Statin drugs can inhibit the production of coenzyme Q10, so if you're taking statins be sure you're also supplementing with coenzyme Q10.

✔ Several studies have demonstrated that statin drugs don't reduce the size of the plaque in the arteries.

I'm a firm believer that inflammation caused by toxins is the major cause of plaque formation in blood vessels and, therefore, a top cause of heart disease. And I'm not the only person to hold this belief. If you want to keep your heart and your circulatory system in good shape, don't immediately get fixated on cholesterol and start reaching for the statin drugs. Start by eating a healthy, detoxified diet; consider the methods of detoxification that I describe throughout this book; and get plenty of exercise.

Supplementing to Help Circulation

Several natural supplements are showing quite a lot of promise in fighting circulatory system ailments. In addition, any supplement that helps to reduce toxicity is a huge step in the right direction. Here are some of the supplements that have shown the most promise thus far:

✔ **Alpha-lipoic acid (ALA):** A powerful antioxidant that reduces blood pressure.

✔ **Chlorella:** Known to reduce blood pressure and help to reduce the levels of heavy metals in the body.

✔ **Coenzyme Q10:** Reverses energy starvation in the heart muscle, which can help prevent abnormal heart rhythms.

✔ **Folic acid:** Reduces blood pressure in women and peripheral vascular disease in men.

✔ **Garlic:** Good in your pasta and also as a supplement. It has a long history of reducing blood pressure and cholesterol.

✔ **Ginseng:** A dynamic supplement with a powerful antioxidant effect. It reduces hypertension, improves cardiovascular function, and improves glucose control.

- ✔ **L-arginine:** Improves the functioning of the cells that line the arteries and also improves exercise tolerance in patients with congestive heart failure.

- ✔ **Lycopene:** An antioxidant that was shown in the *American Journal of Clinical Nutrition* to cut cardiovascular disease by one half. Not bad!

- ✔ **Magnesium:** Lowers blood pressure and subsequent stress on the arteries and heart muscle.

- ✔ **Omega-3 fatty acids:** Reduce your risk for heart disease. (These claims are supported by the U.S. Food and Drug Administration.)

- ✔ **Resveratrol:** An antioxidant found in red wine and grape skins. You can also find it as a supplement in tablet or capsule form. A study in *Cardiovascular Drug Reviews* showed that resveratrol improves vascular cell function and helps to prevent the growth of plaque.

- ✔ **Vitamin C:** A potent antioxidant.

These supplements can be helpful, but you should always work hard to include as many antioxidant-rich foods in your diet a possible. Antioxidants are critical for neutralizing the reactive oxygen species (ROS) that I describe earlier in this chapter. Eat your organic fruits and veggies!

Recognizing the Importance of Exercise

Is there anyone who doesn't agree that exercise is one of the most important things you can do to help keep your body healthy? Exercise has long been recognized and celebrated as a key component in a healthy, happy lifestyle. But in my view exercise still isn't emphasized enough when it comes to its benefits and potential for preventing and treating disease, *especially* cardiovascular disease. I could fill up a chapter with the benefits of exercise for your circulatory system, but here are just a few highlights:

- ✔ Exercise causes temporary increases in blood pressure. I know that I've said several times in this chapter that high blood pressure is one of the worst things for your circulatory system, but the very short-term increases in blood pressure that result from exercise are actually good for you because they keep your blood vessels pliable and strengthen your heart muscle.

- ✔ Exercise reduces blood sugar levels, which in turn helps to reduce the toxic effects of sugar and insulin on your blood vessels and the rest of your circulatory system.

- ✔ Muscles that are being exercised are the only things that can take glucose out of your blood vessels and use it without the presence of insulin. Your brain is affected by blood glucose levels, so exercising is almost as good for the mind as it is for the body!

Making sure you exercise regularly

Many health and medical organizations suggest exercising three to five times per week. That's fine, but I suggest that you should get some kind of exercise every day. If you exercise every day, you of course enjoy additional health benefits, but there's another important factor to consider: Making exercise a normal part of your day is the only way that you can really make a habit out of it, which is a critical step. When exercise isn't part of your daily routine, you're much more likely to dread it and end up putting it off. Before you know it, you're putting it off so much that you're not even exercising three to five times per week.

If you don't exercise at all now, exercising every day will probably seem like a struggle, but you need to force yourself to do it. For the first couple months, you may have to really fight the urge to skip exercising. But for most people, three months is the sweet spot; that's the point by which exercise really becomes a habit. By then it gets a lot easier, and after three months most people say that they miss exercise and feel a lot worse if they don't do it.

When you're exercising, in addition to getting lots of good cardiovascular benefits, you're also working up a sweat. Sweating is one of the best ways to clear toxins out of your body, so you're getting fit and detoxifying at the same time!

Considering a few different types of exercise

You should consider doing several different types of exercise, each of which has unique benefits:

- ✔ **Aerobic exercise** increases your heart rate and your body's need for oxygen. Walking and jogging are common types of aerobic exercise. I recommend walking because of the injuries incurred from jogging. Can you believe that of all the sports activities in the United States (including professional sports), jogging causes the most injuries? If you're already a jogger, please just be careful to stretch, wear appropriate shoes, and take good care of your joints.

    If you don't currently exercise but you want to begin walking, your goal should be to start slow and walk for short periods of time. Over the course of a few weeks (or months, if you're in bad shape now), you should be able to reach the point where you're walking as fast as you can for up to 30 minutes a day. Most people can walk 4 miles per hour when they're walking quickly, so you should be able to walk about 2 miles in a 30-minute walking session.

If you have medical problems, you should contact your physician to make sure that it's safe for you to exercise. If you have a problem with any weight-bearing parts of your body, you may be able to exercise on a bicycle or stationary bike. Some people also like stair climbers. The idea is to find what you can do and keep with it. People with arthritic problems often find that exercise increases their ability to perform activities without pain.

✔ **Resistance training** (or *weight training*) includes a whole variety of maneuvers that involve pushing or pulling on something that doesn't easily move. It's a great way to build strength and muscle tone, which increases endurance in performing daily activities. Resistance training also has beneficial effects on glucose utilization. The amount of resistance used will be different for each person but should be taxing to produce good results. You'll have a harder time working up a sweat with resistance training than with aerobic exercise, but give it a try. You may get to the point where you're pumping iron *and* pumping excess iron (and other heavy metals) out of your body through your sweat!

✔ **Rebounding,** which is a type of exercise that is often overlooked, involves the use of a rebounder or mini trampoline. Some people scoff at this kind of workout, but they shouldn't be so quick to dismiss it. There's a unique process in play with rebounding: As you bounce, you reach a maximum height before you start down. At that instant, you are effectively at zero gravity. When that happens, every blood vessel in your body enjoys minimal effects from blood pressure. At the other end of a bounce, when you're at the bottom and start to come up again, you experience two to three times the force of gravity, and your blood pushes hard against the walls of your blood vessels. This up and down pressure on the blood vessels helps to keep them toned and flexible, which can have extremely positive effects on their health. Rebounding also increases the flow of lymph throughout you body, which is very beneficial for you immune system. Of course, if you're very clumsy and bounce off the mini trampoline and break a lamp, your blood pressure will likely get a real spike, but that shouldn't happen too often after you get the hang of it!

If you want to really see the benefits of exercise, try incorporating all three types I mention here: aerobic, resistance, and rebounding. Set a weekly schedule, and do each method on a different day. You'll get some wonderful circulatory system benefits, but you'll also give virtually every other part of your body a boost, as well. Exercise stimulates the gastrointestinal tract to be more regular, increases *endorphins* (the feel-good chemicals in the brain), helps to defeat depression, and does terrific things for the lungs. If you can work up and maintain a good sweat, you'll also help to flush out toxins from your body, which will take stress off your immune system and help to protect you from illness.

I personally believe that daily exercise and sweating will give you at least ten extra years of disease-free, healthy life (if you combine these efforts with detoxification and a reduction in the amount of toxins you take in, of course).

Recipes for Improved Circulation

A healthy, wholesome, toxin-free diet is key when fighting diseases of the circulatory system and generally working to improve the health of your blood, blood vessels, and heart. Try out some of these tantalizing recipes and rest assured that you're doing wonders for your body while you're delighting your palate.

🍅 Fennel Orange Salad with Sesame Dressing

Fennel is high in *quercetin flavonoids,* which are powerful antioxidants. It also contains *anethole,* which reduces inflammation in the body and can be a great way to fight cardiovascular disease. And both fennel and oranges are very high in vitamin C, which neutralizes free radicals. Fiber, potassium, and *folate* (a B vitamin), which are also present in fennel, help reduce the amount of homocysteine in your blood. Homocysteine levels are considered a risk factor for heart attacks.

Perhaps the most amazing thing about fennel is that while it contains a huge variety of healthy materials, it also tastes wonderful! It's crunchy and sweet with a licorice taste — the perfect complement to juicy and tart oranges.

Preparation time: *20 minutes*

Yield: *6 servings*

2 large bulbs organic fennel, trimmed

4 cups organic watercress, rinsed

4 large oranges, peeled, pith removed, and sliced 1/3-inch thick

3 organic radishes, thinly sliced

2 tablespoons flaxseed oil

2 tablespoons freshly squeezed orange juice

1 tablespoon freshly squeezed lemon juice

2 teaspoons apple cider vinegar

1/4 teaspoon stevia

Pinch cayenne pepper

2 tablespoons sesame seeds

1 Cut the root end off the fennel and cut off the tough green stems, leaving some green attached to the bulb. Pull off the outer skin and discard. Cut fennel bulb in half, then thinly slice it crosswise. Arrange on watercress on a serving platter with oranges and radishes.

2 In small bowl, combine oil, orange juice, lemon juice, vinegar, stevia, and pepper; mix well. Drizzle over salad and top with sesame seeds. Serve immediately.

Per serving: *Calories 129 (From Fat 55); Fat 6g (Saturated 1g); Cholesterol 0mg; Sodium 53mg; Carbohydrate 19g; Dietary Fiber 5g; Protein 3g.*

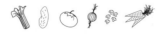

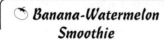 Banana-Watermelon Smoothie

Smoothies are so easy to make, and everyone loves them. They will cool you down on a hot day, and nothing makes a better breakfast when you're a little bit pressed for time.

Watermelon is very high in *lycopene,* an antioxidant that can help reduce the risk of cardiovascular disease. Men who had high levels of lycopene in their body fat were 50 percent less likely to suffer a heart attack. You can only obtain lycopene by eating red or pink fruits and vegetables, like tomatoes, cherries, watermelon, and pink grapefruit.

Preparation time: *5 minutes*

Yield: *3–4 servings*

3 cups cubed organic watermelon	3 tablespoons local organic honey
2 bananas, frozen, peeled, and cut into chunks	1/3 cup plain organic yogurt
2 tablespoons flaxseed oil	1/4 cup freshly squeezed orange juice

1 Combine all ingredients in food processor or blender and process or blend until smooth. Serve immediately.

Per serving: Calories 292 (From Fat 95); Fat 11g (Saturated 2g); Cholesterol 4mg; Sodium 17mg; Carbohydrate 51g; Dietary Fiber 4g; Protein 3g.

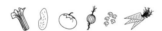

Spicy Black Bean and Spinach Soup

Black beans and spinach contain lots of magnesium, a nutrient essential to lung and heart health. Combined with tomatoes, which are high in lycopene, and flaxseed, which contains lots of omega-3 fatty acids, this soup is like a prescription in a bowl (only tastier and much more natural)!

You can make this soup ahead of time; just leave out the spinach, flaxseed oil, lemon juice, and seeds. Refrigerate up to three days. Gently reheat the soup, and then bring it to a simmer. Add the spinach and let wilt, and then continue with the recipe.

Preparation time: *10 minutes plus overnight soaking time*

Cooking time: *2 hours 45 minutes*

Yield: *6 servings*

2 cups dried organic black beans	*1 tablespoon fresh organic oregano leaves*
6 cups filtered water	*1/4 teaspoon cayenne pepper*
2 organic onions, peeled and chopped	*6 cups organic baby spinach leaves*
6 cloves organic garlic, peeled and minced	*2 tablespoons flaxseed oil*
2 organic jalapeno peppers, minced	*2–3 tablespoons freshly squeezed lemon juice*
4 ripe red organic tomatoes, chopped	*1/3 cup roasted organic pumpkin seeds*
2 large organic carrots, sliced	*1/4 cup roasted organic sunflower seeds*
1 teaspoon turmeric	

1 Look over black beans, picking out any shriveled beans or extraneous matter. Rinse beans well and drain. Place in large bowl; cover with 6 cups water. Cover and let stand overnight.

2 In the morning, drain the beans and place in large pot. Add 1 chopped onion and 3 cloves garlic; cover with 9 cups filtered water. Bring to a simmer; reduce heat to low, cover, and simmer 2 hours until beans are tender.

3 In skillet, heat olive oil over medium heat. Add remaining onion, remaining garlic, and jalapeno peppers; cook 4–5 minutes until tender. Add to black beans along with tomatoes, carrots, turmeric, oregano, and cayenne pepper. Bring to a simmer; simmer 30–40 minutes until vegetables are tender.

4 Stir in spinach leaves; cook and stir until spinach wilts. Remove from heat and stir in flaxseed oil and lemon juice. Serve immediately, garnished with pumpkin and sunflower seeds.

Per serving: *Calories 364 (From Fat 88); Fat 10g (Saturated 1g); Cholesterol 0mg; Sodium 100mg; Carbohydrate 56g; Dietary Fiber 18g; Protein 18g.*

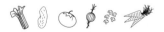

Baked Ginger Salmon with Tomato Coulis and Asparagus

You should eat wild salmon twice a week for your health. This robust and flavorful fish is bursting with omega-3 fatty acids, which are very important to heart health. And adding ingredients high in lycopene and vitamin C, like tomatoes, makes this dish even better for you.

Preparation time: *15 minutes*

Cooking time: *1 hour*

Yield: *4 servings*

4 (6–8 ounce) wild Alaskan salmon steaks

1 tablespoon organic olive oil

1/4 cup minced fresh organic ginger root

2 cloves garlic, minced

2 tablespoons freshly squeezed lemon juice

1/8 teaspoon white pepper

2 red organic tomatoes, chopped

1 yellow organic tomato, chopped

2 cups organic grape tomatoes

1/4 cup finely chopped organic green onions

1/4 cup freshly squeezed orange juice

1 tablespoon flaxseed oil

1 clove garlic, minced

1/2 cup chopped organic flat-leaf parsley

1/2 cup chopped organic basil leaves

1 pound organic asparagus

2 cups filtered water

1 Preheat oven to 350 degrees F. Place salmon on baking dish. In small bowl, combine olive oil, ginger root, 2 cloves minced garlic, lemon juice, and pepper; spread over salmon. Bake salmon for 25–40 minutes until fish flakes with a fork.

2 In medium bowl, combine all the tomatoes, onions, orange juice, flaxseed oil, 1 minced clove garlic, parsley, and basil. Cover and refrigerate.

3 Meanwhile, heat water and asparagus until simmering; reduce heat to low and simmer 5–6 minutes until crisp-tender. Drain.

4 When salmon flakes when tested with a fork, place on serving platter along with asparagus. Serve the tomato mixture on the side.

Per serving: *Calories 343 (From Fat 124); Fat 14g (Saturated 2g); Cholesterol 80mg; Sodium 116mg; Carbohydrate 17g; Dietary Fiber 4g; Protein 38g.*

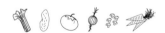

Chapter 14

Using Detoxification to Help Your Body Heal after a Smoking Addiction

*W*ant to shorten your lifespan, ruin your health, and pump yourself full of thousands of dangerous, harmful toxins? All you have to do is take a stroll down to the nearest gas station, pick up a pack of cigarettes, and light up. When it comes to introducing toxins into your body and degrading your health at a rapid rate, very few things can stack up with smoking.

Smoking is involved in one out of five deaths in the United States each year. Direct causes of death associated with smoking include emphysema, bronchitis, chronic obstructive pulmonary disease, and cancer. These are truly agonizing conditions, and they are awful ways to die. Smoking also decreases the amount of life you get to live before you're faced with those sorts of awful diseases: On average, smokers die 13 to 14 years earlier than nonsmokers.

As a society, we pay a great price for the damages done to our fellow citizens by smoking. Medical expenses and time lost from work because of smoking cost us an estimated $193 billion every year. Imagine all the good we could do with that kind of money if we could somehow convince everyone to cut out the smoking habit.

I know you've probably heard plenty of statistics about the dangers of smoking, so I'll stop there and let you know how I'd like to bring detoxification into the smoking conversation. After you've quit smoking, your body begins to heal itself almost immediately. You can do quite a lot of good for your body and make the process much easier if you embrace a few detoxification methods.

I have three goals in this chapter:

- ✔ To give you a very full picture of the amount and range of toxins that you put into your body when you smoke. I think it's important for you to realize just how toxic smoking can be, so you can be even more motivated to quit if you're a smoker now and even less likely to pick up smoking if you're not a smoker.

- ✔ To explain two alternative methods for smoking cessation — acupuncture and hypnosis — that dovetail very nicely with a detoxification lifestyle.

- ✔ To present detoxification techniques that can be a boon for your body as it begins to heal and rebuild after a smoking addiction is defeated.

Before I get started, note that most of the details in this chapter apply to all types of smoking (cigarettes, cigars, pipes, and even secondhand smoke), and many are relevant for users of smokeless tobacco, too.

Realizing the Monumental Toxic Impact of Smoking

About 4,000 chemicals are present in cigarette smoke. As much as I'd like to list all of them here to really emphasize the dangers associated with smoking, I'm afraid I just don't have the space. Instead, I cover a few of the main groups of toxins that enter your body when you inhale tobacco smoke, with the hope that even a small sampling will convince you that smoking is essentially the opposite of detoxification.

Carcinogens

Tobacco smoke contains more than 50 known *carcinogens:* chemicals that cause cancer. Fifty! The carcinogenic effect of smoke is so great that the U.S. Environmental Protection Agency (EPA) has classified tobacco smoke as a group A carcinogen. (That's the most dangerous group.)

What do all these carcinogens do? Well, back in 1964 the U.S. Surgeon General reported that smoking was causative in cancer of the lungs and the larynx (voice box). That was the beginning. Later, smoking was shown to be causative for cancers of the bladder, esophagus, mouth, and throat. The latest releases connect smoking to some kinds of leukemia, stomach cancer, pancreatic cancer, cervical cancer, liver cancer, prostate cancer, and kidney cancer. (Smoking hasn't been shown to be a primary cause in this last group, but it has a high association with these conditions. And let's be honest: Would anyone really be surprised if smoking caused these conditions?)

Carbon monoxide

Carbon monoxide is a dangerous gas that can easily cause death if you're exposed to enough of it. This gas is present in automobile exhaust and in many types of industrial waste. Carbon monoxide is particularly nasty for your health because it attaches to the red blood cells where oxygen is supposed to attach, and it does so about 200 times more effectively than oxygen.

In a heavy smoker, the oxygen-carrying capacity of red blood cells can be reduced as much as 15 percent by carbon monoxide. This is a significant reduction in the ability of your blood to carry oxygen to your tissues. Smoking really does suffocate every last corner of your body.

Nicotine

This toxin is the main cause of physical addiction to smoking. Nicotine does some strange, harmful things to your body, including the following:

- ✔ Constricting blood vessels
- ✔ Increasing blood pressure
- ✔ Decreasing blood flow
- ✔ Causing cold hands and feet
- ✔ Creating chest pain
- ✔ Stimulating the adrenal glands, which affects cardiovascular function
- ✔ Decreasing bicarbonate release from the pancreas, which slows digestion
- ✔ Making blood platelets more likely to clump, increasing the risk of clots

As you'd probably guess, none of these effects is positive or healthy for your body.

Other chemical toxins

Here's a very quick look at just a few of the other chemical toxins lurking in cigarette smoke. All of them are toxic, some are thought to be carcinogenic, and many are very strong irritants:

- **Acetone:** A very strong irritant also found in fingernail polish remover and varnish remover.

- **Acrolein:** An extremely toxic chemical to the lungs.

- **Ammonia:** A strong irritant similar to the ammonia in cleaning fluids.

- **Creosote:** Used to treat railroad ties. It's a toxic component of the tar in cigarette smoke.

- **Hydrogen cyanide:** A deadly toxic poison commonly used as a rat killer.

- **Toluene:** Very toxic and used to make paint and varnish remover.

- **Vinyl chloride:** Used to make vinyl. It causes dizziness, headaches, and fatigue, and long-term exposure can lead to cancer and liver damage.

This list really could go on for pages and pages. But isn't the presence of just one of these materials in cigarette smoke enough to keep you from picking up a pack?

Heavy metals

The presence of heavy metal toxins in our environment is on the rise, and you certainly don't need to add to the problem by smoking. Tobacco smoke is lousy with heavy metals, and the secondhand smoke that comes off the end of a lit cigarette (often called *sidestream smoke*) is particularly bad. For example, there's six times as much *cadmium* — a dangerous heavy metal toxin — in sidestream smoke as in the smoke inhaled by a smoker.

Here are just a few examples of the heavy metals you can find in tobacco smoke:

- **Arsenic:** An extremely toxic, deadly poison.

- **Cadmium:** Often found in large amounts in cigarette smoke; shown to cause a variety of cancers.

- **Lead:** Highly toxic and present in almost all forms of tobacco smoke.

- **Lead 210:** A unique type of radioactive lead.

You need to be spending your time and efforts limiting your exposure to heavy metals and working to detoxify your body, not deliberately adding them to your lungs through smoking.

Choosing a Smoking Cessation Method

Ask anyone who has ever tried to stop smoking: A smoking addiction is one of the most difficult bad habits to quit. Statistics show that 70 percent of smokers want to quit, and 40 percent try to stop smoking every year. Eight out of ten smokers start the habit before they're 18 years old, and 20 percent of high school students smoke. Starting at such an early age makes the actual habit of smoking very ingrained and even more difficult to kick.

The nicotine in tobacco smoke is extremely addictive on a physical level. It has a very significant effect on your brain, stimulating pleasure centers and increasing natural "feel good" chemicals like norepinephrine, dopamine, and serotonin. Nicotine also causes a release of adrenaline from the adrenal glands.

The physical aspects of smoking addiction are bad, but the mental and behavioral aspects can be just as troublesome. Many smokers associate having a cigarette with a time for relaxation and pleasure. They smoke during the good times in their day — maybe when they get off of work or after they eat a good meal. Or they make cigarettes part of several daily rituals like getting in the car, talking on the phone, and taking a coffee break. For these types of smokers, quitting is extra difficult because they associate smoking with so many different facets of their lives.

If you're a smoker and you want to quit, you have lots of options, including the following:

- ✔ **Quitting cold turkey:** This method involves simply dropping the habit all at once, with no real planning or weaning of any kind. Research shows that quitting cold turkey is only about 5 percent effective.

- ✔ **Using nicotine patches or gum:** Many of these options started out as prescription only, but most are now available over the counter. The patches have shown a success rate of over 20 percent, but the gum is quite a bit less effective.

- ✔ **Taking prescription drugs:** A handful of prescription drugs for smoking cessation are on the market. Typically, I'm not a fan of turning to a pill to solve health problems. But in this case you have to weigh the potential benefits of quitting smoking against any ill effects from the prescription. Do some research and talk to your doctor if you're interested.

These are some of the most common methods for kicking the smoking habit, but they're certainly not your only choices. I devote the rest of this section to two smoking cessation techniques that often fly under the radar but happen to fit in very nicely with a detoxification lifestyle: hypnosis and acupuncture. Both are toxin-free, holistic methods for snuffing out the smoking habit. If you're a smoker and you're looking to quit, I recommend taking them into consideration.

Getting help from hypnosis

In 1958, the American Medical Association recognized hypnosis as an appropriate therapy for the treatment of smoking addiction. Since that time, a whole host of hypnosis methods has been developed to help people stop smoking. Many of the practitioners suggest that hypnosis can work for smoking cession because it enhances relaxation, motivation, and self control, which are all key factors for anyone who's trying to stop smoking. Some practitioners use a posthypnotic suggestion to avoid cigarettes. Another method is to use hypnosis to replace the physical motion of reaching for a cigarette with another innocuous motion, such as squeezing your earlobe. I know that method may sound a little odd, but let's face it: Squeezing your earlobe is quite a bit better for your health than inhaling about 50 known carcinogens several times a day.

The data collected on successful smoking cessation through hypnosis varies quite a bit, but most of the numbers point to a success rate of about 20 percent. Some individual practitioners claim much higher success rates, though — some as high as 90 percent.

If you're a smoker and you'd like to really look into using hypnosis to curb the habit, the first step is finding the right practitioner. The key is networking. Start by asking your physician if she knows of a good option. Then ask your friends and family; you may be surprised who has received hypnotherapy before. There may also be a local or state society of hypnotherapy practitioners in your area, so do some online searching to find out. If such a society or organization exists in your area, contact the office and ask for a recommendation. And always evaluate several possibilities before making your choice.

Adding acupuncture to your toolbox

If you're the kind of person who likes health and medical practices that have been around for a while, acupuncture just may be for you. The practice, which involves stimulating specific points on the body with long, thin, metal needles, has been around for about 5,000 years and has become a more and more popular method for smoking cessation in recent years.

The research on the benefits of acupuncture for quitting smoking is scattered and generally weak, so it's tough to wrap any hard numbers around the potential for acupuncture in smoking cessation. I do think the practice has merit, though, and like so many of the other methods for kicking the smoking habit, it's worth considering even if the success rates are fairly low, given the horrendous health effects that smoking causes.

If you want to look into visiting an acupuncturist for help with your smoking addiction, be sure you do lots of research before selecting a practitioner. The difference in the skills of individual practitioners is huge. Some have been trained by masters of this art for years and are very skilled. Unfortunately, others hang out a shingle after only a week-long course.

To be certain your acupuncturist is talented, practiced, and safe, flip back to Chapter 5 and read my suggestions for how to select an alternative practitioner. Focus on vetting credentials, speaking with current and past clients, and confirming affiliations with any trade organizations and other groups.

Sweating Out Cigarette Toxins

If you haven't quit smoking yet, detoxing is crucial. Many of the toxins in cigarette smoke are fat-soluble, and one of the best ways to detoxify for fat-soluble toxins is sweating. (Read all about the detoxification benefits of sweating in Chapter 18.) If you've been a smoker for any extended period of time, you almost certainly have quite a large collection of toxins built up in your body's fat cells. Those toxins are like a ticking bomb: It's only a matter of time until they start fouling up your body's important systems, if they haven't already.

When you've finally snuffed out your last cigarette, you should immediately begin thinking about the ways you can increase the amount of sweating you do for detoxification purposes. That's a surefire way to help your body get rid of the residual fat-soluble toxins that are still hanging around from your days as a smoker.

Sweating is a powerful means of detoxification. It has one-third the detoxification potential of your kidneys, which are world-class detoxification powerhouses. Check out Chapter 18 for a rundown of how you can use sweating to ramp up the amount of toxins that you flush from your body.

Supplementing to Heal Your Body

Before or after you've stopped smoking, your body has to deal with the effects of all the toxins that you inhaled over the months or years you were a smoker. You can play an active role in that process by taking some of the following supplements:

- ✔ **Glutathione** is one of our body's most important antioxidants, and it can help undo some of the damage that smoking did to your body after you've put down the pack. You can find glutathione as a supplement to be taken orally, and you can also boost its effect by pairing it with a melatonin supplement.

- ✔ **Vitamin C** is another extremely important antioxidant, and your body has to use a lot of it to thwart the damaging effects of smoking. It's not uncommon for smokers to have very low levels of vitamin C in their bodies. If you're trying to quit smoking or if you've already been successful in doing so, be sure you're supplementing with lots and lots of vitamin C. You need at least 2,000 mg for good health, but don't hesitate to ramp up your dose to 4,000 mg per day if you've recently stopped smoking. It'll do quite a lot to help your body heal.

- ✔ **Vitamin A,** like vitamin C, is decreased by smoking, so vitamin A supplements are very useful for people who are trying to quit or those who have just kicked the habit.

- ✔ **Green tea, grape seed extract,** and **tryptophan** are all great for former smokers. All three supplements fortify the immune system and replace the important materials in your body that tobacco toxins deplete.

- ✔ **Alpha-lipoic acid (ALA)** deserves a special note. It supports liver function in an amazing way. Smoking puts an incredible toxic strain on the liver, so be sure to take an ALA supplement to help get your liver back in healthy working order.

Counting Calories after You Quit

Weight gain is a common side effect of smoking cessation, and that shouldn't surprise anyone. While you're smoking, your body has to expend about 375 calories each day in an effort to repair the toxic damage that smoking causes. If you stop smoking and you don't also make healthy changes to your diet and exercise routine, you run a real risk for weight gain. In addition to the calories that are no longer needed to repair the harm that smoking causes, recent quitters also often replace the oral habit of smoking with eating. And that new habit sure isn't slowed down by the fact that food tastes a heck of a lot better after you quit smoking.

Putting on a few pounds instead of lighting up multiple times a day is definitely the lesser of two evils, but no one really wants weight gain to be the reward for finally winning the war against smoking. But here's the good news: You can quit smoking and avoid weight gain by making some relatively minor adjustments to your eating and exercising. Focus hard on sticking to the detox diet plans I describe in Chapters 7 and 9, and be sure to get at least 30 minutes of vigorous exercise each day. That should be enough to keep you from adding on a few pounds after you've waved goodbye to a smoking addiction.

Recipes for Helping You Kick the Smoking Habit

When you're trying to stop smoking, or if you recently stopped, eating healthy food is a key way to help your body repair the damage done by smoking. An antioxidant-rich diet will give your body the fuel it needs to fight off smoking-related toxins.

Smoking cessation makes food taste better, so many former smokers find themselves eating quite a bit more than they did when the tar and other nasty materials from smoking were dulling their taste buds. If you quit smoking and find that foods taste a lot better than they did before, be sure you're focusing your meals on healthy food options; that way, if you're tempted to take a few extra bites, at least they'll be bites of the good stuff. Here are a few recipe suggestions for people who are trying to quit smoking or those who have recently won the battle.

☙ Mixed Grain Cereal with Grapefruit Yogurt Topping

Kicking an addiction to smoking is one of the hardest things you can do. Making and eating delicious recipes like this one will help to reduce the negative health effects of smoking after you've quit and make it easier for your body to heal with plenty of calcium, protein, and antioxidants.

Grapefruit contains a compound called *naringin,* which lowers cancer-causing enzyme levels in your body. Paired with vitamin C, this powerful ingredient will help start to counteract the effects of smoking after you've snuffed out your last butt.

Preparation time: *10 minutes, plus overnight soak*

Cooking time: *18 minutes*

Yield: *3–4 servings*

1 cup long-grain organic brown rice	1/2 cup freshly squeezed grapefruit juice
1 cup organic amaranth	2 tablespoons local organic honey
1 cup organic steel-cut oats	1 1/4 teaspoons powdered stevia
1/2 cup organic millet	1/2 teaspoon cinnamon
1/2 cup organic barley	1 cup plain yogurt
1/2 cup flaxseed	1 cup organic grapefruit pieces
2 cups filtered water	2 tablespoons local organic honey

1 *Prepare the grain mixture:* Combine rice, amaranth, oats, millet, barley, and flaxseed in container; mix well. Seal container and store at room temperature up to one month.

2 To use, combine 1 cup of the grain mixture with the water in medium saucepan. Cover and let stand overnight. In the morning, add grapefruit juice, honey, stevia, and cinnamon and bring to a simmer. Simmer, covered, for 12–18 minutes until grains are tender.

3 Meanwhile, combine yogurt, grapefruit, and 2 tablespoons honey; mix well. Serve hot cereal topped with yogurt mixture.

Per serving: Calories 333 (From Fat 51); Fat 6g (Saturated 2g); Cholesterol 8mg; Sodium 35mg; Carbohydrate 64g; Dietary Fiber 6g; Protein 9g.

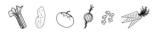

Crunchy Lemon Chicken with Roasted Tomato Sauce

Foods rich in vitamin C, like lemon and tomatoes, help your body heal when eaten with the protein in chicken. You can make the tomato sauce for this meal ahead of time; simply reheat it gently and pour it over the chicken just before you serve the dish. This recipe is special enough for company but easy and delicious enough to prepare for you and your family anytime!

Preparation time: *30 minutes plus 2 hours marinade time and 10 minutes "set" time for the chicken*

Cooking time: *40 minutes for the tomatoes and 15 minutes for the chicken*

Yield: *4 servings*

1/2 cup lemon juice	1 cup grape tomatoes, halved
2 tablespoons honey	1/2 cup chopped organic fresh basil
1/2 teaspoon turmeric	1/4 cup ground organic almonds
1/8 teaspoon cayenne pepper	2 tablespoons ground organic pistachios
4 boneless, skinless organic chicken breasts	1/4 cup organic wheat germ
6 organic plum tomatoes, cut in half	1 teaspoon dried basil leaves
1 organic yellow onion, peeled and chopped	1/4 teaspoon white pepper
3 cloves organic garlic, minced	3 tablespoons organic olive oil
2 tablespoons organic olive oil	1/2 cup organic chicken broth

1 In shallow pan, combine lemon juice, honey, turmeric, and cayenne pepper; mix well. Cut chicken breasts into three strips each, lengthwise; add to marinade. Cover and refrigerate 2–4 hours.

2 Meanwhile, place plum tomatoes, cut side up, in roasting pan. Sprinkle with onions and garlic and drizzle with 2 tablespoons oil. Roast in preheated 400-degree F oven 20 minutes. Add grape tomatoes; return to oven and roast 15–20 minutes longer until tomatoes soften. Remove from pan and place in serving bowl; stir in basil.

3 Remove chicken from marinade; reserve marinade. On shallow plate, combine almonds, pistachios, wheat germ, dried basil, and white pepper. Coat chicken in this mixture. Let chicken stand 10 minutes.

4 Heat 3 tablespoons oil in large skillet. Add chicken; cook, turning once, about 10–12 minutes until chicken is cooked and coating is brown and crunchy. Remove chicken from pan and place on serving plate.

5 Add reserved marinade and chicken broth to pan; boil 2 minutes, stirring to incorporate brown bits from pan. Add tomatoes; heat through. Serve with the chicken.

Per serving: *Calories 458 (From Fat 234); Fat 26g (Saturated 4g); Cholesterol 73mg; Sodium 133mg; Carbohydrate 27g; Dietary Fiber 4g; Protein 33g.*

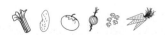

☙ Brown Rice Potato Pilaf

Root vegetables like butternut squash and sweet potatoes help promote lung health with their high antioxidant content. These compounds counter inflammation and help the healing process. They're also high in fiber, which helps you feel full and helps your body remove toxins more quickly.

This dish can be served as a side dish or as a vegetarian main dish. Add whatever dried fruits and nuts you like.

Preparation time: *20 minutes*

Cooking time: *About 1 hour 10 minutes*

Yield: *6 servings*

3 tablespoons organic olive oil

1 organic onion, peeled and chopped

3 cloves organic garlic, peeled and minced

1 organic sweet potato, peeled and chopped

1/2 organic butternut squash, peeled, seeded, and chopped

1 1/2 cups organic brown rice

1 teaspoon turmeric

1/2 teaspoon ground cumin

1/4 teaspoon saffron threads

2 cups filtered water

1/2 cup freshly squeezed orange juice

3 tablespoons freshly squeezed lemon juice

2 tablespoons local honey

1/2 cup chopped organic dried apricots

1/2 cup organic golden raisins

1/4 cup toasted sesame seeds

1 In large skillet, cook onion and garlic in olive oil 4–5 minutes until just tender. Add sweet potato and squash; cook and stir until starting to brown, about 10–12 minutes.

2 Add rice; cook and stir 3–4 minutes longer. Add turmeric, cumin, and saffron to 2 cups water; let stand while rice is sautéing. Add water mixture to rice mixture along with orange juice. Bring to a simmer, cover pan, and lower heat.

3 Cook 40–50 minutes until rice and vegetables are tender. Remove from heat; add lemon juice, honey, apricots, and raisins; fluff with fork. Cover pan again and let stand 5 minutes, then fluff with fork again, sprinkle with sesame seeds, and serve.

Per serving: Calories 429 (From Fat 101); Fat 11g (Saturated 1g); Cholesterol 0mg; Sodium 19mg; Carbohydrate 76g; Dietary Fiber 7g; Protein 7g.

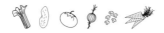

⏱ Herbed Fruit Soup

Many people gain weight after they quit smoking simply because they have nothing to do with their hands. So make lots of good and healthy food that combines nutrients with fiber so you are satisfied.

You can make this soup with any red fruit, including cherries, cranberries, boysenberries, watermelon, and pink or red grapefruit. It can be served warm or cold. If the soup is very thick when chilled, stir in some more orange juice or apple juice until you reach the desired consistency.

Preparation time: *5 minutes*

Cooking time: *40 minutes*

Yield: *6 servings*

2 cups filtered water

2 cups organic apple juice

1/3 cup finely chopped peeled Granny Smith apple

1/4 cup local honey

3 cups organic fresh or frozen raspberries

2 cups organic fresh or frozen red currants

2 cups chopped organic strawberries

3 tablespoons freshly squeezed lemon juice

2 tablespoons fresh thyme leaves

3 tablespoons minced fresh mint leaves

1 teaspoon vanilla

1 In large saucepan, combine water, apple juice, apple, and honey. Bring to a simmer; reduce heat to low and simmer 10 minutes. Add raspberries, currants, and strawberries and bring back to a simmer; cook 20-30 minutes until fruits are very tender.

2 Remove from heat and add lemon juice, thyme, mint, and vanilla. Serve hot, or cool 30 minutes, then chill. Garnish with fresh herb sprigs.

Per serving: Calories 158 (From Fat 7); Fat 1g (Saturated 0g); Cholesterol 0mg; Sodium 6mg; Carbohydrate 40g; Dietary Fiber 8g; Protein 2g.

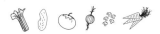

Chapter 15

Drowning Alcohol Abuse

In This Chapter

▶ Recognizing alcohol as a toxin and understanding its dangers

▶ Using detox methods to help your body beat alcohol's effects

Alcohol is the most common toxic chemical ingested today. About two-thirds of adults in the United States drink alcohol, and its effects on our bodies are wide ranging and can be very serious. Drinking alcohol is so common that you can easily forget it's an extremely potent toxin.

My goal in this chapter is to give you a full sense of what this toxin can do to your body. It's not a pretty picture, as you may guess. I then clue you in on some detoxification methods that can both reduce the harmful effects of alcohol and also help you to avoid drinking too much booze.

One quick note before I dive in. You may have read or heard that certain amounts of alcohol can be good for you, and for the most part that seems to be true. Medical research has shown that 2 to 3 ounces of alcohol per day can offer beneficial effects for your cardiovascular system. Also, several types of antioxidants, including flavonoids and resveratrol, are present in certain kinds of alcohol like red wine and dark beer. That's all well and good, and if you consume alcohol on that very limited level, it may boost your health in some ways. But the line between just enough and too much alcohol appears to be very thin; studies have also shown that more than 2 to 3 ounces of alcohol per day have a negative impact on your body.

REMEMBER

Throughout this chapter, I use a very general gauge of quantity when it comes to alcohol. Because alcohol content differs from drink to drink, the line between safe, healthy drinking and unhealthy drinking can be a moving target. Very broadly speaking, you're in the safe zone if you have two drinks per day, and a drink can be loosely defined as a can or bottle of beer, a glass of wine, or a 1.5-ounce serving of 80 proof liquor.

Understanding the Toxic Effects of Alcohol

Make no mistake: Alcohol is a toxin. When you drink an alcoholic beverage, the alcohol is absorbed from your intestines into your bloodstream and taken to your liver. Your liver recognizes it as a toxin and does its best to break down the alcohol in an effort to detoxify it. (About 95 percent of the alcohol you drink is broken down by your liver, and only about 5 percent is removed via your kidneys, sweat, and breathing.)

Your liver is an amazing organ and typically gives alcohol detoxification the ol' college try, but it isn't able to detoxify all the alcohol. If your liver is healthy, it breaks down alcohol at the rate of 2 to 3 ounces per hour. As a result, some alcohol ends up spreading through your body, where it gets widely distributed and produces its toxic effects.

Short-term effects of overconsumption

As you know if you've consumed multiple alcoholic drinks in a short span of time, the level of toxicity is related directly to the amount of alcohol you ingest. The toxic effects of alcohol begin in the brain, and they include the following:

- Aggressiveness
- Alteration in sexual inhibition
- Anesthesia
- Drowsiness
- Euphoria
- Impaired judgment
- Mood changes
- Release of inhibitions
- Sedation

Alcohol's effects on the brain are compounded by the changes it causes in the rest of your body's tissues, from your muscles to your eyes and everything in between. Here are a few of the other common effects of alcohol toxicity:

- Altered depth perception
- Decreased muscle function
- Decreased vision at night

✔ Decreased visual focus

✔ Impaired motor skills

If you've ever consumed too much alcohol, you've likely experienced one or several of these toxic effects. But alcohol toxicity doesn't stop there — not by a long shot. The potent toxic impact of alcohol can continue to cause much more serious effects on your body, including death. Alcohol can effectively paralyze your *diaphragm* — the muscle that is responsible for expanding and contracting your lungs — causing you to stop breathing and die from a lack of oxygen. Your heart can also be damaged, and booze can cause fatal irregularities in your heart's rhythm.

Long-term effects of overconsumption

The types of toxic effects I list in the previous section can result from a single episode involving a large amount of alcohol consumption. But what happens when you consume a lot of alcohol over a long period of time? (I'm talking about years here.) The resultant health problems are even more varied, and they include some very troubling mental conditions.

Long-term exposure to alcohol causes changes in personality that surface as anger, rage, anxiety, depression, fatigue, and lack of self-esteem, as well as self-loathing, intense guilt, and remorse.

Depression is one of the most dangerous mental effects of abusing alcohol over a long period of time. Alcohol abuse can lead to depression, and many people who suffer alcohol-related depression turn to booze as a way to get temporary relief from their depression. That quickly turns into a cycle that can ruin a person's life, and it's very hard break.

The physical impact of long-term exposure to alcohol is centered primarily on the nerves, brain, and liver, and I give each one of these areas attention here. I also give you a glimpse into the serious problems that booze can cause for your sleep patterns. These problems are little known but extremely serious, especially given that most people don't get enough healthy sleep as it is.

Nasty for your nerves

The medical community has been debating for years the damage that alcohol does to your *peripheral nerves,* which are all the nerves that aren't part of your brain or spinal cord. One camp insists that alcohol damages these nerves directly, while the other says that the vitamin and mineral deficiencies that result from drinking alcohol are to blame. Which group is right? Well, for the purposes of detoxification, it doesn't really matter. The point is that everyone agrees alcohol has a nasty toxic impact on your peripheral nerves, and the damage is severe and often long lasting. Here's a short list of the symptoms that you can experience as a result of that damage:

✔ Heat intolerance

✔ Impotence in men

✔ Muscle weakness due to nerve dysfunction

✔ Numbness in the feet, which spreads up the legs

✔ Numbness in the fingers, which spreads up the hands

✔ Pain in the arms and legs

✔ "Pins and needles" sensations in the feet and legs

✔ "Pins and needles" sensations in the hands and arms

✔ Problems with urination, including incontinence, difficulty starting urination, and incomplete emptying of the bladder

Sounds pretty awful, doesn't it? Well, the problems don't stop there. As if the damage to the peripheral nerves isn't enough, alcohol also causes debilitating effects on the *autonomic nerves,* which are the nerves that control your body's automatic functions. Long-term alcohol abuse can really foul up the functioning of those nerves, and the results are painful (both for the drinker and for his family and friends to watch). Here's a quick rundown of what can happen:

✔ Constipation

✔ Decrease in stomach activity

✔ Diarrhea

✔ Difficulty swallowing

✔ Loss of control of heart rate

✔ Radical drop in blood pressure when standing up

✔ Speech problems

✔ Vomiting

Your nerves are extremely complex tissues, and you can do them a huge amount of harm by drinking too much toxic alcohol. Is that extra glass of wine or mixed drink really worth it? If for some reason you aren't convinced, take a look at what alcohol abuse can do to your brain.

Bad for your brain

Long-term alcohol use damages your brain in all kinds of ways. At the top of the list is the killing off of brain cells. The fact that alcohol can destroy your brain's cells should give you a pretty good indication of how bad it is for what many people consider to be the most awe-inspiring and complex structure in the natural world.

In addition to the direct damage that alcohol does to your brain, it also creates vitamin and mineral deficiencies that rob your brain of the materials it needs to take care of even basic functions.

Finally, the damage that alcohol does to your liver (I tackle that topic in the next section) means that it isn't able to detoxify your body efficiently, and many other toxins that would've been broken down in the liver are therefore allowed to roam free in your bloodstream. It doesn't take long for these other toxins to reach your brain and begin affecting it in a very dangerous way.

This triple threat of alcohol's harmful effects on your brain — direct effects, vitamin and mineral deficiencies, and increased general toxicity — often ends in catastrophic damage to brain function. Let me fill you in on just a few of the possibilities:

- ✔ Abnormal emotional function.

- ✔ Dramatic decrease in problem-solving abilities.

- ✔ Loss of function of intelligent behavior.

- ✔ Loss of long-term and short-term memory; amnesia.

- ✔ Loss of the ability to use senses such as sight and smell.

- ✔ *Wernicke-Korsakoff syndrome,* which is triggered by a severe lack of vitamin B1 (also called *thiamine*). Symptoms include confusion, hallucinations, coma, and death if left untreated.

That's just a sampling; the list really could go on for pages.

Lousy for your liver

The burden of detoxifying alcohol in your body falls almost exclusively on your liver, so it's no surprise that alcoholic liver disease affects a large number of heavy drinkers. Three kinds of liver damage result from alcohol toxicity:

- ✔ **Alcoholic hepatitis:** This inflammation of the liver tissue is caused by alcohol and *acetaldehyde,* a very toxic substance that the liver produces when it's trying to break down alcohol. Symptoms include jaundice, fever, abdominal tenderness and pain, nausea, vomiting, and loss of appetite. This condition can be caused by a single drinking binge and can last for years. Thirty-five percent of heavy drinkers develop alcoholic hepatitis.

- ✔ **Alcoholic cirrhosis:** When alcohol cause normal liver tissue to be replaced by scar tissue, *alcoholic cirrhosis* is the result. Liver function is severely hindered by cirrhosis, and the condition is irreversible. Twenty percent of heavy drinkers develop cirrhosis, and it kills tens of thousands of people every year in the United States alone.

✔ **Fatty liver:** When alcohol causes *fatty liver,* the liver's normal cells are replaced with fat cells. The liver becomes enlarged, but its function is greatly reduced.

In addition to these three specific debilitating conditions, alcohol ruins your liver in several other general ways, which create indirect problems with many other parts of your body. When your liver detoxifies alcohol, it creates byproducts that are damaging not only to the liver but also to your body's other tissues. These chemicals are responsible for large scale inflammation. If you check out Chapter 13, which is all about the toxins that harm your circulatory system and how you can limit their effects, you'll realize that most heart disease is caused by inflammation. The harmful chemicals can be countered by antioxidants, but when you add in the taxing effects of all the other toxins we take in on a daily basis, it's really hard to get enough antioxidants to win the war.

Your liver is also an important storage facility. It stores *glycogen* (a storable form of glucose), as well as vitamins B12, A, and D. And your liver's crucial functions don't stop there: Your liver converts fats and glucose to energy, produces cholesterol your body uses to create hormones, and synthesizes critical amino acids. If your liver has to spend all its time detoxifying alcohol, it has limited resources for performing these other vital functions, and your health can completely fall apart as a result.

When taken with alcohol, certain drugs (both prescription and over-the-counter) can cause extreme and irreversible damage to your liver, and even death. At the top of the list are drugs containing acetaminophen, pain killers, anti-anxiety medications, and drugs prescribed to reduce cholesterol.

Stealing healthy sleep

The effect of alcohol on your sleeping patterns merits special attention because the problem is serious and often misunderstood.

Alcohol causes sleepiness. However, when you go to sleep with alcohol in your system, you don't get normal, healthy sleep. Alcohol prevents your body from going into a particular state of sleep when your muscles are completely relaxed and 95 percent of dreaming occurs. You don't need to consume much alcohol for this problem to happen; only about 6 ounces will harm your sleep patterns in a serious way.

After your liver manages to detoxify all the alcohol in your system — remember, that's about 2 to 3 ounces per hour — then your brain rebounds and tries to make up for the lost sleep stages. But it isn't able to do so, and your sleep isn't as restful and rejuvenating as it is when no alcohol is in your system. When you wake up the next day, you'll likely feel tired and unrested. Larger amounts of alcohol cause a proportionately larger effect, and your physical and mental functions can be severely decreased.

Some people use alcohol as a way to help them fall asleep, but that's a very unhealthy and unsafe practice. Alcohol hurts your sleep patterns and prevents you from getting healthy, normal sleep, so drinking it before bedtime is a surefire way to wake up feeling tired and worn down the next day.

If you continue to go to sleep with alcohol in your system over a long period of time, your body eventually develops a tolerance for alcohol that is the definition of addiction. You won't be able to go to sleep without alcohol, and every time you drink to fall asleep you're adding to your body's toxicity. It's an extremely harmful, unhealthy cycle of addiction.

Using Detoxification Techniques against Alcohol

Like many other health issues, alcohol toxicity can be decreased and its effects reduced if you use some basic detoxification techniques. Changing your drinking behavior to mesh with your overall detoxification goals will help you cut out unhealthy alcohol use. And supplementing with a range of vitamins, minerals, and herbs can help you undo some of the damage done by booze. I cover both topics in this section.

Adjusting your drinking behavior

If you realize and understand that alcohol is a toxin, and you're convinced that detoxification should be a top priority in your life (and I hope you are!), you should be prepared to make some changes to your drinking behavior. You want to make choices about alcohol that jibe with your other detoxification efforts. Here are a few tips that fall in line with that way of thinking:

- ✔ Limit your alcohol intake to 2 to 3 ounces per day.
- ✔ Eat something when you're drinking.
- ✔ Don't drink and take any sort of drug at the same time.
- ✔ Eat a diet that contains foods with high vitamin B content.
- ✔ Don't drink by yourself.
- ✔ Seek help from a doctor or other professional if you consistently drink more than 4 ounces per day.

Supplementing to help your body beat alcohol's effects

Alcohol use can easily cause deficiencies of several important vitamins and minerals in your body. If you want to thwart the damaging effects of alcohol, the first step is taking supplements that help to make sure your body isn't being robbed of what it needs to perform. Look for supplements that include the following key vitamins and minerals:

✔ Magnesium

✔ Potassium

✔ Vitamin A

✔ Vitamin B complex (includes B1, B3, B5, B6, B7, B9, and B12)

To help your body recoup the vitamin B that it can lose as a result of alcohol use, be sure to eat plenty of vitamin B–rich foods like bananas, lentils, beans, turkey, peppers, and potatoes.

You can also seek out supplements that will help your liver to cope with the damages associated with alcohol toxicity. Here are the ones I recommend:

✔ **Alpha-lipoic acid (ALA):** This compound is very potent in supporting basic liver function and has been successful in treating liver toxicity that was considered lethal otherwise. Capsules and tablets are the most common supplement forms of ALA.

✔ **Catechin:** A powerful antioxidant compound, catechin can help limit the damage done to your liver by alcohol and other toxins. It also fights intestinal toxins and improves the health of your body's cell membranes. One of the most common supplement forms is green tea extract, so if you're interested look for that supplement in tablet form.

✔ **Milk thistle:** Derived from a plant that is common to many areas of the world, this herbal supplement offers a potent antioxidant power and inhibits an enzyme in the liver that leads to inflammation. You can take it as a capsule or in liquid form.

✔ **N-Acetylcysteine:** In addition to combating liver toxicity caused by alcohol and other toxins, this compound provides antioxidant effects and boosts your immune system, to boot.

✔ **Resveratrol:** Studies have shown this antioxidant to be very beneficial in reducing liver damage. You can find it in tablet or capsule form.

✔ **Vitamin C:** This jack-of-all-trades supplement is a requirement for anyone looking to heal any part of the body (including the liver). Don't think twice about taking as much as 4,000 mg per day.

✔ **Vitamin D:** This old standby is necessary for any detoxification effort.

I've been working with patients on alcohol addiction for decades, and I've seen the terrific effects of these kinds of supplements on many occasions. Some of my patients have had extreme liver toxicity caused by alcohol, and supplements like milk thistle and ALA have helped their livers heal to the point where they were seeing normal liver function within one week of starting supplementation.

Recipes for Helping You Detox from Alcohol

If you're worried that alcohol toxicity is harming your body, you should start detoxifying for alcohol immediately. Your efforts should include changes in your diet that focus on including antioxidant-rich foods and foods that contain plenty of B vitamins.

Here are several tasty recipes that you can make to help steer your diet toward helping you reduce the ravages of alcohol toxicity.

♻ Fruity Peppermint Granita

Fresh herbs like peppermint, chamomile, and lavender may help alcoholics recover and ease withdrawal symptoms. Just the aroma of peppermint helps soothe an upset stomach. Peppermint is combined with fruit juices and frozen to make a refreshing and healthy granita you can eat as a snack or dessert.

Preparation time: *10 minutes*

Chilling time: *5 hours*

Yield: *4 servings*

1/2 cup chopped fresh organic peppermint leaves

1/2 cup filtered water

2 cups freshly squeezed orange juice

1/2 cup freshly squeezed lemon juice

2 tablespoons local organic honey

1/4 teaspoon powdered stevia, to taste

1 Combine all ingredients in a blender; blend until finely minced. Strain mixture through a fine sieve, pressing on mint leaves to extract as much flavor as possible.

2 Pour mixture into 9"x13" pan; the liquid should be about 1/4- to 1/3-inch thick. Freeze for 5 hours, scraping the mixture every hour with tines of a fork to make crystals.

3 When ready to serve, scrape the frozen mixture to fluff up; spoon into glasses, and serve immediately.

Per serving: Calories 98 (From Fat 3); Fat 0g (Saturated 0g); Cholesterol 0mg; Sodium 3mg; Carbohydrate 25g; Dietary Fiber 1g; Protein 1g.

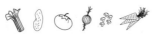

☁ Spicy Eggs with Broccoli Sprout Salad

For recovering alcoholics, L-glutamine is an important nutrient because it has been shown to decrease cravings for alcohol and also make the withdrawal process more bearable. It's found in foods like eggs, wheat germ, dairy products, and oats. But for it to work most effectively, it should be combined with foods rich in niacin. These include celery (especially deep green celery), mushrooms, asparagus, and broccoli.

This dish, commonly known as "Eggs in Purgatory," is delicious for a breakfast or a late supper. The fresh and crisp salad is a nice contrast to the warm and rich eggs.

Preparation time: *20 minutes*

Cooking time: *35 minutes*

Yield: *6 servings*

2 (1/8-inch thick) slices American ginseng root	2 tablespoons extra virgin olive oil
1/4 cup water	1 organic yellow onion, peeled and chopped
3 tablespoons extra virgin olive oil	3 cloves organic garlic, peeled and minced
2 tablespoons freshly squeezed orange juice	1 organic jalapeno pepper, minced
1 tablespoon fresh thyme leaves	4 red organic tomatoes, chopped
2 cups fresh organic broccoli sprouts	1 cup organic or freshly squeezed tomato juice
2 cups organic cherry tomatoes, cut in half	2 tablespoons freshly squeezed orange juice
1 cup sliced organic celery	1/8 teaspoon cayenne pepper
1 cup sliced organic mushrooms	6 eggs

1 In small saucepan, combine ginseng and water; simmer 5 minutes, then cool. Strain liquid into medium bowl; add olive oil, orange juice, and thyme leaves; whisk to combine. Add sprouts, cherry tomatoes, celery, and mushrooms; toss gently and set aside.

2 Preheat oven to 375 degrees F. In large skillet, heat 2 tablespoons olive oil over medium heat. Add onion, garlic, and jalapeno pepper; sauté 5 – 6 minutes until crisp-tender. Add tomatoes, tomato juice, orange juice, and pepper; simmer 5 minutes.

3 Carefully crack eggs onto the simmering sauce, keeping them separated from one another. Bake 15–20 minutes until eggs are just set. Serve egg mixture with sprout salad.

Per serving: Calories 250 (From Fat 152); Fat 17g (Saturated 3g); Cholesterol 213mg; Sodium 109mg; Carbohydrate 17g; Dietary Fiber 3g; Protein 9g.

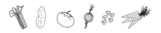

Beef and Cabbage Lentil Salad

Uncooked cabbage is another good source of L-glutamine. Cabbage is also rich in *gluco-sinolates,* which help improve immune function so your body can recover and regain health. Raw vegetables, of course, are central to any detox diet. This combination is fresh and delicious, with lots of crunch and beautiful color.

Lentils are loaded with plenty of folic acid and fiber that are essential for an alcohol detox. Zinc, which helps protect the liver against alcohol, and iron, a nutrient alcoholics may be deficient in, are found in beef. It's important to look for 100 percent organic, grass-fed beef when you're on a detox diet.

This delicious salad will satisfy anyone's appetite. It can be eaten hot or cold; in fact, leftovers are delicious served the next day.

Preparation time: *15 minutes*

Cooking time: *45 minutes*

Yield: *4 servings*

1 pound organic, grass-fed beef ribeye steaks	*1 tablespoon apple cider vinegar*
2 tablespoons freshly squeezed lemon juice	*1 tablespoon local honey*
1 1/2 cups organic French Puy lentils	*1/3 cup extra virgin olive oil*
3 cups filtered water	*2 tablespoons Dijon mustard*
2 cups chopped organic red cabbage	*1 tablespoon minced fresh oregano*
1 organic green bell pepper, chopped	*1/4 teaspoon pepper*
1 organic yellow bell pepper, chopped	*2 tablespoons chopped fresh flat-leaf parsley*
2 tablespoons freshly squeezed lemon juice	

1 Place steaks in shallow pan; sprinkle with 2 tablespoons lemon juice and rub into both sides. Refrigerate while preparing lentils and the salad.

2 Sort lentils and rinse. Drain and combine them with water in medium saucepan. Bring to a boil, lower heat, cover, and simmer until lentils are tender, 23–28 minutes. Drain if necessary and set aside.

3 In serving bowl, combine cabbage, bell peppers, and lentils. In small bowl, combine 2 tablespoons lemon juice, vinegar, honey, olive oil, mustard, oregano, pepper, and parsley. Mix well and pour over cabbage mixture; toss gently to coat. Set aside.

4 Remove the meat from the fridge and let it come to room temperature. Place beef on broiler pan; broil, turning once, 8–12 minutes until desired doneness. Remove from heat, cover, and let stand 5 minutes. Slice beef thinly and arrange over salad; serve immediately.

Per serving: Calories 658 (From Fat 307); Fat 34g (Saturated 9g); Cholesterol 54mg; Sodium 242mg; Carbohydrate 55g; Dietary Fiber 18g; Protein 37g.

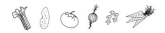

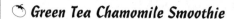

♨ Green Tea Chamomile Smoothie

Green tea and chamomile will help you calm down and regain your composure. Tea is also a wonderful healing food that brings balance to your body. It relieves muscle spasms, boosts the immune system, and fights infection. Along with vitamin C–rich foods like mangoes and oranges, this smoothie is the perfect pick-me-up any time of the day.

Preparation time: *20 minutes*

Cooking time: *5 minutes*

Yield: *3–4 servings*

2 tablespoons organic green tea leaves	1/4 cup freshly squeezed orange juice
1/3 cup filtered water, heated	1/3 cup plain organic yogurt
1 tablespoon dried organic chamomile flowers	2 tablespoons local honey
2 ripe organic mangoes, peeled and cubed	1 frozen banana, peeled and cubed

1 Place tea leaves and chamomile flowers in a small bowl; pour heated water over. Let steep 5 minutes, then strain, reserving liquid. Chill liquid until cold.

2 Combine all remaining ingredients, including the chilled tea, in a blender or food processor. Process until smooth and thick. Serve immediately.

Per serving: *Calories 196 (From Fat 12); Fat 1g (Saturated 1g); Cholesterol 4mg; Sodium 17mg; Carbohydrate 48g; Dietary Fiber 4g; Protein 2g.*

Chapter 16

Enhancing Mental Health with Detoxification

Most of the chapters in this book focus on various aspects of your physical health, but I couldn't write a book about improving your total health with detoxification without a mention of mental health. When you get right down to it, mental health is just as important as physical health. You could be as physically fit and healthy as possible, but if your mind isn't sound, you likely won't lead a meaningful, fulfilling, enjoyable life.

Mental health and physical health are also incredibly interrelated. You can't separate the mind from the body, after all. Decreased mental wellness has a profound effect on physical wellness, and lack of physical health creates mental unrest. Scores of studies show a very high correlation between mental health problems and cardiovascular disease, arthritis, Parkinson's disease, substance abuse, and many other chronic diseases.

The hectic world that we live in today puts a huge amount of stress on our minds, and the influx of toxins — which harm your brain's delicate chemical balance — certainly don't make things any easier. If you're not careful, the combination of a stressful life and elevated toxicity can wear on your mind and end up causing a mental health problem. Depression (or *non-traumatic stress syndrome,* as I call it) is one of the most common conditions caused by increased stress on a number of levels, and it's one that (thankfully) you can avoid or defeat by embracing several methods of detoxification.

Digging into Depression

Depression is one of the most common challenges to a healthy state of mind. The problem isn't a small one. Estimates indicate that 80 percent of people who go to a physician are depressed and 80 percent of people with depression aren't treated. (Keep in mind that chronic illness is a major stressor that can cause depression, and chronic illness is a top reason for physician visits.)

At any given time, almost 19 million people in the United States are living with depression, and the absenteeism cost of that problem alone is about $51 billion per year.

Depression is a very emotionally charged word. Historically, the word conjures images of weakness and an inability to get a grip on life. Many people think that those living with depression should be able to just straighten up and get over it. In fact, studies have shown that 54 percent of people still think that depression is a personal weakness. That's an extremely discouraging statistic, especially because we now know that people who are depressed experience biochemical changes in the brain that can't be changed with all the willpower in the world. We *must* get familiar with the real causes and symptoms of depression because we can't do much about it if we don't fully understand the problem. That's what this section is all about.

Understanding the causes of depression

In my experience, the central cause of all depression is stress. I've never encountered anyone in or outside my practice with depression who didn't have abnormally high stress. Stress is the common thread of depression, to the point where I think we should drop the term depression and call this complex of symptoms *non-traumatic stress syndrome* (NTSS). This term better represents what is actually happening, and it's generally more acceptable to patients as an explanation of their problems. I use the two terms interchangeably, and I think we'd all be better off if more people did the same.

When I use the word "stress," I'm talking about social and mental stress — demanding jobs, big changes to your personal live, and so on — but I'm also talking about physical stress. Not surprisingly, elevated levels of toxins in your body can put a huge amount of physical stress on you, which can help push you toward depression.

Here's another important aspect of depression: It isn't caused by depressing situations. That statement may sound odd to some people, but it's true. Consider this: If depression was caused by depressing situations, every person living on the street would be massively depressed. But that's not the case; some street people are actually happy. And some people who have great jobs and steady paychecks and nice houses are among the most depressed.

All the stressors you face on a daily basis have a negative effect on how your body and mind function. The combined impact can be huge, even without the presence of a major stressful factor. A little bit of stress and toxicity here and there all add up to cause dysfunction and disease. Let me fill you in on some of the details of both mental and physical stress, so you can identify them easily and deal with them if you need to.

Changing brain chemistry

The chemistry of the brain is fabulously complex, and the balance of chemicals that play a role in brain function is a delicate one. You've probably heard of the importance of certain chemicals in the brain called *neurotransmitters,* and for good reason: Most studies indicate that a depletion of neurotransmitters is one of the top contributing factors in people suffering from NTSS. They're not the only important chemicals in your brain, but they're near the top of the list.

What causes a depletion of neurotransmitters? A couple things. The first is stress. Stress causes an increased firing of nerves in the brain, which can't take place without neurotransmitters. Too much stress means too much nerve firing, which uses up your brain's supply of neurotransmitters. That's a pretty simplistic description of a very complicated set of processes, but you get the idea.

The other side of the neurotransmitter problem is a dietary deficiency of essential nutrients that your body uses to make neurotransmitters. If you don't get enough of the right kinds of nutrients, your body isn't able to generate neurotransmitters, and your brain is left wanting.

Environmental toxins — from heavy metals to chemical toxins — can have a major negative effect on your neurotransmitters. Increased exposure to toxins can cause a range of mental health conditions, including (but definitely not limited to) NTSS. Heavy metals are among the worst, with lead and mercury leading the way.

Stress on stress on stress

Mental stress is the kind of stress that you suffer from as a result of events that cause change in your life. Stressors vary from person to person, and they can include almost anything. Here's a list of some of the most common stressors:

- Death of a spouse
- Marital separation or divorce
- Marriage
- Sexual dysfunction
- Loss of a job

- Change in working conditions, including increased responsibility
- Monotony
- Change in financial status
- Personal injury or illness (especially chronic illness)
- Pain
- Change in the health of a family member
- Hormonal changes such as puberty, premenstrual syndrome, menopause, or pregnancy
- New babies or departing children (empty nest syndrome)
- Vacation
- Retirement
- Fear of aging
- Moving or buying a new house
- Excessive time demands of daily schedule
- Difficulty with sleep
- Alcohol or drug abuse
- Imagined changes in life or fear of possible negative changes in life
- Very hot or cold climates
- Chronic allergies

This isn't a complete list, but it does include some of the more common causes of stress. And stress certainly isn't the same for everyone. One person may thrive on having a packed daily schedule, while that same schedule could completely overwhelm another person.

Did anything about that list surprise you? How about the fact that some of those things are traditionally thought of as happy life events? Did you expect, for example, to see "vacation" on the list?

Stressful events or changes don't have to be sad or depressing. Many things that are usually thought of as positive — like marriage or new babies, for example — can create a huge amount of stress. Sometimes happy events are even more stressful for certain people than sad events.

The stress of positive life changes

It's difficult to think of positive life changes as being a cause for depression, but the situation is very real. Not long ago, a 23-year-old woman came to my practice as depressed as anyone I have ever seen. She had just gotten married, and the event was grand at all stages. There were lots of wedding showers; a big, flashy ceremony; and an incredible honeymoon on a Caribbean island. After her marriage, she moved to a new town where her husband lived. They got a new house and started very lucrative, challenging jobs. I could barely hear all the details of her story because she just couldn't stop sobbing. She was afraid that she was going crazy because she couldn't function and she wanted only to stay in her bedroom and cry.

All the recent events in her life were positive and happy, but they all involved big changes in her daily life, which created stress. Stories like hers are very common, but they're often ignored and the resulting conditions untreated because many people can't understand how it's possible to be depressed with so many good things happening in life.

Seeing the symptoms

The symptoms of depression are wide ranging, and they can sometimes be difficult to identify. The problem is further complicated by the fact that all psychiatric diagnoses are manmade. The same isn't true in other areas of medicine. Take orthopedics: A broken leg is a broken leg. That sort of diagnosis isn't subject to personal opinion, and it isn't likely to change over time. But psychiatric diagnoses just aren't as clear cut because the symptoms and conditions can be a moving target. For a mental health condition to be identified, a group of psychiatrists sit down and decide on the symptoms that make up that illness. The symptoms and their order of importance may change over time and can be subject to social pressures. These types of diagnoses aren't an exact science by any means.

Depression diagnoses are a classic example. Psychiatrists have developed a group of symptoms that they lump together and call depression. How does it work? It's actually pretty simple. You must have five or more of the following symptoms during the same two-week period, and those symptoms must be accompanied by a depressed mood or a loss of interest in pleasure:

- ✔ A depressed mood for most of the day, nearly every day.

- ✔ Markedly diminished interest or pleasure in all or almost all activities most of the day, nearly every day.

- ✔ Significant (more than 5 percent) weight gain or loss without dieting, or change in appetite nearly every day.

✔ Insomnia or *hypersomnia* (constant sleepiness) nearly every day.

✔ A feeling of restlessness nearly every day.

✔ Fatigue or loss or energy nearly every day.

✔ Feelings or worthlessness or guilt nearly every day.

✔ Diminished ability to think or concentrate.

✔ Recurrent thoughts of death.

To me, the logic of that kind of diagnosis is a little flawed. For example, what happens if you have only four of the symptoms (not the required five), but your symptoms are severe? I'm also not convinced that these symptoms cover all the bases of depression or NTSS. I have a few other things I look for when I'm figuring out if a person may be suffering from the condition. Here are the other questions I ask:

✔ Do you feel depressed, sad, and melancholy?

✔ Have you lost interest in hobbies?

✔ Are there things that used to be fun that are not fun now, like keeping the house clean or doing routine maintenance on the car?

✔ When you get home do you see several things that need to be done but you can't decide what to do? Do you just sit down or have to force yourself to get up and do those things?

✔ Is your overall motivation to do things decreased?

✔ Does it take you a long time to go to sleep?

✔ While you are waiting to fall asleep does your mind go on fast forward hopping from topic to topic?

✔ Do you wake up frequently during the night?

✔ Do you wake up early?

✔ Could you sleep much longer if you had a chance?

✔ Do you have trouble with focus? If you are doing something boring does your mind wander?

✔ Are you having trouble with your memory?

✔ Is your sex drive decreased?

✔ Have you developed new pains?

✔ Do little things seem to hurt worse than they used to?

✔ Do you have trouble making decisions about small things?

✔ When was the last time you felt so full of joy you thought you would jump out of your skin?

✔ Are you easily frustrated?

✔ Do you get angry over things that didn't bother you before?

✔ Do you lose your temper or hold it in more than you used to?

✔ Do you feel overwhelmed?

✔ Do you ever feel that if you could just run away everything would be better?

✔ Do you ever think of suicide?

As you can see, NTSS can include many different changes in behavior. In my view, when a patient answers yes to several of these questions, it can be a definite cause for concern. When your neurotransmitter levels are depleted, you soon start to exhibit some of the behaviors in these two symptom lists, which can further elevate your stress levels, creating an escalation in your NTSS that can turn dangerous very quickly.

If you or someone close to you begins experiencing some of the symptoms I list in this section, get professional help right away.

Analyzing Autism Spectrum Disorders

While depression or NTSS has become extremely common, another set of complex biochemical changes in the brain has reached epidemic status: autism spectrum disorders (ASD). Autism now affects 1 in every 91 children born in the United States, and that statistic doesn't include children with ADD or ADHD. In my opinion, ASD is a continuum that runs from ADD on one end to profound autism at the other.

Fingering the cause

The cause of autism spectrum disorders? Toxins, and a variety of biochemical alterations that affect the brain as a result of increased toxicity.

It has taken many years for even the basic causes of autism to be identified. Over the decades, the disorders have been attributed to everything from inattentive mothers to psychiatric disorders. But the root of the problem is a biochemical disorder that involves the kind of toxicity I discuss in many areas of this book. As with any controversial disease or condition, plenty of naysayers refute this line of thinking, but the evidence is growing and enforcing it more and more every day.

Figuring out the best treatments

Effective treatment for ASD requires a range of efforts, the scope of which is too broad to cover in this chapter. The best treatments involve clearing up the gut to get rid of yeast, parasites, abnormal bacteria, and viruses; detoxifying heavy metals; making dietary changes that focus on wholesome, organic, healthful food; supplementing with the essential vitamins, minerals, amino acids, antioxidants, and essential fatty acids; and eliminating wheat and milk products.

We don't have all the answers, but data collected by the Autism Research Institute has shown these changes to be effective in improving the behaviors and life of children on the spectrum. Seventy-four percent of parents of ASD children report that their children are improved after having heavy metals removed; 72 percent are improved after receiving methyl-B12 injections; and 65 percent show improvement after being on a gluten-free, casein-free diet.

If you or someone you know suffers from an autism spectrum disorder, be sure to talk to your doctor about the importance of detoxifying and avoiding toxic influences. For more information, visit the Web sites of the Autism Research Institute and Defeat Autism Now! (www.autism.com) or Generation Rescue (www.generationrescue.org).

Busting Stress and Anxiety through Detoxification

The stress put on our bodies and minds as a result of changes in our lives and the presence of toxins can lead to behavioral changes, including depression or non-traumatic stress syndrome (NTSS). That's the bad news, and you can read all about it in this chapter's earlier sections. The good news is that you can harness the power of a few detoxification techniques to curtail stress and head off these types of mental conditions at the pass.

The toxins that you bring into your body through environmental exposure and food decrease its ability to conduct the normal chemical reactions that need to take place millions of times each day throughout your many systems to keep you healthy. Your brain — with its delicate balance of neurotransmitters and other vital biochemistry — is no exception, so it's easy to see how increased toxicity can throw off your brain's regular functioning.

If you want to stop this trend before it begins to have devastating effects on your brain health and mental state, or if you want to slow or reverse a condition that you're already suffering from, start by employing some of the basic detoxification measures that I describe in detail in Part II of this book. For example:

- ✔ Undertake basic bowel detoxification against yeast, abnormal bacteria, and parasites.
- ✔ Conduct a heavy metal evaluation and detoxification if necessary.
- ✔ Make smart dietary choices (which I discuss in the next section).
- ✔ Supplement to ensure the proper intake of key nutrients.
- ✔ Make sure you sweat heavily on a daily basis through exercise.

That's a quick rundown, but I also want to make sure you get a full sense of how you can focus on a few detoxification standards to improve your mental health. So please keep reading!

Beefing up your brain

Elevated levels of stress and toxins can give your brain and its delicate chemical balance a real beating. But you don't have to simply roll with the punches; you can do a number of things to help knock out those damaging effects.

Antidepressant drugs do have a place in the treatment of depression, particularly when the symptoms are life-threatening or when a patient refuses to use more natural measures. However, it's unfortunate when the latter happens, because natural measures are effective in most cases. I am often able to effectively treat NTSS in my patients when I put them on a regimen of supplements that provide them with the building block chemicals their bodies use to make neurotransmitters. In many cases this kind of treatment works even when antidepressant prescription drugs have failed.

Here are some of the supplements that have really worked for my patients. (It's also worth noting that solid scientific studies support the idea that these substances are helpful in treating depression.)

- ✔ **Folic acid:** This vitamin is required for the development of nerve tissue in the developing brains of babies in the womb, and it's also necessary for the production of a naturally occurring and very important compound in your brain called S-Adenosyl methionine. (You may want to call that one by its nickname, Sam-E, and you can read more about it in this list.)
- ✔ **Inositol:** This compound, found in most of your body's cells, is involved in *cell signaling,* which is transmitting information between cells. (That's right, your cells talk to each other!) Studies have shown that inositol is as effective as antidepressants in treating depression.

✔ **Omega-3 fatty acids:** I talk about these crucial substances quite a lot throughout this book. Omega-3s have been shown to produce antidepressant effects in multiple studies, and you can get them in fish oil or through supplementing.

✔ **Phosphatidylcholine:** In addition to being a real mouthful to pronounce, this one is part of the chemical mix that results in acetylcholine, which is a major neurotransmitter in the brain.

✔ **S-Adenosyl methionine:** Also called Sam-E, this chemical is a precursor of serotonin and dopamine, which are two of the most important neurotransmitters.

I've found these substances to be really useful in treating NTSS in my patients. Another added benefit is that they have no side effects, and they're not known to cause any toxicity.

The substances I list in this section are terrific at helping to boost the brain and fight off NTSS, but don't try to use them on your own to treat that condition. Be sure to consult a physician who's familiar with these kinds of treatments before starting any kind of regimen.

Managing stress with what's on your plate

You can't do much good cutting out the stress that threatens your mental state if you aren't committed to good health, and you're going to have a very hard time achieving good health if your diet isn't good. If you haven't already done so, take a few minutes to look through Chapters 6 and 7 so you can understand what you need to include in your diet to give yourself the best possible foundation for health. It all starts with your diet.

In addition to the general food choices and eating behaviors I describe in Chapters 6 and 7, you really want to focus on a few diet specifics in order to reduce the stress you're putting on your body and mind. In particular,

✔ **Don't eat anything white.** That includes sugar, sugar substitutes, and flour, for starters. Cauliflower is an exception.

✔ **Avoid processed foods.** Processed foods are lousy with toxins, and they don't provide you with any of the nutrients your body really needs. Be sure to read food labels and don't eat anything with ingredients you can't pronounce.

✔ **Cut out the trans fats.** This step is critical in any healthy, detoxified diet.

✔ **Load up on B vitamins.** Get B vitamins with lean beef (100 percent organic, of course), lentils, bananas, avocado, clams, oysters — even octopus!

Using natural supplements to stave off stress

Natural supplements — particularly those that are herb-based — have been used for thousands of years to help boost mental health and relieve stress. Most of these are available at your local vitamin or health food store, and several have been verified by a variety of scientific data over the years. Here's the cream of the crop:

- **Chamomile:** I recommend chamomile tea as a delicious way to reduce anxiety and aid sleep.

- **Kava kava:** Used for centuries as a calming supplement, the root of the kava kava plant — available at health food stores in capsules and liquids — can also be very effective in reducing anxiety and decreasing the effects of depression.

- **Lemon balm:** Part of the mint family, this herb has shown some effectiveness in treating anxiety when taken as a tea or in capsule form.

- **Passionflower:** Made from a common plant found in the southeast region of the United States, this supplement can be found in capsule or liquid form.

- **Rhodiola:** Europeans have embraced this herbal supplement for many years, and it's starting to see an increase in popularity in the United States. Use it to help relieve depression symptoms and to bust stress and anxiety.

- **Skullcap:** This herbal supplement has a funny name, but its capacity for decreasing stress is serious business.

- **St. John's wort:** You may have read reports that St. John's wort's potential for treating depression isn't quite as impressive as everyone once thought, but I'm still a firm believer that it can be a very powerful means for helping those with mild to moderate depression. Most negative studies on St John's wort focused on patients with major depression.

- **Valerian root:** Many people know this supplement as a useful remedy for insomnia, but it's also good for relieving stress. It comes in liquid or tablet form.

Considering a few other ways to deal with stress

Today, you can find a stressor just about everywhere you look. Most of us live in a hectic, frenzied environment where big changes happen all the time, and it can be difficult to keep up and prevent stress from really wearing us down. You need to tackle the wide variety of stressors with an equally varied arsenal of stress-busting methods. Many of these methods are completely toxin free, so I support them enthusiastically. I'll start with some quick ones and then get into a little more detail on exercise and sauna:

- ✔ **Personal time:** This sounds so simple, but when was the last time you turned off your phone, pushed back from the computer, and asked the kids to play quietly by themselves for an hour or so? You need to find time in your daily life to relax and clear your mind. Try a bubble bath or some deep breathing, or maybe just find a comfortable corner of your home and dive into a good book for an hour or so. (Just make sure the book isn't a spy thriller or a horror novel — remember that we're trying to eliminate stress here, not create it!)

- ✔ **Sex:** Sex is one of our most basic methods for stress and anxiety relief. Do whatever you need to do to maintain a healthy sex life.

- ✔ **Yoga:** You can read study after study that supports the use of yoga for stress relief. It's also great for your physical health, so roll out the mat and get started!

- ✔ **Meditation:** This practice has also been used for stress relief and enhanced mental clarity for thousands of years. It doesn't require any fancy equipment or expensive memberships — just a little time and some quiet.

- ✔ **Journaling:** So many people don't take the time to reflect on their days. You need to savor your accomplishments and work thoughtfully through your problems, and writing in a journal is a great way to do so. Few other methods are as effective for getting feelings and concerns off your chest.

Exercise

I'll tout the benefits of exercise as long as I have breath in my lungs, but special consideration needs to be given here to the mental health benefits of regular exercise. Getting 30 minutes of exercise each and every day is a terrific way to enhance your health in a way that isn't possible through any other means, and it's also a proven way that you can boost your mind. Here are just a few of the ways that exercise can help your mental state:

- ✔ **Endorphin release:** These "feel good" neurotransmitters are released when you exercise, and they're great at elevating your mood.

- ✔ **Decreased anxiety:** This wonderful effect is due to a combination of physical and mental factors.

- ✔ **Increased stamina:** More stamina means more energy, which allows you to accomplish more without fatigue.

✔ **Sense of accomplishment:** Whether you're walking briskly for a few blocks or running a marathon, you're doing something good for your body and mind. That feeling of accomplishment can really boost your sense of self worth.

✔ **Improved pain threshold:** Constant pain can have a devastating effect on your mental health, and exercise helps your body deal with pain much more effectively.

✔ **Decreased impotence:** Especially in men, exercise can help thwart impotence, which helps you unlock more of the stress-busting benefits of a healthy sex life.

✔ **Increased fun:** Going out for a jog with your spouse or playing a few good-spirited sets of tennis with a buddy can be a lot of fun, and it's tough to argue that having fun puts you in a better, healthier state of mind.

Exercise every day! Just 30 minutes of daily physical activity will have a fantastic effect on your health — both physical and mental. Check out Chapter 13 to figure out which kinds of exercise will work best for you.

Sauna

Many of the toxic chemicals that put stress on your body and harm your brain function are packed away in fat cells. You can flush out these toxins by spending time in a sauna, because the intense sweating works to shuttle the toxic chemicals out through your skin. Doing so will help to decrease your toxic load, and it's also extremely relaxing. What's better for eliminating anxiety and stress than sitting in a nice hot sauna with a fluffy towel and a big bottle of water? Sauna is truly a great way to reduce the physical and mental causes of stress. I explain all your options for sauna in Chapter 18.

Recipes for Improving Your Mental Health

Diet is an important aspect of mental health. The chemical processes that take place in your brain are complex and wondrous, and they require a lot of key nutrients. The recipes here are chock-full of healthy ingredients that will help to give your brain the good stuff it needs. They're also fun to make, and whipping up something tasty in the kitchen can be a pleasant, stress-busting experience!

Stir-Fried Beef and Peppers

Beef is high in vitamin B12, which is necessary for your healthy brain function. It's also high in protein which, when eaten with vitamin C, helps your body heal. Peppers are one of the best sources of vitamin C on the market. They're sweet, crisp, and inexpensive too.

Serve this delicious stir-fry on hot cooked quinoa or brown rice mixed with a little extra virgin olive oil and chopped flat-leaf parsley.

Preparation time: *10 minutes, plus marinade*

Cooking time: *15 minutes*

Yield: *4 servings*

2 tablespoons apple cider vinegar

2 tablespoons freshly squeezed lemon juice

2 tablespoons organic tamari sauce

2 tablespoons local honey

1/2 cup organic beef broth

1/4 teaspoon pepper

1 pound grass-fed organic beef sirloin

2 tablespoons organic olive oil

1 yellow organic onion, peeled and sliced

4 cloves organic garlic, peeled and minced

2 tablespoons minced organic fresh ginger root

1 organic red bell pepper, sliced

1 organic yellow bell pepper, sliced

1 organic green bell pepper, sliced

1 In shallow container, combine vinegar, lemon juice, tamari, honey, beef broth, and pepper; mix well. Add beef; cover and marinate 4–8 hours.

2 When ready to cook, remove beef from marinade; reserve marinade. Slice beef into 1/3-inch slices against the grain. Prepare all vegetables.

3 Heat wok or skillet over high heat until hot. Add oil, then beef; stir-fry 3–5 minutes until beef is browned; remove from wok. Add onion, garlic, and ginger root; stir-fry 2–3 minutes until tender. Add peppers; stir-fry 2–3 minutes until crisp-tender.

4 Return beef to wok along with marinade. Stir-fry 3–4 minutes until sauce is slightly thickened and coats food. Serve immediately.

Per serving: *Calories 288 (From Fat 114); Fat 13g (Saturated 3g); Cholesterol 63mg; Sodium 532mg; Carbohydrate 19g; Dietary Fiber 2g; Protein 25g.*

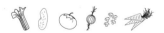

Edamame Salmon Wraps

Omega-3 fatty acids, found in salmon, are essential to brain health. Other foods rich in this essential nutrient are soybeans and flaxseeds. Magnesium, another nutrient critical to brain function, is found in green leafy vegetables. And citrus fruits are rich in vitamin C.

How to put these nutrients all together in a delicious and easy recipe? These wrap sandwiches have all these ingredients, so eat up for better brain health.

Preparation time: *10 minutes*

Cooking time: *11 minutes*

Yield: *4 servings*

1 cup freshly shelled organic soybeans (edamame) or frozen organic edamame

2 cups filtered water

1 pound wild Alaskan salmon fillets

2 tablespoons freshly squeezed lemon juice

3 tablespoons organic olive oil

3 tablespoons freshly squeezed orange juice

1 tablespoon local honey

1 tablespoon Dijon mustard

1 tablespoon fresh thyme leaves

1/8 teaspoon pepper

2 organic oranges, peeled and sectioned

2 tablespoons organic flaxseed, ground

4 leaves organic dark romaine lettuce, torn

4 organic whole wheat 10-inch tortillas

1 Place soybeans in medium saucepan; cover with water. Bring to a simmer; simmer 2–3 minutes until tender. Drain and set aside.

2 Place salmon on broiler pan; drizzle with lemon juice. Broil 6 inches from heat source until cooked through, about 6–8 minutes. Cool and break salmon into large pieces.

3 In medium bowl, combine olive oil, orange juice, honey, mustard, thyme, and pepper; mix well. Add salmon and stir gently, then add soybeans, oranges, and flaxseed.

4 Line tortillas with lettuce leaves, add salmon mixture, and roll up. Cut each wrap in half and serve immediately.

Per serving: *Calories 496 (From Fat 186); Fat 21g (Saturated 3g); Cholesterol 53mg; Sodium 339mg; Carbohydrate 43g; Dietary Fiber 7g; Protein 33g.*

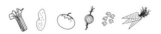

↺ Mixed Nut Snack

Snacks are an integral part of any healthy diet. When you snack, make it as delicious and healthy as possible. Nuts, which are high in good dietary fats and protein, are helpful to your brain's dopamine and serotonin levels. Dopamine is made from the amino acid *tyrosine,* and serotonin is made from the amino acid *tryptophan.* Almonds, pecans, walnuts, sunflower seeds, and pumpkin seeds all have lots of tryptophan. And cashews and pistachios are high in tyrosine.

You can use any of your favorite nuts in this recipe. Just be sure to buy 100 percent organic, unsalted varieties. Enjoy this delicious snack in moderation, with the knowledge that you're healing your brain and body as you eat.

Preparation time: *5 minutes*

Cooking time: *25 minutes*

Yield: *12 servings (1/2 cup each)*

1 1/2 cups organic unsalted slivered almonds	1 teaspoon ground turmeric
1 1/2 cups organic broken pecans	1 teaspoon ground cinnamon
1 cup organic unsalted cashew halves	1/8 teaspoon cayenne pepper
1 cup shelled organic unsalted pistachios	1/2 cup unsalted shelled sunflower seeds
2 tablespoons organic almond oil	1/2 cup unsalted pumpkin seeds
1 tablespoon curry powder	

1 Preheat oven to 350 degrees F. Combine all the nuts on a rimmed baking sheet.

2 In small bowl, stir together oil, curry powder, turmeric, cinnamon, and cayenne pepper. Drizzle over nut mixture and toss to coat. Bake 15 minutes, then add sunflower and pumpkin seeds; stir gently.

3 Bake 10 minutes longer, stirring twice during baking time, until nuts are fragrant and crisp. Cool completely and store in airtight containers at room temperature.

Per serving: *Calories 388 (From Fat 317); Fat 35g (Saturated 4g); Cholesterol 0mg; Sodium 4mg; Carbohydrate 13g; Dietary Fiber 6g; Protein 11g.*

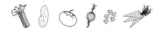

Part IV
Maintaining Healthy Detoxification Habits

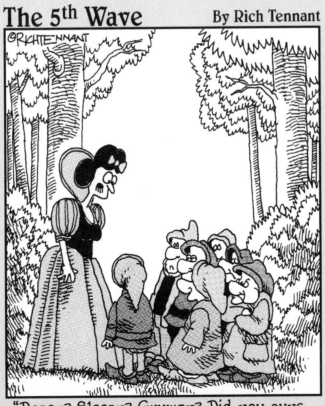

The 5th Wave — By Rich Tennant

"Dopey? Sleepy? Grumpy? Did you guys forget to take your supplements again?"

In this part . . .

*I*f you want to kick-start a detoxification effort or continue one that's already in motion, you need to do two things. This part includes details on both.

First, you have to make sure you're getting the important substances your body needs to stay healthy. That's what Chapter 17 is all about. Second, you have to be willing to try a range of things that can detoxify your body. Chapter 18 shows you how, from chelation to acupuncture and all points in between.

Chapter 17

Supporting Healthy Body Chemistry

Chemical reactions are the basis for all your body's myriad functions and processes. Everything the human body does — from passing gas to thinking up a complex theory of quantum physics — is based on chemical reactions. Science doesn't even know how many chemical reactions are occurring constantly in your body. To give you an idea of how big a picture I'm talking about here, consider that vitamin C is involved in at least 1,700 reactions that take place in the body. That's just one vitamin! The knowledge that we have of basic body chemistry is in its infancy, at best.

Here's what we do know: Your body absolutely has to have a number of substances in order to conduct all the necessary chemical reactions to keep you healthy and functioning normally. These substances — vitamins, minerals, essential fatty acids, and essential amino acids — are the focus of this chapter, along with another class of substances called antioxidants that can do wonders to improve your overall health.

With toxic influences assaulting your body all the time, it's critically important that you get enough of these vital substances so your body can function properly and carry out its natural detoxification processes successfully.

Whenever you experience increased stress on your body, such as with illness, chronic disease, or pregnancy, you must pay special attention to make sure you get all the essential nutrients.

Valuing Vitamins

In total, your body has to have 13 vitamins. Four of those vitamins (A, D, E, and K) are *fat-soluble,* which means they can be stored in your body. It's possible (although unlikely) to get too much of the fat-soluble vitamins, to the point where they become toxic. The other vitamins (B vitamins and C) are *water-soluble,* meaning that any excess amounts are removed easily through the urine.

Although the fat-soluble vitamins can be toxic if you consume vast amounts of them, it's virtually impossible to reach that level of toxicity through diet and difficult even with supplements.

The U.S. Food and Drug Administration (FDA) sets recommended daily allowances (RDAs) for vitamins, but RDAs are only the amounts you must get each day to avoid diseases associated with vitamin deficiencies. You should get much higher levels of the essential vitamins if you want to enjoy maximum health.

Vitamin A

Your body gets vitamin A from substances called *carotenoids,* which are commonly found in foods like carrots, squash, spinach, kale, and sweet potatoes. You can also get vitamin A from dairy foods, eggs, liver, and fish liver oil. Researchers estimate that as many as one-third of all Americans don't get enough vitamin A, and deficiencies can cause some rough stuff. Not getting enough vitamin A can lead to night blindness, skin dryness, decreased mucus membrane secretions, and increased susceptibility to bacterial infections. The FDA recommends that you get 900 micrograms of vitamin A per day, but I suggest getting 7,500 micrograms.

The B vitamins

The B vitamins are a whole group of vitamins that have similar chemical structures but play different roles in your body's many chemical reactions. You may hear these vitamins referred to as *B-complex* vitamins. Call them whatever you want — just make sure you're giving your body plenty of them for optimum health!

Vitamin B1

Sometimes called *thiamine,* vitamin B1 is required for carbohydrate metabolism and for the production of substances in your body that regulate your nerves. Foods that are richest in B1 include organ meats (liver, heart, and kidney), lean meats, eggs, leafy green vegetables, berries, nuts, and legumes.

If you don't get enough vitamin B1, you can suffer from *beriberi,* which is characterized by muscular weakness, swelling of the heart, and leg cramps. Severe cases can result in heart failure and death. The RDA for vitamin B1 is 1.2 milligrams per day, but I recommend getting about 20 milligrams daily.

Vitamin B2

Ever heard of riboflavin? That's another name for vitamin B2. Like vitamin B1, B2 is necessary for the metabolism of carbohydrates, but it also helps your body to metabolize fats and proteins used in the respiratory tract. You can get vitamin B2 in your diet by eating liver, dairy products, meat, dark green vegetables, and mushrooms. If your body runs low on B2, you can end up with skin lesions and sensitivity to light, among other problems. The FDA says you should get 1.3 milligrams per day, but I think you should get 20 milligrams.

Vitamin B3

Vitamin B3 goes by a few other names that you may have heard of: niacin, nicotinic acid, and niacinamide. Your body needs it to produce energy, and it's also handy for decreasing cholesterol. Your body can make B3 from the amino acid tryptophan, but you can also get it in the food you eat. If you want to up the amount of vitamin B3 you're getting, try to eat more dried beans, peas, nuts, liver, poultry, and meats. Vitamin B3 deficiencies cause *pellagra,* which is a condition marked by a variety of skin-related symptoms as well as mental confusion, depression, swollen tongue, and diarrhea. I think adults should get 65 milligrams per day, but the FDA's RDA for vitamin B3 is a paltry 16 milligrams each day.

Vitamin B5

Also known as *pantothenic acid,* vitamin B5 helps you convert food to energy, and it's important for the creation of adrenal gland steroids, antibodies, bile, red blood cells, and neurotransmitters. You can find B5 in a really wide variety of foods, from fish to sweet potatoes. A lack of vitamin B5 can result in numbness, as well as reduced amounts of the important substances that vitamin B5 helps your body to make. The RDA is 5 milligrams per day; I think you should get more like 200 milligrams each and every day.

Vitamin B6

Vitamin B6 wears many hats when it comes to your health. You need it to absorb and use amino acids, and it's also critical for the formation of red blood cells. How can you tell if you're not getting enough vitamin B6? Some of the symptoms include cracks at the corners of the mouth (ouch!), smooth tongue, convulsions, dizziness, nausea, anemia, and kidney stones. Some delicious food sources of vitamin B6 include avocados, spinach, green beans, bananas, and whole grains. The daily dose recommended by the FDA is 1.5 milligrams per day, but I advise you to set your sights on about 20 milligrams.

Vitamin B7

A couple aliases for vitamin B7 are *biotin* and *vitamin H.* Generally speaking, vitamin B7 helps convert food to energy, and it's required for making proteins and fatty acids. On a more tangible level, you need it for healthy hair, skin, fingernails, and toenails. If you're looking for a good dietary source, turn to broccoli, sweet potatoes, cheese, kidney beans, sunflower seeds, nuts, and salmon.

Long-term use of antibiotics can cause vitamin B7 deficiency. If you've recently taken a round of antibiotics, focus on getting plenty of B7 through your diet and supplements.

The RDA for vitamin B7 is 30 micrograms; I suggest getting about 1,000 micrograms instead.

Vitamin B9

This vitamin is very important. Vitamin B9 (also known as *folic acid*) is unusual because it is stored in the liver. You absolutely have to have it for the formation of many proteins, including *hemoglobin,* which is the substance that shuttles oxygen around your body in your blood. You can get vitamin B9 in organ meats (liver, kidney, heart), leafy green vegetables, legumes, nuts, and whole grains. In adults, deficiencies can cause anemia.

Vitamin B9 (folic acid) is essential for developing fetuses, particularly for the development of brain tissue. If you're pregnant or you know someone who's pregnant, make sure there's plenty of vitamin B9 to go around!

If you ask the FDA, you should get 400 micrograms of vitamin B9 per day. But if you ask me, upwards of 800 micrograms is a better daily dose.

Vitamin B12

Vitamin B12 is a must-have for the formation of red blood cells and proteins, and also for the functioning of the nervous system. You definitely don't want to run short on this vitamin, so be sure to get it in your diet (liver, fish, meat, eggs, and milk are a few good sources) or through the use of supplements. Not getting enough vitamin B12 can result in anemia, nerve problems, and intestinal conditions. The FDA and I differ greatly in the amount of vitamin B12 you should get on a daily basis. They say 2.4 micrograms; I say 500 micrograms.

Vitamin C

It's difficult to overstate the importance of vitamin C (also called *ascorbic acid*) for your health. As I mention earlier in this chapter, at least 1,700 chemical reactions in your body require vitamin C, and it's probably involved in many more reactions that haven't yet been identified. Vitamin C is also an essential ingredient in the formation of *collagen,* which is the material that holds all your body's tissues together. Vitamin C is critical for healing; your body simply can't heal itself without plenty of vitamin C.

A vitamin C deficiency can cause a condition called *scurvy,* which leads to hemorrhages, loosening of teeth, and problems with long bone development in children. Interestingly, all mammals make vitamin C except humans and gorillas. Dogs, for instance, make about 35,000 milligrams per day. Because humans aren't able to make vitamin C, you have to make sure you get plenty in your diet and through supplements. The FDA recommends 90 milligrams per day, but that's laughable. I get as much vitamin C in my diet as I can, and I also take 2,000 milligrams per day in supplements. If I'm not feeling well, I up that number to 6,000 milligrams per day.

If you're in need of a good natural laxative, try taking 8,000–10,000 milligrams of vitamin C in a day.

You don't have to walk very far down the produce aisle to find good sources of vitamin C. Some of the best are citrus fruits, strawberries, cantaloupe, pineapple, broccoli, Brussels sprouts, tomatoes, spinach, kale, green peppers, cabbage, and turnips.

Vitamin D

Vitamin D plays several important roles in your body. It's essential for healthy bones, and it also helps to keep your immune system at its best. You can get vitamin D through food sources, but it's almost impossible to get as much as you need through diet. If you drank ten tall glasses of vitamin D–fortified milk every day, you would have only minimal vitamin D levels.

So how do you get vitamin D? It's simple: Get some sun. It may sound hard to believe, but your skin actually produces vitamin D when it is exposed to the ultraviolet rays in sunlight. There are some catches, though. Glass blocks the rays in sunlight that make vitamin D, so you can't get sunlight through a glass window and expect your skin to produce vitamin D. People with darker skin produce less vitamin D than people with paler skin given the same amount of sunlight, so if you have a dark skin tone you may need to get a bit more sunlight for the desired effect.

Thirty minutes of sunlight a day will provide enough vitamin D for some people, but getting that amount can be hard to accomplish year round, particularly for people living in the high latitudes. If you can't get that amount, be sure to supplement accordingly. Also keep in mind that sunscreen pretty much eliminates the vitamin D production process in your skin tissue. It's good to get some sun; just don't allow yourself to burn.

Vitamin D deficiencies are serious business. A lack of vitamin D can cause a variety of health conditions, from osteoporosis to rickets to an increased risk of diabetes and infections. Deficiencies are easily treated, but treatment for severe deficiencies can take several months.

Most medical labs can test for vitamin D levels, so if you think you may not be getting enough, I'd recommend going in for a test.

The RDA for vitamin D is 5–10 international units per day. I think you should be getting 2,000–5,000 international units for top-notch health.

Vitamin E

When some of your body's cells — particularly muscle and red blood cells — are developing, vitamin E is an important part of the action. This vitamin is also a potent antioxidant, and you'd be hard pressed to get too many antioxidants. (More on those substances later in this chapter.) Leafy green vegetables are a great place to find vitamin E, and you can also get it from vegetable oils, wheat germ, and liver.

If you supplement this vitamin, keep in mind that four natural forms of chemical compounds called *tocopherols* are used to make vitamin E supplements. Find a product that has all four types, and make sure the supplement is all natural (rather than synthetic).

Vitamin E is one of the fat-soluble vitamins, so your body does store excess amounts instead of flushing them out with your urine, but it's pretty tough to get so much vitamin E that it has a toxic effect. The RDA is 15 milligrams, and I suggest getting between 200 and 400 milligrams each day. (A big difference, I know, but it's an important vitamin!)

Even though the RDA is relatively low, a recent study showed that 90 percent of Americans get less than 15 milligrams per day. That's a disturbing statistic, especially given the important role that vitamin E plays in good health.

Vitamin K

The last essential vitamin I cover in this chapter is vitamin K. This one is necessary for blood clotting, which means that deficiencies can cause bleeding problems. Good dietary sources of vitamin K include alfalfa, fish liver oils (cod liver oil is a classic example), leafy green vegetables, egg yolks, soybean oil, and liver. As with all the other vitamins, I think the FDA's recommended daily allowance is pitifully low. They suggest getting 120 micrograms, but I think you should have about 1,000 micrograms every day.

Because of its role in the blood clotting process, vitamin K is used medically to reverse excessive doses of *warfarin,* a drug that's administered to make blood less likely to clot. Some physicians will tell patients taking warfarin that they shouldn't eat any leafy green vegetables because of the effect that the vitamin K can have on their warfarin regimen. (It's hard to believe that a doctor would suggest that her patients not eat leafy green vegetables, but it really happens.) I think a better route is to stick to a regular, healthy, detox diet with lots of leafy green vegetables and then adjust the warfarin doses to the amount of vitamin K that you're getting from your diet. That's definitely not something you want to try to accomplish on your own, though, so if you're taking warfarin make sure you have a good talk with your doctor about the situation before making any changes.

Making Room for Minerals

Like vitamins, minerals have a variety of functions in the body. Probably most significant is the role that minerals play in the formation of enzymes that make possible a lot of different (and crucial) chemical reactions. You can't enjoy normal body function without the presence of several essential minerals in adequate amounts, and in this section I give you an idea of what you need and how much of it you should try to get every day.

If you've read any of the previous sections on vitamins, you already know that many of the FDA's recommended daily allowances are, in my opinion, way too low. The same goes for some minerals, although the FDA and I do agree for a few of them.

It's pretty tough to take in minerals to the point where they're toxic unless you have kidney problems. If your kidneys are functioning normally, you'd have to really make a concerted effort to get toxic amounts of minerals through your diet, and doing so would even be hard to accomplish with supplements. It's much more likely that you're not getting enough minerals; mineral deficiency has become more and more common due to the depletion of the soil used to grow vegetables (an important source of minerals) and also the heavy processing of food, which has a nasty way of ruining minerals.

Calcium

As far as minerals go, calcium has always seemed to maintain a pretty high profile. You can ask schoolchildren why they need calcium, and many of them will be able to tell you that you've got to have it for strong bones and teeth. That's exactly right, but calcium also does quite a few other things for you. It helps control your blood pressure, for example, and ensures normal nerve function.

It probably comes as no surprise that milk and dairy products are among the most common dietary sources of calcium, but many people are shocked to find out that you can get just as much (or more, in some cases) calcium from leafy green vegetables like kale, as well as broccoli, almonds, cashews, sesame seeds, whole grains, and seafood.

If you don't get enough calcium, your risk for osteoporosis and other bone conditions goes way up, as does the chance that you'll suffer from problems with your nerves.

How much calcium do you need to get every day? The FDA recommends 1,000 milligrams, but I say double it. You can get quite a lot of calcium from vegetables, especially if they're 100 percent organic. But most people can't get enough calcium in their diets, so supplementing is important.

When choosing a calcium supplement, try to get calcium hydroxylapatite. This form is far superior to calcium citrate, and especially to calcium carbonate, which blocks other minerals from being absorbed and is often contaminated with lead.

You can't absorb calcium without vitamin D, so if you try to boost your intake of calcium without ensuring that you're getting enough vitamin D, you're really just spinning your wheels. I recommend getting at least 2,000 to 5,000 international units of vitamin D each day.

Iron

We should all aspire to be iron men or iron women. Iron does some really critical things in your body, including metabolizing other nutrients and helping to regulate your immune system. But iron's most well known contribution to your health is its presence in *hemoglobin,* which is the amazing protein in your red blood cells that carries oxygen throughout your body.

Given that you can't survive without iron, you may be shocked to learn that almost 60 percent of Americans are iron deficient. Low levels of iron can result in anemia. Iron deficiencies are common among vegetarians and also among pregnant or menstruating women. To make sure you're getting enough iron, focus on eating meats, leafy green vegetables, apricots, nuts, seeds, kelp, and cherries.

Iron absorption is increased when you're getting plenty of vitamin C, so if you're worried about an iron deficiency, make sure your diet and supplement regimen includes lots of vitamin C. (That's a good rule anyway because vitamin C is such an important nutrient.)

Iron is one of the few nutrients for which the FDA's daily recommended allowance is on par with what I think people should be getting. The RDA is

8 milligrams per day, and if you're getting that much you should be in good shape, especially if you're also getting all the other essential nutrients in sufficient amounts.

Iron is also more likely to cause toxicity if you're getting too much of it, and it's possible that extremely high levels of iron can help to cause cardiovascular disease, so do your best to stick to that 8 milligrams per day level.

Zinc

This one may bring up the rear on any alphabetical list of important minerals, but zinc deserves some attention. Zinc is involved in wound healing, and it supports normal immune function. You also need it for proper food digestion. If you don't get enough zinc, your immune system will suffer, and you can also end up with chronic fatigue symptoms. Boost your zinc intake by eating seafood, vegetables, pumpkin seeds, mushrooms, and brightly colored fruits.

The FDA and I are on the same page when it comes to the amount of zinc you should get each day; shoot for about 11 milligrams and you should be fine. That's more than most Americans can say; as many as two-thirds are zinc deficient. Losing your sense of taste is one sign of zinc deficiency; if you have that problem, try some zinc.

Sodium

Sodium is very important in controlling fluid levels in the body. It's also involved in blood pressure control, heart function, and the basic functions of your nerves and muscles. Sodium is added to a lot of the foods we eat, so getting enough of it isn't usually a problem. Good natural sources of sodium are kelp, coconuts, carrots, and dried fruits. If your kidneys are working well, sodium toxicity shouldn't be an issue, and the FDA and I agree that you should aim to get about 1,500 milligrams of sodium per day.

Potassium

If you want healthy blood pressure, normal heart function, and sharp senses (and who doesn't?), you need to make sure you're getting enough potassium. Some of the best food sources are apricots, tomato puree, raisins, and figs; each of these has two to three times as much potassium as bananas. Potassium can also be found in green leafy vegetables, citrus fruits, avocados, legumes, and sunflower seeds.

Potassium deficiencies are common when people take diuretics or consume too much alcohol, caffeine, or sugar. The RDA for potassium is 4,700 milligrams per day, and I agree that should do the trick.

Magnesium

Magnesium is an extremely important mineral, and I think it's often overlooked in medicine today. What does it do for you? Well, it's critical for normal nerve and muscle function, immune function, temperature regulation, and digestion, for starters. If you don't get enough magnesium through diet or supplementing, you'll probably suffer from muscle cramps and an irregular heartbeat, which in some cases can be fatal. And low magnesium levels can help to cause low potassium levels. A whopping 70 percent of Americans don't get enough magnesium.

As important as magnesium is, many labs don't test for it because it's rarely found to be low in the blood. The problem is that magnesium can be dangerously low in the body's tissues, and a blood test won't reveal that fact.

A wholesome, healthy diet will include many of the major sources of magnesium, including nuts, green veggies, seafood, beans, organic whole grains, and fruit. The RDA is 420 milligrams per day, but 1,000 milligrams is a healthier dose in my opinion.

Phosphorus

When it comes to normal sensory function and a healthy brain, phosphorus is key. This versatile mineral also works with calcium to maintain strong bones and teeth. Get phosphorous in organic whole grains, molasses, kelp, seeds, lentils, and dairy products. The FDA and I agree that 700 milligrams is a healthy amount, and low phosphorus levels aren't very common at all.

Manganese

Manganese doesn't get a lot of attention, but that doesn't mean it's not an important mineral. You need it for maximum immune function, and it also works as an antioxidant. Foods like eggs, green tea, kelp, blueberries, and avocados contain quite a bit of manganese. The RDA for manganese is a paltry 2.3 milligrams per day, but I strive to get about 500 milligrams per day instead.

It's very difficult to take on toxic levels of manganese through diet and supplementing, but a small portion of the population ends up with manganese toxicity in another way: through welding. Many of the materials used in welding contain very high amounts of manganese, and as a result welders are exposed to a huge amount of it. If you weld, or if you know a welder, it's a good idea to get tested for manganese toxicity. Left unchecked, very high amounts of manganese in the body can have negative effects on the brain.

Copper

Another dynamic mineral, copper plays a part in making hemoglobin, supports immune function, helps in the production of neurotransmitters, and is required for the development of connective tissue and nerve linings. You can get copper in beef, but if you're not a meat eater, seek out copper sources like seafood, nuts, seeds, lentils, and mushrooms. A daily intake of 900 micrograms is recommended by the FDA, but you'll be healthier if you double that amount.

Iodine

Iodine is essential for thyroid function, and your thyroid helps to control your energy levels. (Flip back to Chapter 11 for a lot of useful information on how toxicity can affect your energy.) If you don't have enough iodine, your thyroid can't operate, and you can end up with out-of-whack energy levels, weight gain, dry skin, constipation, profound fatigue, and much more. You can get iodine in fresh vegetables and in seafood, as well as in kelp and *dulse* (a sea vegetable). The RDA is 150 micrograms per day, but you'll be better off if you bring in about 1,100 micrograms instead.

Selenium

Without selenium, your immune system couldn't work properly. Your cell membranes would go haywire. It's also been shown to have antioxidant effects, and it can help protect against certain kinds of cancer. About 60 percent of Americans don't get enough selenium, and you can avoid joining their ranks by eating whole grains, onions, garlic, broccoli, sesame seeds, and Brazil nuts. I think you should get 100 micrograms every day, which is about double what the FDA recommends.

Chromium

Chromium is necessary for your body to manage insulin successfully, and if you're not getting enough chromium you could very well be putting yourself at a greater risk for diabetes. Organic vegetables are an excellent source, but you should probably look to supplement for chromium as well, because in my opinion you should take in about 500 micrograms per day. (The RDA is only 30 micrograms.)

Molybdenum

You're better off not trying to pronounce this one — just make sure you're getting enough of it in your diet. Molybdenum is needed for an enzyme that controls *uric acid,* which is a waste product that can affect your kidney health. The best food sources are navy beans, lentils, black-eyed peas, kidney beans, and some tree nuts. I concur with the FDA's recommendation that you need to get 45 micrograms of molybdenum each day.

Embracing Essential Fatty Acids

Your body uses many different types of fatty acids in its huge range of chemical reactions, and you're able to manufacture the vast majority of those fatty acids. But a couple of essential fatty acids cannot be made by your body, so you have to get them through your diet and through supplementing. Those two essential fatty acids are omega-3 and omega-6, and they're absolutely necessary for good health.

Omega-3 fatty acids

Seven different kinds of omega-3 fatty acids exist, but the ones to keep an eye on are alpha-linolenic acid (ALA), eicosapentaenoic acid (EPA), and docosahexaenoic acid (DHA). ALA can be broken down into the other two, but that's not an incredibly efficient process so you're better off making sure that you get plenty of all three types. The best food sources for EPA and DHA are in the seafood category: fish, oysters, and crab. You can get ALA from a wider range of foods, including the following:

- ✔ Canola oil
- ✔ Flaxseeds or flaxseed oil
- ✔ Soybean oil
- ✔ Tofu
- ✔ Walnuts

Omega-3s are commonly called *fish oils,* and fish is an excellent source, but you can also get the oils from beef. The only catch is that the beef has to be completely grass fed. Cattle raised on feed lots and fed grains and other unnatural things don't contain omega-3s.

The majority of Americans don't get enough omega-3 fatty acids. Some estimates state that up to 85 percent of the population has an omega-3 deficiency, and that's a big time problem when you consider all the conditions that are related to low omega-3 levels, including the following:

- ✔ Increased memory loss
- ✔ Increased risk of Alzheimer's
- ✔ Depression, bipolar disease, and schizophrenia
- ✔ Insufficient amount of neurotransmitters
- ✔ Increased blood pressure
- ✔ Increased risk of heart disease, including atherosclerosis, angina, heart attack, and stroke
- ✔ Arthritis
- ✔ Ulcerative colitis

To avoid health problems associated with a lack of omega-3 fatty acids, you should aim to get about 2–3 grams per day through diet and supplementing. If you're already suffering from some of those problems, up the dose to 4–5 grams every day. Omega-3 supplements usually contain fish oils, and as with all fish products there's a chance for mercury contamination, so make sure your fish oil supplements have been independently tested for mercury.

It's extremely important that pregnant women and babies get enough omega-3 fatty acids, which are critical for growth and development.

Omega-6 fatty acids

Omega-6 fatty acids are important for intercellular signaling, which is to say that your cells need omega-6s to create the chemicals they use to communicate. (Sounds bizarre, I know, but it's true.)

While people are very commonly omega-3 deficient, it's actually pretty rare that someone doesn't get enough omega-6s. That's because omega-6s are present in beef, corn oil, and soy oil, which are abundant in the diets of most Americans. When a person's omega-6 levels are too high compared to omega-3s, inflammation can result.

Assisting with Amino Acids

Amino acids are the building blocks for protein, and proteins are required for life. There are eight *essential amino acids;* your body can't produce them on its own, which means you have to get them through your diet. Twelve other amino acids are called *conditionally essential* because if you don't get enough of the essential amino acids, you have to get some of the other 12 in your diet.

I won't devote too much space here to a discussion of the essential amino acids, because people rarely end up with essential amino acid deficiencies. That's because you get plenty of amino acids if you eat meat, eggs, poultry, or fish. Most people eat at least one of those things, and many people eat all of them, so for them amino acids aren't terribly hard to come by.

Vegetarians and vegans sometimes find it harder to secure all the essential amino acids, and in those cases I recommend bringing plenty of quinoa, buckwheat, hempseed, and amaranth into the diet. All are good sources of essential amino acids, and they're very easy to include in your diet because they're versatile, delicious foods. (If you've never had them, I definitely encourage you to branch out and give them a try, even if you eat meat.)

I go into some additional detail about amino acids in Chapter 7, so please flip back there if you'd like to read more.

Adding in Antioxidants

Antioxidants are beneficial chemicals that help to neutralize toxins in your body. Considering that the toxic load most people are exposed to continues to rise with each passing year, antioxidants are becoming more and more important for overall health. Some antioxidants have specific actions on different parts of the body, and some have a more general effect, but all of them are helpful.

People can produce antioxidants in their bodies, and the level at which they're able to do so is a genetic factor. You can't do much about your genes, but you can make sure you're getting plenty of antioxidants through diet and supplementing.

Here are some of the antioxidants that you should try to include in your diet and supplement regimen, and the doses that I think are the most beneficial:

✔ **Glutathione:** This is the most important antioxidant our body produces. It can be supplemented at 3,000 milligrams per day.

✔ **Alpha-lipoic acid:** ALA is extremely effective for detoxing the liver. Take 800–1,600 milligrams per day.

✔ **Silymarin:** Often called *milk thistle,* this one increases glutathione and can really boost your liver health. Take 100 milligrams per day.

✔ **N-acetylcysteine:** It offers liver protection and helps boost pancreas function in diabetes. Take about 600 milligrams per day.

✔ **Selenium:** I discuss this mineral earlier in the chapter. It improves thyroid function, increases glutathione, decreases the effects of mercury, and is shown to decrease cancer in rats. Try to get about 100 micrograms each day.

✔ **Melatonin:** This one stabilizes sleep and reconstitutes glutathione. Aim to get 3–12 milligrams per day.

✔ **Sulforaphane:** Also called *broccoli seed extract,* this potent multipurpose antioxidant increases glutathione and has anticancer properties. Use 500 milligrams daily.

✔ **Resveratrol:** This exciting new antioxidant has anticancer properties and offers improvement in blood sugar control for diabetics. Thirty milligrams per day will do the job.

✔ **Coenzyme Q10:** This is a required enzyme for the production of energy inside every cell in your body. It also has antioxidant properties. You can supplement with 100–200 milligrams per day.

✔ **Vitamin A:** This vitamin has strong antioxidant properties. Take 7,500 micrograms per day.

✔ **Vitamin C:** Another vitamin that offers excellent antioxidant effects, Vitamin C also suppresses cancer growth in high doses. Take 2,000 milligrams per day, and up that number to between 4,000 and 8,000 milligrams if you're sick.

✔ **Lycopene:** It decreases the risk for prostate cancer in men.

✔ **Beta-carotene:** This precursor to vitamin A packs a healthy antioxidant punch. Shoot for about 25,000 micrograms per day.

✔ **Vitamin D:** I talk about vitamin D in my section on vitamins earlier in this chapter, but it's also worth noting that it works wonders as an antioxidant. Take 2,000 to 5,000 international units each day. Have your doctor check your level.

Chapter 18

Trying a Few Other Kinds of Detoxification

*T*he human body is a wonderful machine. It is designed to heal itself and correct almost anything that goes wrong, so long as it has all the nutrients it needs and is not poisoned. Unfortunately, in the last 50 years or so we have been getting poisoned by the environment and many foods. Fortunately, we do have available some really good options to boost the body's ability to get rid of toxins.

Because toxins and nutritional deficiencies are major factors in acute and chronic disease today, we need to look at ways to increase our detoxification efforts. That's what this chapter is all about.

Sweating It Out in a Sauna

If you're really interested in detoxifying your body, you can't ignore the usefulness and practicality of saunas. Using a sauna is a wonderful way to rid your body of toxins.

Saunas certainly aren't a new invention. They've been around for thousands of years, and their use developed independently in many different societies throughout human history. The Romans had their baths (called *thermae*), the Japanese their hot springs (called *onsen*), and the Aztecs their sweat lodges (called *temescalli*). All were based on the same idea: Humans spend time in a hot environment and sweat heavily to produce curative and restorative effects on health.

Why are saunas so effective at removing toxins? The concept is simple: Saunas make your body sweat at a very high level, and sweating helps to flush toxins from your body. Most of the toxins you're exposed to are *fat-soluble,* which means your body is able to tuck them away in your fat cells in an effort to get the toxins away from your organs and other vital parts. But fat-soluble toxins are released during times of stress or illness, and they then travel through your bloodstream, causing harm to organs and important tissues. After that, some of them end up right back in your fat cells, where they can persist for years. After the toxins reach your fats cells, the only way to detoxify them is to sweat.

Your sweat glands are capable of removing one-third as much toxic material as your kidneys, and many of the toxins that are removed through sweating aren't removed by the kidneys or broken down by the liver. These two facts alone give you a terrific idea of the importance of detoxification through sweating.

Before the advent of air conditioning, humans in most parts of the world were subjected to a kind of sauna every year for several months during summer. That helped to keep the toxins — which were much lower at that point anyway — to a minimum.

Without the natural detoxification caused by sweating in the continuous summer heat, humans must find another way to sweat enough to flush out the accumulated toxins. Saunas are the answer.

Understanding the many benefits of sauna

Saunas have been around for thousands of years for a reason: They're great for your health. Your body benefits several ways from spending time in a sauna regularly, and I give you a feel for these advantages in the next couple of pages.

Flushing out toxins

Saunas are great for flushing out the toxins that build up in your body's fat cells. Your kidneys are detoxification powerhouses, and the intense sweating you can enjoy while spending time in a sauna can clear out about one-third of the toxic material that your kidneys remove from your bloodstream. That is no small contribution to a detoxification effort.

Multiple studies have shown that saunas are effective in removing solvents, organic chemicals, PCBs, pharmaceuticals, and heavy metal toxins from the human body.

L. Ron Hubbard's sauna protocol

In the 1970s, L. Ron Hubbard developed a sauna protocol to help drug addicts heal from their addictions. His theory was that even after addicts stopped taking drugs, drug residue was sequestered in fat cells. Like any other toxin, the drug residue would be released occasionally during times of stress. Those releases would trigger the flashbacks and cravings that plague addicts who are trying to keep moving away from their addictions.

Hubbard's protocol uses a dry sauna for three to five hours per day, for an average of 34 days.

It involves exercising before sauna and even during the sauna. Integral to the program are the use of vitamin B3 (an essential vitamin, also known as *niacin*) in increasing dosages, cold-pressed oils with omega-3 and omega-6 essential fatty acids, phosphatidylcholine, and a few other vitamins and supplements. Not only are recreational drug residues removed during the program, but fat-soluble residues of numerous environmental toxins, heavy metals, and even pharmaceutical drugs are flushed out as well.

Consider a very dramatic example of the detoxification power of saunas related to the 2001 terrorist attacks on the World Trade Center in New York. As you may imagine, the people at Ground Zero were exposed to massive amounts of toxins. Firemen and other rescue workers were exposed to toxins ranging from solvents to heavy metals, and the exposure lasted as long as the cleanup effort. Mercury was one of the biggest problems; there was enough mercury in the fluorescent light bulbs in buildings that were destroyed to poison every person in Manhattan.

To help these heroic individuals fight off the dangerous health effects of the toxins they'd been exposed to while helping to save lives and clean up Ground Zero, an intense sauna program was implemented. The program was based on one designed by L. Ron Hubbard. (You can read about Hubbard's sauna program in the nearby sidebar.) A total of 822 people who were exposed to toxins as a result of the events of September 11, 2001 were treated with frequent, long sauna sessions over a period of weeks. The results have been truly remarkable; an overwhelming majority of the program participants have reported major improvements in the toxin-related ailments they were suffering from as a result of their exposure to toxins at Ground Zero.

Enjoying the other benefits of sauna

The health benefits of using a sauna don't stop at detoxification, although they do fit in with the core values of a detoxified lifestyle. For instance, the high temperatures of a sauna can give your immune system a boost. The number of white blood cells that fight infections increases as much as 58 percent with the levels of increased temperature you get in a sauna. And that's just the beginning. Your T cells (another important part of your immune system) and antibodies can increase by as much as 2,000 percent. Also, a lot of microbes just can't take the heat; many of them die off at temperatures of 104 degrees Fahrenheit. Sauna treatments are often used to help people suffering from the common cold, and the success levels are high.

Increased temperatures also help your body to secrete *endorphins,* which are the "feel good" chemicals in your brain. Endorphins also make great painkillers, so it's very common for people suffering from chronic and acute pain to get quite a bit of relief from sitting in a sauna.

Studies have shown sauna to be effective in reducing the symptoms of a range of conditions, from arthritis to chronic fatigue syndrome to fibromyalgia. Research has also supported the use of sauna to help with glaucoma, anorexia, chronic obstructive lung disease, diabetes, obesity, hypertension, and atherosclerosis. If all that weren't enough, saunas can even help people quit smoking and kick drug addictions. Pretty incredible, huh?

If you spend time in a sauna, your cardiovascular system will also thank you. Here are just a few of the benefits you can get from regular sauna sessions:

- Stronger heart muscle contractions
- Improved function of the cells that line your arteries, which are extremely important in helping to keep cardiovascular disease at bay
- Reduced incidence of abnormal heart beats
- Lower blood pressure resulting from a healthy enlarging of the blood vessels
- Increased blood plasma and number of red blood cells, which helps with oxygen distribution and increases exercise tolerance
- Increased fat metabolism, which leads to weight loss

In addition to that last bullet point, a second mechanism for weight loss is also related to saunas. When you sweat heavily in a sauna and flush the toxins out of your fat cells, that process allows the fat cells to reduce in size, which can be a big help with weight loss. I'm a firm believer that toxins imbedded in fat cells are a major contributor to the obesity epidemic in the United States.

Getting a feel for the three different kinds of sauna

If you read any of the last few pages, you're probably pretty excited about using saunas to improve your health. I'm happy to report that you have three excellent sauna options to choose from: wet saunas, dry saunas, and far-infrared saunas.

No matter which type of sauna you choose to enjoy, here are a few sauna basics to keep in mind:

- ✔ Wear as little clothing as possible when in a sauna. Enjoying a sauna in the buff is a great idea, but if you're in a public place, you need to find out if that's appropriate before going *au naturel.*

- ✔ When you first start using a sauna, limit your sessions to 20 minutes or less. Gradually work your way up to sessions of 30 to 40 minutes. Do two sessions each day for maximum detox.

- ✔ Drink lots of water while in the sauna. About 10 to 20 ounces every 30 minutes is a good general rule.

- ✔ Make sure you're relaxed while in the sauna to maximize the experience. Saunas are a great place to meditate — just be sure you don't fall asleep!

- ✔ Shower immediately after you're done, taking care to brush the skin thoroughly to remove the toxins you just flushed out with your sweat.

- ✔ If you can, try to rest for 15 minutes after your sauna session.

- ✔ Saunas are a great way to start or end your day, so don't be afraid to go for a sauna session first thing in the morning or in the evening.

I'm convinced that saunas should be a part of all our lives. Our exposure to toxins makes saunas a necessity if we're going to keep our bodies healthy.

Saunas can be hazardous to your health if you have certain conditions, especially heart disease or high blood pressure, so be sure to talk to your doctor before beginning any sauna program. I go into more detail on who shouldn't sauna a little later in this section.

Wet saunas

A wet sauna is exactly what it sounds like: a space with elevated temperatures and also elevated amounts of water vapor in the air. If a dry sauna is like the weather in Phoenix, a wet sauna is like the weather in sultry New Orleans.

The steam in a wet sauna is usually generated by pouring water on volcanic rocks that are heated by electric or gas heaters. Some saunas use wood fires to generate heat, but they're not common. Temperatures in a high humidity wet sauna generally range from 150 to 190 degrees Fahrenheit.

One of the problems with wet saunas is that it's harder to evaluate the amount of sweating you accomplish because the water vapor condenses on your skin and creates excess moisture. Wet saunas can also be difficult to keep clean because mold is likely to grow in the warm, moist environment. Finally, some people find that the extremely high levels of water vapor can bother their nose and sinuses.

Dry saunas

Dry saunas are extremely common because they're easier to construct and maintain, and you don't have to deal with the mess that the water in a wet sauna creates. Mold is much less of a problem, as well, and many people cite that as one of the main reasons they prefer dry saunas. Temperatures in a dry sauna can reach up to 200 degrees Fahrenheit! That's plenty to generate a very healthy sweat and help to move toxins from your fat cells out through your skin.

Far-infrared saunas

Far-infrared saunas may sound a little space age, and truthfully they've only started catching on in popularity in recent years. At its core, the technology is pretty simple: Far-infrared saunas have a specialized heater that produces energy in the infrared spectrum. Feel free to dig up your high school physics books to read up on the details of the infrared spectrum if you'd like, but for this discussion you just need to know that infrared energy heats up your body without heating up the air around you. It can sound a little discomforting to some people, but the practice really is safe. If you read about it, you'll find that some people absolutely swear by it. Many users contend that far-infrared saunas penetrate the body better than wet or dry saunas, producing a more thorough and heavier sweating effect.

Here are a few advantages of far-infrared saunas:

- There aren't any hot surfaces, so there's nothing that can burn your skin.
- Lower heat ranges (100–130 degrees Fahrenheit) are easier on patients with cardiovascular problems.
- Far-infrared saunas are more energy efficient.
- The warm-up time is only about 5 to 10 minutes, compared to 30 minutes or more with a wet or dry sauna.
- Far-infrared saunas are portable, easy to assemble, and less expensive.
- Some reports indicate that you sweat two to three times more than you do in wet or dry saunas.
- Recent studies have shown that sweat from traditional saunas is 97 percent water, but sweat generated using far-infrared saunas is about 85 percent water and about 15 percent other materials, such as heavy metals, sulfuric acid, sodium, ammonia, uric acid, and fat-soluble toxins.

Knowing who shouldn't sauna

Saunas are safe for most people, but you shouldn't use one if you have any of the following health conditions:

✔ Adrenal suppression (meaning that your body doesn't respond to heat)

✔ Anemia

✔ Hemophilia

✔ Hyperthyroidism

✔ Recent *myocardial infarction* (heart attack)

✔ Unstable *angina pectoris* (chest pain or discomfort)

Also, you should avoid using a sauna or at least use extreme caution if any of the following is true:

✔ You're pregnant.

✔ You have acute joint injuries.

✔ You have enclosed infections.

✔ You have artificial joints.

✔ You have silicone implants.

✔ You're menstruating.

✔ You're taking medication that can be removed through sweat.

Capitalizing on Chelation

Chelation is another detoxification process that can be very useful as you work to rid your body of the harmful toxins that can have long-term damaging effects on your health. Generally speaking, *chelation* is a term used to describe the chemical attraction of one substance to another substance. The word *chele* means "claw-like," and you can think of chelation as one substance acting as a claw that grips another substance in your body. The basic idea is that you introduce a substance — called a *chelating* agent — to your body, where it binds to toxic material and is flushed out with your urine.

When it comes to detoxification, the most basic and well-known form of chelation is the use of the drug ethylenediaminetetraacetic acid — you're better off referring to it as EDTA — to remove lead from the body's systems. EDTA was developed by the Germans before World War II to remove lead from clothing dyes. It was later found that EDTA could be given to people with lead poisoning, and the chemical would remove the lead from their bodies. After the war, EDTA was brought to the United States and patented by a pharmaceutical company for its usefulness in treating lead poisoning. Further research showed that EDTA removed not only lead but also chromium, iron, mercury, copper, zinc, cadmium, cobalt, aluminum, manganese, magnesium, and calcium.

Since then, the effectiveness of chelation using EDTA has come under fire. Many traditional physicians are skeptical about the usefulness of EDTA, even though it has been identified as a potent antioxidant that has been shown to produce beneficial effects in many studies. Millions of people have received chelation therapy to remove heavy metals from their bodies, and the results have been overwhelmingly positive.

The effectiveness of EDTA in removing heavy metal toxins has been disputed over the years, but no matter what you hear, keep in mind that it is an FDA-approved drug that has been used safely for more than 60 years.

Several different types of chelation are commonly used today: natural, oral, rectal, transdermal, and intravenous. Each method has its advantages and potential problems, and I fill you in on the range of options over the next few pages.

Natural

Natural chelation involves the use of a substance that occurs naturally to draw toxic materials out of the body. The natural substances are many and varied, but one prime example is glutathione. *Glutathione* is a natural antioxidant that has been shown to work well in the removal of heavy metals. Most people take it orally, in capsule form. Glutathione is thought to remove multiple toxins from your body, and you can increase its effectiveness by taking melatonin supplements at the same time.

Another common substance used in natural chelation is chlorella. *Chlorella* is a single-celled, freshwater algae that has been shown to attach to heavy metals in the intestines. From there, the mix of chlorella and heavy metal toxins is removed from the body with the feces. I would certainly place chlorella in the "might help, and can't hurt" category, and I would recommend taking it on a regular basis if you're interested in natural chelation.

If you want an extremely natural form of chelation, try incorporating more cilantro into your diet. Cilantro is an herb in the parsley family that has been shown to help remove heavy metals from the intestines. Many people find it delicious even without considering its detoxification properties!

Oral

Oral chelation involves the use of chemical chelating agents that can be taken orally to help reduce the amount of toxins that are floating around in your body. Two of the most common chemical chelating agents taken orally are dimercaptosuccinic acid (DMSA) and sodium 2,3-dimercaptopropane-1-sulfonate (DMPS). Taking something orally is extremely easy because you can eat it or drink it with few issues, but DMSA and DMPS have been called into question recently because many people believe they aren't absorbed very well by the body when taken orally. Also, if you have existing stomach or bowel problems, the absorption rate is even weaker.

Rectal

If you're looking around for chelation options, you'll probably run across rectal suppositories that include EDTA. (You can find such products easily on the Internet.) All I can say is buyer beware! EDTA and DMSA can be given rectally, but the absorption rate is very poor and the results are extremely hard to evaluate. If you go this route, don't expect much!

Transdermal

Like rectal suppositories used for chelation, transdermal chelation doesn't produce the best of results. Absorbing a chelating agent through the skin doesn't really work all that well. I don't recommend the transdermal method of chelation. If this method appeals to you and you decide to pursue it, just don't plan on the best possible results, especially when it comes to reducing heavy metal toxicity.

Intravenous

When it comes to chelation, intravenous administration of chelating agents is the gold standard. IV chelation offers exact dosages that aren't affected by varying rates of absorption, and it really removes all the variables that are present with oral, rectal, and transdermal options.

As you can imagine, the intravenous chelation method must be done by a qualified professional, so if you're very serious about removing toxins — particularly heavy metal toxins — from your body using chelation, ask your doctor about your options for chelation with intravenous chelating agents, but don't expect a traditional physician to have any knowledge or respect for chelation.

DMPS

When administered via IV, DMPS is a slam dunk for removing mercury from the human body. It has a long, illustrious history of success and safety. It hasn't been approved by the FDA but is approved to be imported and used legally, and pharmacies that offer compounding can prepare it for IV use.

EDTA

If you want to harness the power of chelation to remove any toxin other than mercury, EDTA administered through IV is one of the best ways to go. It has a 60-year history as a safe and effective means for removing a wide range of toxins, particularly the heavy metal toxins that are so prevalent in our environment today.

Advocating Acupuncture

Acupuncture is an ancient method of improving health and healing, and it fits in extremely well with a general effort to make your body perform at a higher level without the introduction of potentially harmful toxins. The origins of acupuncture are in Asia, where acupuncture is a part of traditional Chinese medicine. Variations also come from Tibet, Vietnam, and Korea. At this point, more than 3 million adults and 150,000 children in the United States receive acupuncture treatments each year.

In broad terms, acupuncture involves the use of extremely small, sharp needles that are inserted into the skin at specific points that have been shown to produce a range of effects on the body. In total, more than 2,000 acupuncture points on the body can be stimulated individually or, more commonly, in groups.

The needles aren't the extent of acupuncture treatment, however. Several variations exist, including the use of mild electric currents in the needles. Some practitioners choose to apply pressure to certain points instead of actually inserting needles. Some others embrace a variation of acupuncture called *auriculotherapy*, which is based on the concept that acupuncture points on the ears can be stimulated to produce effects across the entire body.

A trained, talented acupuncturist will assess your health history, as well as any symptoms of current conditions, to figure out which abnormalities in your health are causing you the most harm. He then stimulates the acupuncture points on your body that will help to relieve you of your conditions.

Here are just a few conditions that are commonly treated using acupuncture:

- ✔ Allergic rhinitis (allergies to dust, dander, or pollen)
- ✔ Chemotherapy side effects
- ✔ Depression
- ✔ Dysentery
- ✔ Headache
- ✔ Hypertension
- ✔ Nausea and vomiting (including morning sickness)
- ✔ Primary dysmenorrheal (painful periods)
- ✔ Rheumatoid arthritis
- ✔ Sciatica
- ✔ Sprains
- ✔ Stroke

The most accepted use of acupuncture in the United States is for the treatment of pain. Acupuncture is used to treat fibromyalgia, carpel tunnel syndrome, lower back pain, menstrual cramps, myofacial pain, neck pain, osteoarthritis, tennis elbow, and postoperative dental pain.

Acupuncture is safe and, when practiced correctly, has no harmful side effects. The big challenge is to find someone who is skilled in the art. You should check the credentials of anyone you're thinking of seeing for an acupuncture treatment. Training varies from weekend courses to thousands of hours of training. I once checked the credentials of an alternative practitioner who was the president of two national organizations, which seemed very impressive at first. The problem was that he was the only member of both organizations.

Mixing in Meditation

Meditation dovetails extremely well with other detoxification measures. It has taken many forms across the centuries, and many different cultures and religions use it. I don't have the space here to explain all the various types of mediation, but you should try to embrace some general principles related to the practice as you endeavor to lead a detoxified life.

In general, meditation practices are mental disciplines in which a person attempts to reach beyond reflective thought to grasp a deeper state of consciousness, relaxation, and awareness. If practiced effectively, meditation results in a marked reduction in stress that can improve your health on every possible level.

Many religions utilize meditation as an integral part of the belief system, but meditation doesn't have to be related to any religion. Every person needs to seek out the form of meditation that suits him or her best, but you need to keep an open mind and realize that you stand to gain quite a lot just through clearing your mind and focusing your thoughts for a few minutes each day.

Part V
The Part of Tens

The 5th Wave   By Rich Tennant

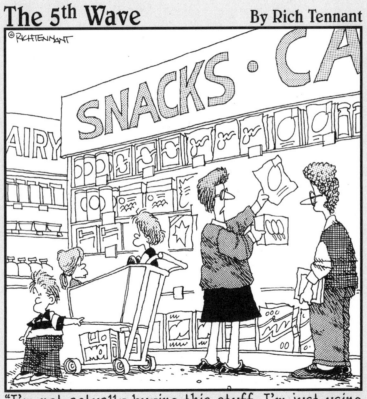

"I'm not actually buying this stuff, I'm just using it to hide the fruit, legumes and greens until we get checked out."

In this part . . .

Most readers really like this part of a *For Dummies* book. It features a few sets of lists that can help you latch on to some detox details without diving too deep into any one area. This is a great place to whet your appetite for detoxification and detox dieting, and to gain some quick, easy know-how that you can apply right away.

Chapter 19

Ten Foods to Leave at the Store

*W*hen you're grocery shopping, do you feel like you have a very good sense of what kinds of foods you should put into your cart and, eventually, into your body? If not, that's one of the first skills you should develop as you work on the many ways that you can detoxify your body and strive for maximum health.

In Chapter 6, I fill you in on what you shouldn't be eating. In Chapter 7, I focus on all the kinds of foods that should fill your shopping cart, your pantry, and your stomach. If you're interested in some detailed information on detox diet food choices, those are the chapters for you. However, if you want to get some quick, basic information on the foods that you should definitely leave on the grocery store shelf, you've come to the right place. Read on to find out which foods you should eat very, very sparingly or — if you're really serious about detoxification and building good health — not at all!

Milk

Cow's milk can seem like a harmless food, and millions of dollars are spent each year to make you think that it's healthy. But the truth is that most of the milk you find in grocery store refrigerators can be harmful to your health. Most milk is heavily processed: It's spun, heated, separated, and reconstituted, for starters. The majority of the healthy proteins that can be found in milk are destroyed during all the processing steps. How different is the milk at the grocery store from natural cow's milk? One research project gave grocery-store-bought milk to newborn calves, and all of them died before they reached 2 months of age.

Here's some more food for thought: A 12-year Harvard study of 80,000 nurses showed that the nurses who drank the most commercially produced milk also had the most bone fractures. That certainly doesn't jibe with the message that comes from milk proponents, who insist that we need to drink milk to get the calcium and vitamin D we need. That's simply not the case. You can get all the calcium and vitamin D necessary for strong bones (and more) from vegetables, sunshine (for the vitamin D), and supplements.

Some people can't imagine life without cow's milk. If you're among them, please find a good, clean source of whole, raw milk. Chances are you can get a tip if you ask around at your local health food store.

If you want to drink milk but you're not dead set on drinking cow's milk, try substitutes like rice milk, almond milk, and soy milk. (However, if you go with the soy milk option, remember that almost all soy products have been created using genetically modified soybeans.)

Many brands of commercially produced milk contain antibiotics and hormones. If you want to drink cow's milk, make completely sure that the brand you buy states clearly on the label that the milk doesn't contain these toxic substances.

Margarine

It always breaks my heart when I hear about someone who has decided to give up butter in favor of margarine in order to lose weight and stay healthy. Given the amount of fat present in butter, a lot of people avoid it. But *please* don't start eating margarine as a substitute. It's unhealthy and in many cases can contain trace amounts of toxins.

About halfway through the 20th century, people began eating margarine as a butter substitute for health reasons. We're now at the point where Americans eat twice as much margarine as they do butter. The problem is that margarine isn't healthy. More often than not it contains hydrogenated oils and trans fats, and you don't want either of those things in your system.

What's more, margarine is made using processes that involve toxins, and I have a hard time believing that margarine makers are able to remove all the toxins from the finished product. Two of the toxins commonly used to make margarine are *hexane* — a nasty petrochemical solvent — and nickel, which is a very harmful heavy metal toxin.

Before you reach for the margarine, consider using very small amounts of 100 percent organic butter instead. The butter may not be as good for you as many of the other foods out there, but it's always better for you than margarine.

Corn Oil

If you look in most people's pantries, you're likely to find a bottle of corn oil. If the same goes for you, do yourself a favor and get rid of that bottle!

Corn oil is an extremely common cooking and baking ingredient, but it's flat-out not good for you. In addition to being loaded with plenty of bad fats, most corn oil is hydrogenated and made using genetically modified corn. I won't get into the nitty gritty details of genetically modified food products here, but please flip back to Chapter 6 if you want the scoop.

If you're looking for healthy oil alternatives to corn oil, consider using 100 percent organic coconut oil and hempseed oil. Find them at a nearby health food store or online.

Artificial Sweeteners

In my opinion, very few products are as detrimental to detoxification and a detox diet lifestyle as artificial sweeteners. If you could get a dime for every food product in the average grocery store that contains an artificial sweetener, you could easily be reading this book on a big, beautiful boat someplace sunny (with a nice glass of 100 percent organic carrot juice by your side!).

I cover the details of artificial sweeteners in Chapter 9, so flip back there if you want to read up. For the purposes of this list, I'll just say that you should do everything you can to cut artificial sweeteners and any products that contain artificial sweeteners out of your diet. You're much more likely to live a healthy, detoxified life if you can make that important step.

You should avoid artificial sweeteners at all costs and do your best to limit your intake of sugar. But what's left to use for sweetening foods and drinks? Try using *stevia,* which is an extremely low calorie, natural sweetener that comes from a plant and has been used in other cultures without negative health impacts for decades.

Artificially Colored Foods

When it comes to foods that have been colored, I like to imagine what it would be like to go back in time a few centuries and offer some of these food items to the people of that era. Can you imagine trying to get an early American settler, for example, to drink a fluorescent blue liquid and eat a neon pink snack cake?

The chemicals used to make most food colorings are a murderer's row of harmful toxins, and you don't want them in your body. Many food coloring products are made of coal tar — the same stuff used on our streets. Don't eat foods that have been colored! To make sure you're making wise choices, always check ingredients lists. When in doubt, do a simple logic check: Is the bright green gummy snack in front of you really that color because of natural factors? Probably not. Skip it.

Olestra

In the 1980s, scientists cooked up a new substance that was touted as a terrific replacement for fat. The idea was simple: The olestra molecule had some of the characteristics of fat, but it was too big to be absorbed by the human digestive system so it didn't end up in your body and didn't cause weight gain and all the other problems commonly attributed to fat.

Sound too good to be true? It is. At its very best, olestra is simply a fake, unnatural fat. At its worst, it makes absolutely no contribution to weight loss and can cause a disgusting anal discharge condition. Not good.

What's more, olestra doesn't do any of the positive things that good fats can do for your body, like helping you to absorb important vitamins (vitamins A, D, E, and K). Leave olestra and any products that contain olestra on your grocery store shelves.

Tuna

Tuna is a delicious, easy-to-find fish, and you can get it in all kinds of forms — from a gourmet tuna steak at a fancy restaurant to a big vat of tuna salad at a corner grocery store and deli. Unfortunately, more often than not, tuna contains the deadly toxin mercury. Because of that disturbing trend, I have to suggest you avoid eating tuna whenever possible.

If you're used to eating tuna and you want to continue making fish part of your diet, try using wild Alaskan salmon instead. That variety of fish traditionally scores very low when it comes to mercury levels, and it also happens to taste great and works in a huge range of delicious recipes. (For a good example, check out the recipe for Crunchy Curried Salmon Wraps in Chapter 9!)

Soy

When I tell my patients that they should consider avoiding eating soy or buying soy food products, they sometimes look at me in disbelief. Most people think of soy as harmless or even healthy, and in a perfect world that might be true.

The problem is that an overwhelming amount of the soy and soy products available in the United States come from genetically modified soybeans. And if you know anything about soy, you know how impossible it is to get away from the stuff. It's everywhere!

What if you want to keep soy and foods that contain soy in your diet? Make sure that the soy you eat is 100 percent organic and that it doesn't come from a genetically modified soyce . . . er, source.

Processed Meats

It doesn't take a natural foods specialist to realize that processed meats are a bad idea. Just looking at some potted meats can make you wonder how it ever makes sense for someone to eat those materials. But lots of people do eat potted meat, along with other processed meats like lunchmeat and hot dogs.

Just to set the record straight, here's what's wrong with processed meat: It offers little or no nutritional value and can be full of toxins. All the various chemical and mechanical techniques used to make processed meat rob it of whatever nutrients it had to begin with, and just about every processed meat product on the market contains a toxin called *sodium nitrite.* It's a chemical used as a preservative, and after it's in your body it can go through a chemical reaction or two to create *nitrosamines,* which are compounds that many people believe cause cancer (particularly liver cancer).

Animal Fats

What's an animal fat? You guessed it: any fat that comes from an animal. Animal fats are not bad if they come from clean animals. And fats (oils, really) that come from fish are quite good for you. But most animal fats available in your grocery store are rotten for your body's systems; they often contain toxins because substances like antibiotics, hormones, and steroids are used on many commercially raised animals.

To get the good types of fats into your diet, focus on vegetable fats (more commonly referred to as *vegetable oils*). The best varieties to use are coconut oil, flaxseed oil, olive oil, and hempseed oil. (Make sure you pick out 100 percent organic oils if possible.)

Chapter 20

Ten Ways to Tell That Your Detox Diet Is Working

Say you've made the decision to start on a detoxification diet. You get the necessary equipment; clean the processed and toxin-filled food from your fridge and pantry; replace it with wholesome, natural, organic food; and work hard to improve your eating habits. These steps aren't easy to take, so if you complete them successfully, congratulations are in order!

But enough with the congratulations — how do you know when this diet is really working? How do you know when the healthy choices you're making start to have a positive effect on your body?

That's the topic I tackle in this chapter. Read on to get the scoop on ten wonderful ways that you can tell your efforts to implement and stick to a detox diet are paying off and helping to create a healthier you.

You Lose Some Weight

When your body contains high levels of toxins, it relies on a natural process that isolates the toxic materials and tucks them away where they can't do any harm to your important organs and tissues. That process involves toxins being absorbed and stored for long periods of time in fat cells. Many people don't know it, but fat cells can be storehouses for toxins, particularly heavy metals and chemical toxins. After toxins end up in fat cells, another natural process takes place. That process causes fat cells to grow and expand in an effort to dilute the toxins. Put these two processes together, and toxins can not only result in an abundance of fat cells but also a growth in the size of those fat cells.

So what happens to those fat cells when you embark on a detoxification diet? When you drastically cut down on the amount of toxins you take in with your food and water, and when you also make a concerted effort to eat the kinds of foods that boost your body's efforts to rid itself of toxins, the result is an overall decrease in the amount of toxic materials present in your body. And when the toxin levels go down, your body no longer needs the multitude of growing fat cells necessary to sequester all those toxins, so your body begins to do away with them. This nifty sequence of events is one of the main reasons why detox dieting is such a great way to help you reach your ideal weight. (It also doesn't hurt that detox diets focus on healthful, low-fat foods, which can only give you another step down the path of healthy weight management.)

You Don't Get Sick as Often

With all the foreign substances that can end up in your body, it's safe to say that your immune system, which your body relies on to fight infection and disease, has plenty to deal with. Even in the purest, cleanest environments, harmful materials end up in your bloodstream and in your body's organs and tissues. When that happens, your immune system comes to the rescue. It's an extremely complex and effective natural machine, and you want to keep it in the best possible condition so it can thwart the dangerous advances made by bacteria, parasites, viruses, and toxins.

The immune system is complex and kind of fragile. Its many unique parts must work together in order for you to enjoy maximum immunity, and these parts can be thrown out of whack or even destroyed if they're exposed to certain materials, including toxins. In relatively low amounts, toxins can be a disruption to your immune system, and when toxic levels are high the effects can be devastating. Your body can quickly lose the ability to defend itself against foreign invaders.

You may not notice a huge effect on your immune system when you first start a detox diet, but after a while you may be pleasantly surprised by how resilient you are against infections. You may dodge the bullet when the rest of the people in your office catch a nasty cold, for example. The reason is that a decreased toxic load takes away a major threat to your immune system, and all those wonderful, efficient parts of your body are able to work together to keep you healthy and feeling great.

Your Gas Doesn't Smell as Bad

Okay, this one may catch you off guard. But it's true! Sticking to a detox diet will go a long way toward preventing the creation of foul-smelling gas in your intestines. Allow me to explain.

When your intestines are at their healthiest, you have a balance of bacteria that features a normal amount of good, beneficial bacteria and only trace levels of bad bacteria. At their worst, the good bacteria don't have any effect on you at all, and at their best they can help you digest certain foods that you wouldn't be able to digest on your own. Bad bacteria, however, can do all sorts of nasty things to your body, including causing disease, robbing you of key nutrients, and even contributing to really bad-smelling gas.

How can you make sure your intestines contain the right amounts of good bacteria and very little amounts of bad bacteria? Go on a detox diet. Making wise food choices will help to create an environment in your intestines that helps good bacteria to succeed and makes it hard for harmful bacteria to get a foothold. And that will work wonders if you're one of the many people who suffer from offensive, foul-smelling gas.

You Have More Energy

Want to put some pep in your step? Go on a detox diet. A noticeable (and extremely pleasant) increase in energy levels is one of the first things that my patients mention when they've been on a detoxification diet for a few weeks. Why does that happen? There are several reasons, but an important one is the ability of your thyroid gland to work as it's supposed to. Your thyroid gland is responsible for regulating your metabolism, which is the root of your energy levels. The thyroid can be a fickle gland, and it's prone to acting up when you have too many toxins — particularly mercury — in your bloodstream and elsewhere in your body.

When your thyroid goes on the fritz, it can do lots of bizarre and unpleasant things to your body, including wreaking havoc on the amount of energy you have. (Read all about that subject in Chapter 11.) If you want to enjoy healthy, comfortable amounts of energy — not too much, not too little — work toward detoxifying your body and put a detox diet at the very top of your priority list.

Your Skin Looks and Feels Better

Sweating is one of the most effective and important methods for detoxification. When your body is overrun with toxins and you sweat them out constantly, your skin can really improve. Sweat is good for your skin and can make you look and feel very healthy. Sweating also increases the natural oils on the skin that keep the skin soft and moist.

Slashing the amount of toxins in your body using a detox diet helps to limit the toxins that you sweat out onto your skin. When you combine that effort with a careful skincare regimen and a commitment to drinking plenty of purified water, you're bound to end up with softer, healthier skin.

You can also use a sauna to help sweat out the toxins that are already in your body — see Chapter 18 for details. Just be sure that you take a good, long shower after you're done so toxins go down the drain and don't stay on your skin.

Your Food Allergies Improve

If you're one of the millions of people who suffer from food allergies, you know how annoying, frustrating, and even dangerous they can be. Some food allergies are relatively easy to deal with — it's pretty easy to avoid eating oysters if you're allergic to shellfish, for example. But others are a real pain. If you're allergic to gluten (a common substance in many grains), you know exactly what I'm talking about.

If certain foods give you fits and you want to improve the situation, get started on a detox diet right away. Dodging toxins and eating foods that help to flush them from your body will help to prevent a condition called *leaky gut syndrome* that can contribute to the occurrence and severity of food allergies. Leaky gut syndrome occurs when toxins irritate and inflame your intestines, and as a result the intestines accidentally allow dangerous materials to pass through your intestinal wall into your bloodstream. Many people believe that leaky gut syndrome can play a big part in causing food allergies. If you can cut way down on your toxicity, you'll keep your intestines healthy and make leaky gut syndrome much less of an issue.

Your Blood Pressure Decreases

One out of every four Americans suffers from *hypertension,* commonly known as high blood pressure. This condition contributes to stroke, heart attack, and kidney failure, among other problems, and the unhealthy diets and abundance of toxins that are so prevalent in our world today are only making matters worse.

If you or someone you're close to suffers from hypertension, I strongly suggest a detoxification diet. It's a little known fact that several toxins can have a harmful effect on your blood pressure. Lead is the worst of the bunch, and it also happens to be one of the most common toxins. Cut out those toxins and take an active approach to flushing them out of your body, and you're almost certain to lower your blood pressure and help keep it down at a healthy, comfortable level.

Your Bowel Movements Are More Regular

People sometimes cringe when it comes time to talk about bowel movements, but the truth is that they're an important part of your health and you need to pay attention to them. Regular, comfortable bowel movements are a sign that your digestive system is working as it should, and that should be a goal for everyone.

Toxins have a negative impact on your bowel movements. They can cause lots of intestinal problems from constipation to diarrhea and everything in between. The results can be malnutrition, dehydration, and increased toxicity, just to name a few.

A detox diet greatly reduces the amount of toxins that enter your body, which helps improve the quality and regularity of your bowel movements. Also, a detox diet provides you with plenty of fiber and other food substances that contribute to healthy bowels and bowel function.

Your Mental State Improves

Quite a bit of evidence suggests that detoxification and the avoidance of toxins can help your brain and the rest of your nervous system operate on a higher, healthier level. Of course, some folks also like to refute that idea.

You could spend half a lifetime sorting through the studies and research results trying to figure out the exact, quantitative effect of toxins on your neurological system and your mental health. Before you go off and do that, consider this: Nearly every patient I've ever helped to start and follow through with a detoxification diet has reported that his or her mental state has improved by leaps and bounds. Detox diets make people feel calmer and more at ease, and they also help people think more clearly and avoid the "brain fog" that makes it hard to excel at work and enjoy personal time.

You Live a Long, Healthy Life

Okay, okay, so this one takes a little bit more time for you to see the results. But if you make the commitment to maintain a detox diet for life — and don't be mistaken, that's the kind of timeline we're talking about here — you'll be less likely to suffer from the diseases that now afflict so many people as they age. These diseases include Alzheimer's, Parkinson's, multiple sclerosis, and many different forms of cancer. Going on a detox diet and following a detox protocol is probably the best chance you have to avoid facing these illnesses. And a detox lifestyle will positively affect every other aspect of your health in the meantime.

Chapter 21

Ten Supplements to Take Daily

In This Chapter

▶ Getting sufficient vitamins

▶ Making sure minerals are on your list

▶ Adding other supplements to your regimen

*T*he best way to get the important substances you need (vitamins, minerals, essential fatty acids, antioxidants — the list goes on and on) is through a balanced, wholesome, nutritional diet (one that is 100 percent organic whenever possible). But the fact is that many people have a very hard time eating enough of the right kinds of foods to get the substances they need in the correct quantities. That's why I recommend that you strongly consider using supplements to increase the amounts of critical materials your body must have to perform at its very best.

This chapter gives you ten suggestions for supplements that you can take every day to improve your health. I know it may seem overwhelming to think about taking ten (or more) different supplements each day, but keep in mind that doing so can be a real benefit to both your body and mind. Plus, it may help you to live longer and healthier. That said, if you know that you're getting a good amount of some of these substances in your diet and you're interested in keeping the amount of supplements you're taking relatively low, you can adjust your supplement regimen accordingly. For example, if you eat plenty of oily, cold-water fish, you may not need to supplement with omega-3 fatty acids. Think about your diet, and supplement in an appropriate way to make certain you're giving your body what it needs.

Here's one very important note to keep in mind when you're thinking about supplements: The daily recommended allowances for vitamins, minerals, and other substances that you see on food labels don't mean a whole lot. These guidelines show you the minimum amounts necessary for your body to keep on keepin' on, but they don't tell you what amounts you need for your body to go above and beyond that base level.

One more thing: If you want advice on how to select supplements, flip back to Chapter 5.

Multivitamin

A good, comprehensive multivitamin should be the foundation for your supplement regimen. Your body absolutely must have 14 vitamins in order to function properly, and chances are you don't get all 14 in the amounts you need from your diet. It is possible to get all your vitamins from food, but you have to eat a diet that is much healthier than most people even aspire to. (You have to eat loads and loads of produce — mostly vegetables — and choose only 100 percent organic varieties.) For more information about all the vitamins you need, flip back to Chapter 17.

Some people take a once-a-day multivitamin. While that's definitely better than taking nothing at all, the pill probably doesn't include high enough doses of each of the vitamins you need. How do I know? If a once-a-day vitamin contained adequately high doses of all 14 essential vitamins, it would have to be at least as big as a golf ball. Most of the multivitamins that offer comprehensive vitamin coverage require you to take several pills a day. Four capsules or pills a day is a pretty standard number.

A range of good brands and reasonably priced options is available. You want to find a company that does third-party analysis (see Chapter 5). Most of the better products are not sold over the counter and must be purchased through an integrative physician or a pharmacy that is involved in natural wellness.

Make sure the multivitamin you choose includes a good calcium source, and make sure that it comes as calcium hydroxyl apatite and not calcium carbonate. You don't necessarily have to understand the differences between the two; just make sure your multivitamin includes the former and not the latter.

Multimineral

In total, you need to supply your body with 16 different minerals if you want it to perform at an optimal level. I won't list them here — check out Chapter 17 for a rundown — but rest assured that getting anything less than all 16 means a compromise for your health.

Multimineral supplements are easy to find, and in many cases you can find multivitamin/multimineral combination supplements. These options can be tricky, and you need to make sure that if you choose to go that route you buy an option that includes all 14 vitamins and all 16 minerals. (That's quite a lot!)

When you're picking out a multimineral supplement, go with one that contains *chelated* minerals. I'll spare you all the boring details of the process that creates chelated minerals. But keep in mind that unless you're getting chelated minerals, you're probably paying for minerals that end up in your toilet instead of in your body's important systems.

Don't take a multimineral supplement that comes from a clay source. These products are not chelated, and they contain silver, tin, and nickel. In some cases they even list lead as an ingredient!

Omega-3 Fatty Acids

You've probably heard or read about omega-3 fatty acids in the news recently. The importance of this essential fatty acid has been getting a lot of press, and for good reason. It's one of those substances that your body has to have to survive and thrive, and despite all the wonderfully complex chemical processes your body can do, it can't manufacture omega-3 fatty acids.

The best dietary source of omega-3s is organic beef. Fish is the next best source. You should eat fish as part of a healthy diet, but unless you're eating wild Alaskan salmon or one of the other few types of fish that don't commonly contain high levels of mercury, chances are you're getting a very unhealthy dose of toxins along with your omega-3 fatty acids.

To steer clear of mercury but still get your omega-3s, supplement with liquid fish oil or a capsule or softgel. Take one gram twice a day to get what you need.

Resveratrol

Resveratrol is a powerful antioxidant, and I recommend that everyone get a dose of it each day. Resveratrol has developed a much higher profile since a Harvard Medical School study a few years ago showed a pretty dramatic increase in the health and lifespan of mice when they were given resveratrol in addition to their diets. If you read up on this antioxidant, you'll probably see that it is present in red wine, and that's the truth. (It's also present in grape skins.) But if you wanted to get a significant dose of resveratrol from red wine alone, you'd have to glug a few hundred bottles of the stuff per day, and that would kill you long before you got to enjoy any benefits of resveratrol.

The good news is that you can buy resveratrol supplements at many health food stores and at any good vitamin retailer, either in person or online. You'll see it listed either as resveratrol or *red wine extract*. I recommend getting 30 milligrams per day, which should be rather easy given the breadth of supplement options on the market.

Vitamin C

If you take a good multivitamin, you're probably getting a good amount of vitamin C each day. But don't think for a second that you're getting all that your body needs to really be able to operate on a high level.

I recommend taking a 1,000-milligram vitamin C supplement twice each day. I know that sounds like a lot, but if you've read much of this book, you know that I believe very firmly that vitamin C is a huge boon for your good health. Even though it's present in lots of fruits and vegetables, it can still be difficult to get enough of the stuff in your diet. Hundreds (perhaps thousands) of vitamin C supplement options are available, so do some research and talk to your integrative doctor to find out which ones are right for you.

When you're fighting an illness, take 8,000 milligrams of vitamin C each day instead of the usual 2,000 milligrams.

Vitamin B Complex

The term *vitamin B complex* refers to all the B vitamins: B1, B2, B3, B5, B6, B7, B9, and B12. Several of the B vitamins have other commonly used names — *riboflavin* and *niacin* are two good examples — and you can read all about those names, as well as my dosage recommendations, in Chapter 17.

The range of important functions that the vitamin B complex plays in your body is staggering, and I wouldn't even attempt to cover all the details here. Just know that if you want to be healthy and live a long, comfortable life, you'd better plan on getting plenty of B vitamins.

I think it's a good idea to take a vitamin B complex supplement in addition to your multivitamin every day. You can find such a supplement that will give you what you need in only one dose per day. Check out Chapter 17 to get my recommendations on how much of each of the B complex vitamins to get every day.

Magnesium

Several solid studies done over the course of the last few years have shown very strong connections between high levels of magnesium intake and the avoidance of cardiovascular illness. People who get plenty of magnesium — in their diets and through supplementing — commonly have a lower heart disease risk.

In addition, magnesium is involved in about 300 different biochemical reactions that take place in your body, so you can see why it's a good idea to make sure you're getting enough of it. To be certain, take a supplement that gives you 600 milligrams per day.

Sulforaphane

Not everyone has heard of sulforaphane, and that's too bad. It's been making headlines on a pretty regular basis lately, and I hope that continues, because I think everyone should be taking it as a supplement regularly.

Recent studies have indicated that sulforaphane helps to thwart some kinds of cancer and can slow tumor development. Other studies show that sulforaphane reduces the amount of *H. pylori* bacteria in the stomach, and that bacterium causes stomach lining inflammation and ulcers. If those aren't good reasons to take sulforaphane each day, I don't know what are.

You can get sulforaphane in supplement form in two ways: broccoli seed extract or straight sulforaphane. If you go with the latter, shoot for 500 milligrams per day. If the former is your preferred sulforaphane supplement, try to get 30 milligrams every day.

Vitamin E

Like vitamin C and the vitamin B complex, vitamin E is something that will almost certainly be included in your multivitamin regimen but probably not in high enough amounts. You can see continuing health benefits of supplementing with vitamin E up to 800 milligrams per day, so don't be afraid to get that much.

What are some of the health benefits of taking additional vitamin E? First, vitamin E has powerful antioxidant effects, and if you check out Chapter 5 you'll know how important antioxidants are to your total health. But vitamin E does all sorts of other good things for your body as well, from boosting your immune system to keeping your blood vessels in tip-top shape.

Do yourself a huge favor, and don't scrimp on the vitamin E.

Alpha-lipoic Acid (ALA)

You'll often see alpha-lipoic acid referred to as *ALA*. It's a top-notch antioxidant that helps your body fight disease and keeps your various cells functioning at a high level.

I always suggest to my patients that they take an ALA supplement, and I recommend finding a capsule form that provides about 800 milligrams per day. That number has been shown to offer many health benefits without being overwhelming or wasteful in the body. You can find ALA supplements at any good health food store and at your local vitamin retailer.

Chapter 22

Ten Common Detoxification Pitfalls

*Y*ou know what they say about the best-laid plans, don't you? Unfortunately, that old chestnut extends to the best-laid detoxification plans. Even if you're completely sold on the idea that you need to correct your current dietary blunders with a healthy detox diet and take additional steps to detoxify your body, you have plenty of chances to slip up on the road to your new, improved, detoxified life.

I've been helping patients with their detoxification efforts for decades, and by now I know where many of them go wrong. From these many, many years of hindsight, I offer the material in this chapter, which clues you in on ten of the most common ways that your detox endeavors can go astray. These pitfalls pertain to both detox dieting and general detoxification.

I want you to succeed in your quest to rid your body of toxins and keep them out, so I don't pull any punches here. My hope is that if you can see potential pitfalls coming, you'll be more likely to sail smoothly past them on your way to a longer, healthier, detoxified life.

Keeping Unhealthy Food in the House

When you start out on any detoxification endeavor, particularly a detox diet, one of the very first steps you should take is to clear out all the toxin-laden, processed, and generally unhealthy food from your kitchen. You can read all about the kinds of food you should avoid in Chapters 3 and 6 of this book.

Don't hang on to any of it — clear out the cabinets, the pantry, the fridge, and the freezer. (And don't forget your secret stash of cookies or snack cakes!) If you have unhealthy food in your home, it will continually tempt you. Eventually, you'll probably end up caving to that temptation, so it's always best to clear out the bad foods from the get-go.

When the unhealthy and toxic foods are out of your home, restock your kitchen with wholesome, healthy foods like the ones I describe in Chapter 7. The change may seem like a bit of a shock at first, but before long you won't miss all the nasty and unhealthy foods you used to eat because you'll feel so good from eating nutritious, toxin-free foods.

Not Reading Labels

Want to avoid eating and drinking toxins? If so, you have to abide by this extremely important (yet wonderfully simple) rule: Always read labels. You can't really know what's in the food you eat and the beverages you drink unless you read the labels, particularly the ingredients lists. If you take the time to examine a label, you'll know right away if a food or drink contains toxic or otherwise questionable ingredients, and you'll know to steer clear of it and opt for a toxin-free alternative.

If you've tried to really examine and analyze food labels in the past but you've been caught up in all the jargon and confusing information, check out Chapter 3. In that chapter, I give you the full rundown on how you can be smart about labels in order to keep toxin-filled foods away from you and your family. For now, let me quickly clue you in on the three things you should always do when you're evaluating a label:

- ✔ Don't buy a food that has ingredients you've never heard of or can't pronounce.

- ✔ Pay special attention to the order in which ingredients are listed on the label. They're supposed to be listed in decreasing order of amounts included.

- ✔ Keep an eye out for different variations of the same toxin.

What's *not* included on a label can be just as important as what is clearly listed. For example, if you're shopping for organic food and you don't see "100% organic" on the label, you know there's always a chance that the food contains or was produced using some sort of toxic materials.

Eating Out

If I told you that every restaurant or eatery out there served food that contained toxins, I'd be lying. A handful of restaurants pride themselves on providing natural, organic, wholesome food, and if you're lucky enough to live in an area where one of these establishments is located, I fully support you going there to eat.

That said, the vast majority of restaurants don't have much of a commitment to serving up toxin-free food. If you make a plan to eat out, you're likely making a plan to have a side of toxins with your meal. The people running these restaurants aren't bad; they usually are just not focused on what foods and additives are toxic.

You can have nearly total control of the quality and toxicity of the food you eat in only one place, and that's at home. Prepare your own food whenever you can. If you find yourself in a situation where you know you won't be able to make your food and eat at home, either pack some food from your kitchen or do plenty of research ahead of time to discover nearby restaurants that can accommodate your desire to eat healthy and toxin-free.

Eating Too Fast and Not Chewing Enough

So many people act like they're in a competitive eating match when they have a meal. Don't be one of them! If you shovel down your food and don't take the time to chew it properly, you're putting your digestive system at a huge disadvantage. Leisurely eating, with lots and lots of chewing, is an extremely important first step in any healthy digestive process (see Chapter 9).

When you eat slowly and chew your food thoroughly, you break everything down into a nice food slurpy, which is just perfect for your stomach. Doing so allows your stomach to carry out its critical functions and prepare your food for the intestines, which is really where the digestive magic happens.

If you swallow your food before you've chewed it into a semi-liquid and soaked it thoroughly with your saliva, you get the delicate digestive dance off on the wrong foot. The results can range from poor nutrient absorption to increased toxicity.

Washing Food Down with Drinks

This one always surprises my patients, so don't feel like you're alone if my advice catches you off guard. Ready? Don't drink liquids when you eat a meal. Sound crazy? It's actually the healthiest way to eat. Let me explain why.

When you drink beverages while eating a meal, you dilute two important digestive liquids: your saliva and your stomach acid. Watering down your saliva compromises its ability to start breaking down your food, and it makes the food you swallow less slick and more likely to irritate your esophagus. Diluting your stomach acid is even worse. Your stomach acid is a marvel of nature; it's so powerful that it can destroy many toxins — especially biologic toxins like bacteria, viruses, and parasites. When you drink a lot of liquids with your food, your stomach acid is diluted, which makes it a lot more difficult for the acid to penetrate your food and get to all the toxins that may be lurking in it. You need your stomach acid to be robust in terms of quantity and acidity, and having a beverage with your meal is a real hindrance to both.

Want to make sure your saliva and stomach acid are able to work at the highest possible level? Don't drink liquids when you're eating. Wait at least one hour after a meal, and then feel free to have a big, refreshing glass of clean, purified water.

Not Doing an Annual Bowel Cleanse

In Chapter 4 I write extensively about all the amazing things your bowels do to absorb what your body needs and keep out the toxins and other materials that can be a serious drag on your body's many complex systems. The last time I checked, bowels weren't included on any list of the world's natural wonders, but I think it's time we reevaluate that omission.

Your bowels are wonderfully effective, but in the toxic environment in which we live today, you need to do everything you can to keep your bowels in healthy working order. That includes getting a bowel cleanse once each year. The bowel cleanse process helps to ensure that your bowels aren't being negatively affected by a range of toxins. It also helps to make sure that your bowels are able to operate as they should, which in turn helps many aspects of your health from your weight to your immune function.

A bowel cleanse is really a relatively simple process, and it's one that people used to go through all the time just a few decades ago. To get a rounded view of the available bowel cleansing techniques, check out Chapter 5.

Not Exercising 30 Minutes per Day

Our bodies are built for activity, and it's always a shame to me when people don't realize and embrace that fact. No matter your age or physical condition, regular exercise is a key way that you can keep your body functioning as it's supposed to. If you don't exercise, you're simply asking for trouble.

I'm not talking about running a marathon or bench-pressing 300 pounds here. For most adults, just 30 minutes per day of vigorous exercise — enough to get you up near your target heart rate — can make a tremendously positive impact on your overall health. Yet many people don't do it, and as a result we're more overweight and prone to diseases than ever before.

Besides the well-known and well-documented reasons to exercise, here are two other important benefits that you stand to enjoy if you can commit to engaging in physical activity for just a half hour every day:

- ✔ **Better sleep:** Study after study has proven that exercising during the day — particularly in the morning — helps to regulate your sleep cycle and make your body ready to shut down for sleep when bedtime rolls around. With so many people living extremely busy lives these days, who can afford not to get quality sleep?

- ✔ **Detoxification through sweating:** A good 30-minute exercise session will get you sweating, and sweating is one of the most effective ways to detoxify your body. You can excrete all manner of toxins with your sweat, from chemicals to heavy metals. Just be sure you take a good shower when you're done exercising so those toxins don't sit around on and irritate your skin.

Not Sweating Enough

Working up a good sweat is a fantastic way to get toxins out of your system. Your sweat glands are great at removing toxic materials from your body, and you should take advantage of their talents.

Not long ago — back before air conditioning and before people started settling into sedentary lifestyles — just about everyone on earth spent a good portion of the year sweating quite a bit every day. Unless you live in a very cold area, you can imagine what it would be like in the heat of summer if air conditioning weren't widely available. In those days, people were detoxifying their bodies all the time. But fast forward to the present day, when people don't sweat nearly as much and the toxic load in our environment has been greatly increased. We need to sweat more than ever before.

You should strive to sweat often in the interest of aiding your body's natural detoxification processes. Here are three ways you can do just that:

- ✔ **Exercise regularly.** I cover this topic in the previous section.

- ✔ **Spend time in a sauna.** This is a great way to work up a sweat, and I recommend it for anyone who is in good physical condition. Three types of sauna are available: wet, dry, and infrared. For details, have a look at Chapter 18.

  Consult your doctor before beginning to use a sauna. People who suffer from blood pressure problems, cardiovascular disease, or epilepsy should not use saunas. Pregnant women should also avoid saunas.

- ✔ **Drink plenty of water.** Your body can sweat effectively only if you're very well hydrated. To make sure you're getting the most out of your sweat, drink plenty of purified water. (Have a look at Chapter 3 for information on how to ensure your water is clean and toxin free.)

Not Supplementing

Unless you eat a completely healthy, 100 percent organic diet that is made up of huge amounts of fresh vegetables, you're more than likely not getting all the critical nutrients and other materials your body needs to perform at its very best. I encourage you to strive for the best diet you can achieve, but if your diet isn't perfect, you can always add to the vitamins, minerals, essential fatty acids, essential amino acids, and other key substances you need through supplementing.

I talk a lot about supplementing in this book, and I really do recommend it for just about everyone. Some people question the effectiveness of supplements, but I've always found them to be an extremely useful way to augment a healthy diet for both me and my patients.

Some people choose not to supplement because they think doing so will be too much of a hassle, or they think it'll be expensive, or they don't really know which supplement choices to make when they're faced with an intimidating (and enormous) wall of options at their health food or vitamin store. But supplementing can be easy, cost-effective, and confusion free if you know how to go about it, and I'm happy to help you figure out the ins and outs. Start with my explanation on how to pick out supplements in Chapter 5, and then consider my list of recommended supplements in Chapter 21.

Drinking Inadequate Amounts of Water

As far as we know, there's one substance that all life requires: liquid water. Your body needs it, in the truest sense of the word "need." Therefore, you should drink plenty of water every day — not just when it's hot out, or when you're exercising, or when you've recently eaten a lot of salty food. (You shouldn't be doing that last one anyway, of course.) Drink water steadily throughout the day, and you'll not only keep your body healthy on a general level, but you'll assist your body in its quest to rid itself of toxins.

When you're well hydrated, your lymph system — a sort of secondary circulatory system that excels at flushing toxins out of your cells and tissues — is at its best. Your digestive system is also on top of its game when there's plenty of water to go around, and you don't have to read too many pages of this book to realize how important your digestive system is in getting the right materials in your body and keeping the wrong materials (toxins) out.

A good general rule is to drink enough water to keep your urine clear. At the same time, beware of toxin-emitting plastic water bottles. Flip back to Chapter 3 for ways to make sure the water you drink is pure and toxin-free.

Index

● *N* ●

● *O* ●

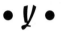

Business/Accounting & Bookkeeping

Bookkeeping For Dummies
978-0-7645-9848-7

eBay Business
All-in-One For Dummies,
2nd Edition
978-0-470-38536-4

Job Interviews
For Dummies,
3rd Edition
978-0-470-17748-8

Resumes For Dummies,
5th Edition
978-0-470-08037-5

Stock Investing
For Dummies,
3rd Edition
978-0-470-40114-9

Successful Time
Management
For Dummies
978-0-470-29034-7

Computer Hardware

BlackBerry For Dummies,
3rd Edition
978-0-470-45762-7

Computers For Seniors
For Dummies
978-0-470-24055-7

iPhone For Dummies,
2nd Edition
978-0-470-42342-4

Laptops For Dummies,
3rd Edition
978-0-470-27759-1

Macs For Dummies,
10th Edition
978-0-470-27817-8

Cooking & Entertaining

Cooking Basics
For Dummies,
3rd Edition
978-0-7645-7206-7

Wine For Dummies,
4th Edition
978-0-470-04579-4

Diet & Nutrition

Dieting For Dummies,
2nd Edition
978-0-7645-4149-0

Nutrition For Dummies,
4th Edition
978-0-471-79868-2

Weight Training
For Dummies,
3rd Edition
978-0-471-76845-6

Digital Photography

Digital Photography
For Dummies,
6th Edition
978-0-470-25074-7

Photoshop Elements 7
For Dummies
978-0-470-39700-8

Gardening

Gardening Basics
For Dummies
978-0-470-03749-2

Organic Gardening
For Dummies,
2nd Edition
978-0-470-43067-5

Green/Sustainable

Green Building
& Remodeling
For Dummies
978-0-470-17559-0

Green Cleaning
For Dummies
978-0-470-39106-8

Green IT For Dummies
978-0-470-38688-0

Health

Diabetes For Dummies,
3rd Edition
978-0-470-27086-8

Food Allergies
For Dummies
978-0-470-09584-3

Living Gluten-Free
For Dummies
978-0-471-77383-2

Hobbies/General

Chess For Dummies,
2nd Edition
978-0-7645-8404-6

Drawing For Dummies
978-0-7645-5476-6

Knitting For Dummies,
2nd Edition
978-0-470-28747-7

Organizing For Dummies
978-0-7645-5300-4

SuDoku For Dummies
978-0-470-01892-7

Home Improvement

Energy Efficient Homes
For Dummies
978-0-470-37602-7

Home Theater
For Dummies,
3rd Edition
978-0-470-41189-6

Living the Country Lifestyle
All-in-One For Dummies
978-0-470-43061-3

Solar Power Your Home
For Dummies
978-0-470-17569-9

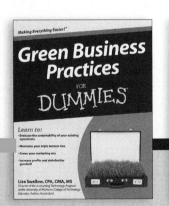

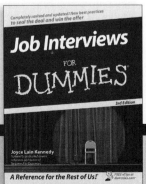

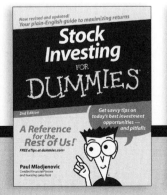

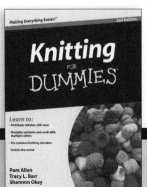

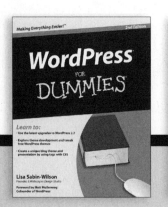
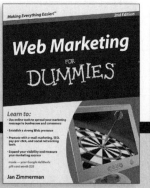
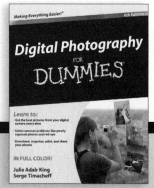
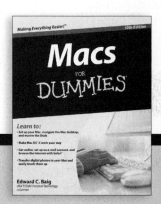

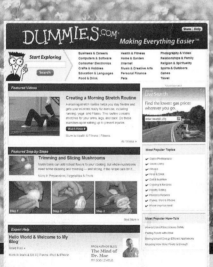

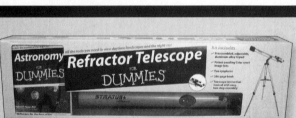
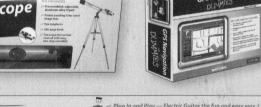
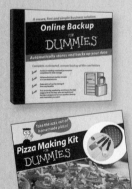
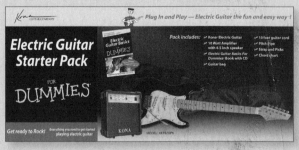
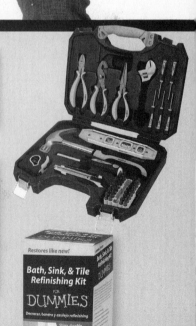
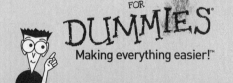